Emergency Surgery: Advanced Techniques

Emergency Surgery: Advanced Techniques

Edited by Gideon Allen

hayle medical
New York

Hayle Medical,
750 Third Avenue, 9th Floor,
New York, NY 10017, USA

Visit us on the World Wide Web at:
www.haylemedical.com

ISBN: 978-1-63241-772-5

The publisher's policy is to use permanent paper from mills that operate a sustainable forestry policy. Furthermore, the publisher ensures that the text paper and cover boards used have met acceptable environmental accreditation standards.

Printed in China.

Cataloging-in-Publication Data

Emergency surgery : advanced techniques / edited by Gideon Allen.
p. cm.
Includes bibliographical references and index.
ISBN 978-1-63241-772-5
1. Surgical emergencies. 2. Medical emergencies. 3. Surgery--Technological innovations.
4. Surgery, Operative. I. Allen , Gideon.
RD93 .E57 2019
617.026--dc23

Table of Contents

Preface ... IX

Chapter 1 **Hospital tests and patient related factors influencing time-to-theatre in 1000 cases of suspected appendicitis** ... 1
Suzanne Beecher, Donal Peter O'Leary and Ray McLaughlin

Chapter 2 **Safety in selective surgical exploration in penetrating neck trauma** ... 6
Frederico Teixeira, Carlos Augusto Metidieri Menegozzo, Sérgio Dias do Couto Netto, Renato S. Poggeti, Francisco de Sales Collet e Silva, Dario Birolini, Celso de Oliveira Bernini and Edivaldo Massazo Utiyama

Chapter 3 **Elevated white blood cell count, decreased hematocrit and presence of macrohematuria correlate with abdominal organ injury in pediatric blunt trauma patients** ... 13
Yehuda Hershkovitz, Sergei Naveh, Boris Kessel, Zahar Shapira, Ariel Halevy and Igor Jeroukhimov

Chapter 4 **Occult fractures of the proximal femur: imaging diagnosis and management of 82 cases in a regional trauma center** ... 19
Bogdan Deleanu, Radu Prejbeanu, Eleftherios Tsiridis, Dinu Vermesan, Dan Crisan, Horia Haragus, Vlad Predescu and Florin Birsasteanu

Chapter 5 **Emergency General Surgery: evolution of a subspecialty by stealth** ... 25
L. Pearce, S. R. Smith, E. Parkin, C. Hall, J. Kennedy and A. Macdonald

Chapter 6 **One year experience of swine dermal noncrosslinked collagen prostheses for abdominal wall repairs in elective and emergency surgery** ... 30
Giulia Montori, Federico Coccolini, Roberto Manfredi, Marco Ceresoli, Luca Campanati, Stefano Magnone, Michele Pisano, Elia Poiasina, Gabriela Nita, Fausto Catena and Luca Ansaloni

Chapter 7 **Geriatric Assessment as a qualification element for elective and emergency cholecystectomy in older patients** ... 38
Jakub Kenig, Piotr Wałęga, Urszula Olszewska, Aleksander Konturek and Wojciech Nowak

Chapter 8 **Critically ill patients with acute cholecystitis are at increased risk for extensive gallbladder inflammation** ... 45
Marios Papadakis, Peter C. Ambe and Hubert Zirngibl

Chapter 9 **The learning curve of single-port laparoscopic appendectomy performed by emergent operation** ... 51
YongHun Kim and WooSurng Lee

Chapter 10 **The importance of open emergency surgery in the treatment of acute mesenteric ischemia** 57
Mansur Duran, E. Pohl, K. Grabitz, H. Schelzig, T. A. Sagban and F. Simon

Chapter 11 **Poor prognostic factors in patients who underwent surgery for acute non-occlusive ischemic colitis** 63
Minsu Noh, Song Soo Yang, Seok Won Jung, Jae Ho Park, Yeong Cheol Im and Kyu Yeol Kim

Chapter 12 **Retrospective one-million-subject fixed-cohort survey of utilization of emergency departments due to traumatic causes** 72
Nan-Ping Yang, Dinh-Van Phan, Yi-Hui Lee, Jin-Chyr Hsu, Ren-Hao Pan, Chien-Lung Chan, Nien-Tzu Chang and Dachen Chu

Chapter 13 **Etiology, treatment outcome and prognostic factors among patients with secondary peritonitis at Bugando Medical Centre** 81
Amri Mabewa, Jeremiah Seni, Phillipo L. Chalya, Stephen E. Mshana and Japhet M. Gilyoma

Chapter 14 **Severe mutilating injuries with complex macroamputations of the upper extremity – is it worth the effort?** 88
Katrin Stanger, Raymund E. Horch and Adrian Dragu

Chapter 15 **Wells criteria for DVT is a reliable clinical tool to assess the risk of deep venous thrombosis in trauma patients** 97
Shrey Modi, Ryan Deisler, Karen Gozel, Patty Reicks, Eric Irwin, Melissa Brunsvold, Kaysie Banton and Greg J. Beilman

Chapter 16 **The selection of diagnostic modalities in the management of pelvic fracture patients requiring transfers** 103
Chih-Yuan Fu, Shang-Ju Yang, Chien-Hung Liao, Being-Chuan Lin, Shih-Ching Kang, Shang-Yu Wang and Yu-Pao Hsu

Chapter 17 **In-hospital costs of an admission for adhesive small bowel obstruction** 110
Pepijn Krielen, Barend A. van den Beukel, Martijn W. J. Stommel, Harry van Goor, Chema Strik and Richard P. G. ten Broek

Chapter 18 **Clinical prediction score for superficial surgical site infection after appendectomy in adults with complicated appendicitis** 118
Pinit Noorit, Boonying Siribumrungwong and Ammarin Thakkinstian

Chapter 19 **Delta neutrophil index as an early predictor of acute appendicitis and acute complicated appendicitis in adults** 125
Dong Hyuk Shin, Young Suk Cho, Gyu Chong Cho, Hee Cheol Ahn, Seung Min Park, Seung Wook Lim, Young Taeck Oh, Ji Woong Cho, Sang O. Park and Young Hwan Lee

Chapter 20 **Thoracic trauma severity contributes to differences in intensive care therapy and mortality of severely injured patients: analysis based on the TraumaRegister DGU** 131
Jörg Bayer, Rolf Lefering, Sylvia Reinhardt, Jan Kühle, Jörn Zwingmann, Norbert P. Südkamp and Thorsten Hammer

Chapter 21 **Getting the invite list right: a discussion of sepsis severity scoring systems in severe complicated intra-abdominal sepsis and randomized trial inclusion criteria** 140
Matti Tolonen, Federico Coccolini, Luca Ansaloni, Massimo Sartelli, Derek J. Roberts, Jessica L. McKee, Ari Leppaniemi, Christopher J. Doig, Fausto Catena, Timothy Fabian, Craig N. Jenne, Osvaldo Chiara, Paul Kubes, Yoram Kluger, Gustavo P. Fraga, Bruno M. Pereira, Jose J. Diaz, Michael Sugrue, Ernest E. Moore, Jianan Ren, Chad G. Ball, Raul Coimbra, Elijah Dixon, Walter Biffl, Anthony MacLean, Paul B. McBeth, Juan G. Posadas-Calleja, Salomone Di Saverio, Jimmy Xiao and Andrew W. Kirkpatrick

Chapter 22 **Acute care surgery: a means for providing cost-effective, quality care for gallstone pancreatitis** 151
Patrick B. Murphy, Dave Paskar, Richard Hilsden, Jennifer Koichopolos and Tina S. Mele

Chapter 23 **Should ambulatory appendectomy become the standard treatment for acute appendicitis?** 159
Benoit Gignoux, Marie-Cecile Blanchet, Thomas Lanz, Alexandre Vulliez, Mo Saffarini, Hugo Bothorel, Maud Robert and Vincent Frering

Chapter 24 **Advanced gallbladder inflammation is a risk factor for gallbladder perforation in patients with acute cholecystitis** 167
Stefan Jansen, Maciej Stodolski, Hubert Zirngibl, Daniel Gödde and Peter C. Ambe

Chapter 25 **Implementation and adoption of advanced care planning in the elderly trauma patient** 173
K. Verhoeff, P. Glen, A. Taheri, B. Min, B. Tsang, V. Fawcett and S. Widder

Chapter 26 **Outcomes following repair of incarcerated and strangulated ventral hernias with or without synthetic mesh** 179
Sameh Hany Emile, Hesham Elgendy, Ahmad Sakr, Waleed Ahmed Gado, Ahmed Aly Abdelmawla, Mahmoud Abdelnaby and Alaa Magdy

Chapter 27 **Laparoscopic cholecystectomy for acute calculous cholecystitis: a retrospective study assessing risk factors for conversion and complications** 188
Petra Maria Terho, Ari Kalevi Leppäniemi and Panu Juhani Mentula

Chapter 28 **Vacuum-assisted closure (VAC) systems and microbiological isolation of infected wounds** 197
Valerio Cozza, Gilda Pepe, Marco Cintoni, Flavio De Maio, Giuseppe Tropeano, Sabina Magalini, Gabriele Sganga, Giovanni Delogu and Daniele Gui

Chapter 29 **Urine flow rate monitoring in hypovolemic multiple trauma patients** 201
Evgeni Brotfain, Yoram Klein, Ronen Toledano, Leonid Koyfman, Dmitry Frank, Micha Y. Shamir and Moti Klein

Chapter 30 **Role of intraoperative cholangiography for detecting residual stones after biliary pancreatitis: still useful?** 207
Abdelrahman Abdelaal, Moamena El-Matbouly, Ibnouf Sulieman, Ahmad Elfaki, Tamer El-Bakary, Sherif Abdelaziem, Salahdin Gehani, Adriana Toro and Isidoro Di Carlo

Chapter 31 **Differentiation in an inclusive trauma system: allocation of lower extremity fractures** **213**
F. S. Würdemann, D. P. J. Smeeing, S. Ferree, F. Nawijn, E. J. M. M. Verleisdonk, L. P.H. Leenen, R. M. Houwert and F. Hietbrink

Chapter 32 **Low values of central venous oxygen saturation ($ScvO_2$) during surgery and anastomotic leak of abdominal trauma patients** **223**
Andres Isaza-Restrepo, Jose F. Moreno-Mejia, Juan S. Martin-Saavedra and Milciades Ibañez-Pinilla

Permissions

List of Contributors

Index

Preface

This book has been an outcome of determined endeavour from a group of educationists in the field. The primary objective was to involve a broad spectrum of professionals from diverse cultural background involved in the field for developing new researches. The book not only targets students but also scholars pursuing higher research for further enhancement of the theoretical and practical applications of the subject.

Emergency surgery is the surgical intervention that is performed without delay to prevent permanent disability or death. It may be performed along with life-saving resuscitation efforts. An acute illness which poses an immediate risk to a person's life or long-term health is called a medical emergency. Some of the cardiothoracic cases in which an emergency surgery often takes place include cardiac tamponade, pneumothorax and acute airway obstruction. Other cases in which an emergency surgery is required include acute appendicitis, peritonitis, bowel obstruction, urinary retention, retained abortion, paraphimosis, acute subdural hematoma, aortic dissection, among others. The topics included in this book on emergency surgery are of utmost significance and bound to provide incredible insights to readers. It strives to provide a fair idea about this discipline and to help develop a better understanding of the latest advances within this field. As this field is emerging at a rapid pace, the contents of this book will help the readers understand the modern concepts and applications of the subject.

It was an honour to edit such a profound book and also a challenging task to compile and examine all the relevant data for accuracy and originality. I wish to acknowledge the efforts of the contributors for submitting such brilliant and diverse chapters in the field and for endlessly working for the completion of the book. Last, but not the least; I thank my family for being a constant source of support in all my research endeavours.

Editor

Hospital tests and patient related factors influencing time-to-theatre in 1000 cases of suspected appendicitis

Suzanne Beecher*, Donal Peter O'Leary and Ray McLaughlin

Abstract

Background: Acute appendicitis is increasingly being managed in the setting of a dedicated emergency theatre. However understanding of hospital factors that influence time-to-theatre (TTT) is poor. Thus, the aim of this study is to identify factors that influence TTT and to observe the effect of prolonged TTT on patient outcome.

Methods: A retrospective review of an electronic prospectively maintained database was performed over a 2 year period. Factors thought to influence TTT were highlighted. A delay was defined as TTT >8 hours. Data analysis was performed using SPSS 20.

Results: 1,000 cases of suspected acute appendicitis were identified. Median age was 19 years. Appendicectomy was performed in 90.7%. 68.1% underwent laparoscopic appendicectomy. Overall mean TTT was 12 hours, 27 minutes. There was a significant association between delayed TTT and female gender ($p = 0.017$), older age ($p = 0.001$), pre-operative radiology (<0.001), normal WCC ($p < 0.001$), normal neutrophils ($p < 0.001$) and histological non-perforated appendix ($p < 0.001$). However, on multivariate analysis, younger age, a neutrophilia and presence of a perforation had a shorter TTT. Delayed TTT did not affect outcome variables including post operative collection (3.59% v 4.38%, $p = 0.528$), readmission rate (6.54% v 5.72%, $p = 0.403$) and length of stay (3.1 days v 3.34 days, $p = 0.823$).

Conclusions: This study highlights key hospital factors that influence TTT in patients with suspected appendicitis. Identification of these influential factors adds greatly to our understanding of patient prioritisation. Finally, TTT delays greater than 8 hour do not appear to affect short-term patient outcomes.

Keywords: Appendicitis, Delay, Time, Factors, Appendicectomy, Appendectomy, Outcome, Readmission, Complications

Introduction

Acute appendicitis is recognised internationally as the most common acute surgical emergency requiring surgical intervention [1]. Acute appendicitis is increasingly being managed in the setting of a dedicated emergency theatre [2,3]. Provision of dedicated emergency theatre facilities has resulted in improved patient outcomes including a shorter length of stay and improved morbidity and mortality rates [4,5].

There is much debate surrounding the timing of appendicectomy performance at present [6]. In order to avoid out of hours appendicectomies being performed, delays may be encountered [7]. Recent published data has noted that delays up to 24 hours do not appear to increase the complexity of appendicitis or associated morbidity [8,9]. On this basis it appears delays less than 24 hours may not adversely affect patient outcome, however timely intervention is still warranted in specific groups for control of sepsis and pain [10,11].

Provision of timely intervention is very much dependent upon an efficient emergency theatre [12]. Despite having dedicated emergency theatres, delays are still encountered on a daily basis between the time when a decision is made to go to theatre and the time of intervention with costly implications [13]. A lack of capacity to facilitate emergency cases for all surgical specialties presumably is the main factor contributing to delays

* Correspondence: suzub@hotmail.com
Department of Surgery, Galway University Hospital/National University of Ireland (NUI), Galway, Republic of Ireland

however there is a paucity of information within the literature pertaining to the factors that influence the time to theatre (TTT) in patients with suspected acute appendicitis. Identification of these factors would greatly enhance our understanding of TTT in suspected acute appendicitis and aid the organisation of emergency surgery services.

Thus we wished to identify the hospital and patient related factors that influence TTT in patients with suspected appendicitis, paying particular attention to patient, procedure and histological factors. We then wished to examine the effect of delayed TTT on short term patient outcomes following appendicectomy.

Methods

An electronic prospectively maintained emergency theatre database was used to identify patients with suspected appendicitis between 31st December 2011 to the 31st December 2013.

Data collected included patient gender, patient age, patient identification number, operation, time added to list, operation start time and operation finish time. We also noted the surgical approach used, either laparoscopic or open. Blood parameters were recorded including White Cell Count (WCC), neutrophils and C-reactive protein (CRP). Use of additional radiological diagnostic modalities pre-operatively was recorded. Outcome variables including length of stay, post-operative collection, conversion to open, readmission and perforation rates were recorded. We did not gather data relating to wound infections as outpatient management of these complications would have provided incomplete and inaccurate data.

The time at which the patient was added to the emergency theatre list represented the time that the decision was made to go to theatre at the time of surgical admission in the Emergency Depatment. A delayed time to theatre for the operative management of acute appendicitis of >8 hours was defined by priority targets for emergency theatre access in emergency surgery guidelines and publications. We thus defined a delayed appendicectomy as >8 hours following the decision to intervene. Out of hours was defined as an operation start time outside the hours of 9 am to 5 pm.

A univariate analysis was performed to identify factors associated with a delayed TTT. Significant factors were then entered into a multivariate analysis and analysed using a logistic regression model to identify independent factors which influenced TTT. Statistical analysis was performed using SPSS version 20.0. A p-value <0.05 was considered statistically significant. Ethics approval was received for the ethics committee at University Hospital Galway.

Results

1000 cases of suspected acute appendicitis were identified from our prospectively maintained emergency theatre electronic database and we subsequently performed a detailed analysis of these cases.

Patient demographics and operative details are outlined in Table 1. The median patient age was 19 years. Of the 1000 patients who had clinical evidence of appendicitis, appendicectomies were performed in 90.7% of patients, with the majority of patients (68.1%) undergoing laparoscopic appendicectomy. In patients who were <12 years, open appendicectomy was more frequently performed (62.5%).

Of the 907 appendicectomies performed, pathology was detected in 730 cases, providing a negative appendicectomy rate of 19.6%. Table 2 details the histopathology findings on the resected appendixes. Acute appendicitis was found in 65.5% specimens. 11.8% of patients had a perforated appendix. A carcinoid tumour was detected in 1%.

We next looked at factors influencing TTT, as highlighted by Table 3. The overall mean time to theatre was 12 hours, 27 minutes. A number of factors were found to be significant on univariate analysis. Younger patients were brought to theatre quicker than older patients ($p = 0.001$). Male patients endured a shorter time awaiting surgery ($p = 0.017$). Patients with abnormal blood parameters, particularly those with a raised neutrophil count on presentation, were also brought to theatre faster than those with normal parameters ($p < 0.001$). Those operated on within 8 hours were more likely to have their appendix removed ($P = 0.035$).

Table 1 Patient demographics & operative details

Total		N = 1000	
Demographics			
	Age* (range)	19 (2–78)	
	Males	435	
	Females	565	
	Total Patients ≤12 years	264	
	Females ≥16 years	360	
	Pregnant Patients	4	
Operative details			
	Laparoscopy Only	93	
	Appendicectomy	907 90.7%	
	Laparoscopic Appendicectomy	618	68.1%
	Open Appendicectomy	228	25.1%
	Conversion to Open	18	2%
	Right Hemicolectomy	3	0.33%
	Unknown	40	4.4%

*Median.

Table 2 Histopathology from appendicectomies performed

Appendicectomies			N = 907
Pathology			730
	Acute appendicitis	603	
	Suppurative/Gangrenous	107	
	Enterobius Vermicularis	323	
	Carcinoid	9	
	Faecolith	199	
	Faecolith + appendicitis	93	
	Faecolith − appendicitis	106	
No pathology			177

Retrospectively, those with histopathological confirmation of a perforated appendix had also been brought to theatre more rapidly than those without ($p < 0.001$). Pre-operative radiology increased TTT by 52% in those patients who underwent either an ultrasound or CT scan ($p < 0.001$).

On multivariate analysis, younger age, a raised neutrophil count and the presence of a perforation were found to be independent factors influencing TTT.

Table 4 displays the impact of theatre delay in those who had histologically confirmed appendicitis. Interestingly, there was no significant difference between any of the outcome variables examined with or without an 8 hour delay.

Table 5 compares outcomes of those operated on during working hours and those operated on out of hours. Time of the day did not have a significant impact on TTT. There was no significant difference in the outcomes for appendicectomies performed out of hours.

Discussion

Organisation of emergency surgery services requires a greater understanding of the factors influencing how we prioritise use of limited resources within the emergency setting. This study identifies three key factors which influence the TTT for patients with suspected appendicitis. These patient related factors provide useful parameters on which to prioritise patients with suspected appendicitis appropriately for emergency theatre.

Understandably, younger aged patients were identified as having quicker access to theatre. Our emergency theatre prioritisation system ensures children <12 years of age in need of an emergency operation are given high priority and invariably have their intervention in a timely manner. This is to the detriment of older patients but is necessary in the setting of limited theatre resources. Interestingly, a neutrophilia was found to be the only blood parameter found to influence TTT. A neutrophilia indicates an acute inflammatory response and would be in keeping with an acute appendicitis and appears to represent a good marker of the clinical severity of the appendicitis and the timing of appendicectomy. Histological confirmation of a perforated appendix was the final factor that influenced TTT. Although presence of a perforation is a factor that is determined retrospectively, these patients would have more advanced clinical signs and signs of sepsis. This indicates that clinical exam is indispensible in deciding who should be operated on urgently. Altogether, these patient related factors highlight

Table 3 Factors influencing TTT

	<8 Hours (447)	≥8 Hours (553)	Univariate p-value	Multivariate p-value
Patient age (mean)	20.6	23.4	0.001	0.027
Gender (N)				
Male	212	223		
Female	235	330	0.017	0.552
Radiology Pre-op (N)	81	180	<0.001	0.836
Ultrasound	60	148	<0.001	0.192
Abnormal bloods (N)				
WCC	304	284	<0.001	0.750
Neutrophils	311	284	<0.001	0.022
CRP	290	297	<0.001	0.160
Operation type (N)				
Diagnostic laparoscopy	32	61		
Appendicectomy	413	488	0.035	0.824
Perforation (N)				
Yes	66	41		
No	349	451	<0.001	0.01

Table 4 Impact of theatre delays on patient outcomes for those with appendicitis

	Theatre <8 hrs (N = 306)	Theatre ≥8 hrs (N = 297)	*P*-value
Perforation	66 (21.5%)	41 (13.8%)	0.008
Conversion to open	6 (1.96%)	11 (3.7%)	0.148
LOS* (*range*)	3 days (1–12)	3 days (1–20)	0.488
Readmission	20 (6.54%)	17 (5.72%)	0.403
Collection	11(3.59%)	13 (4.38%)	0.528

*Median.

the factors that influence our decision making when prioritising patients for an appendicectomy in the setting of a multi-speciality emergency theatre. It is clear that clinical prioritisation influences TTT with young age, increased neutrophils and presumably clinical signs suggesting perforation resulting in the surgeons being more proactive in prioritising these cases. It is also clear that while there were no clear increased complications in the group with longer TTT it is important to realise that this is not the same as saying all patient can wait. The lack of increased complication rate in the delayed group may be as a result of sicker patients being prioritised to earlier theatre times.

This study highlights the patient related factors which influenced TTT. It is likely there are other non-patient related organisational factors which also have a bearing on TTT such as staffing levels for example. However these would difficult to measure and would vary from institution to institution. The lack of influence of pre-operative radiology on TTT was surprising. However, the decision for theatre would not have been taken until after the radiological investigation, thus although the overall length of stay was delayed, the TTT by definition was not. Interestingly the time of day does not impact on TTT.

Delaying TTT beyond the 8 hour time frame does not appear to affect the short-term outcome for patients with acute appendicitis within this study. Although this time-frame was defined by published guidelines and recent studies, we also analysed this data looking at different time-points including 8,12,16 and 24 hours [2,12]. There was no difference noted in patient short-term outcome at any of these time-points. This is consistent with findings from a recent meta-analysis and systematic review which demonstrated delays up to 24 hours in selected patients may be feasible as studies have shown that a delay within this window is not associated with increased rates of complex pathology [6]. Thus there may be scope to extend the recommended TTT within current emergency surgery guidelines, however those with clinical signs of perforation, neutrophillia and younger age were prioritised in this study which may suggest the subgroups that need early surgery.

Table 5 Subanalysis of appendicectomies performed out of hours

	Working hours	Out of hours	P value
Time to theatre*	10:43	14:23	0.215
Length of stay*	3 days	3 days	0.481
Readmission (N)	29	33	0.804
Morbidity (N)	30	39	0.406

*Mean, hh:mm.

Conclusion

This study highlights key 'patient related' factors that influence TTT in patients with suspected appendicitis. Identification of these influential factors adds greatly to our understanding of patient prioritisation in the setting of a dedicated emergency theatre. Finally, TTT delays greater than 8 hour do not appear to affect short-term patient outcomes.

Competing interests
The authors declare that they have no competing interests.

Authors' contributions
SB collected the data & drafted the manuscript. DPO'L performed the statistical calculations & edited the manuscript. RML edited the manuscript. All authors read and approved the final manuscript.

References

1. Owings MF, Kozak LJ. Ambulatory and inpatient procedures in the United States 1996. Vital Health Stat. 1998;13:1–119.
2. Model of care for acute surgery. RCSI. 2013. https://www.rcsi.ie/files/surgery/20131216021838_Model%20of%20Care%20for%20Acute%20Surger.pdf.
3. Uranues S, Lamont E. Acute care surgery: the European model. World J Surg. 2008;32:1605–12. New South Wales.
4. Diaz Jr JJ, Norris PR, Gunter OL, Collier BR, Riordan WP, Morris Jr JA. Does regionalization of acute care surgery decrease mortality? J Trauma. 2011;71:442–6.
5. Hsee L, Devaud M, Civil I. Key performance indicators in acute surgical unit: have we made an impact? World J Surg. 2012;36:2335–40.
6. United Kingdom National Surgical Research Collaborative. Safety of short, in-hospital delays before surgery for acute appendicitis: multicentre cohort study, systematic review, and meta-analysis. Ann Surg. 2014;259(5):894–903.
7. Leff DR, Aggarwal R, Rana M, Nakhjavani B, Purkayastha S, Khullar V, et al. Laparoscopic skills suffer on the first shift of sequential night shifts: program directors beware and residents prepare. Ann Surg. 2008;247:530–9.
8. Teixeira PG, Sivrikoz E, Inaba K, Talving P, Lam L, Demetriades D. Appendectomy timing waiting until the next morning increases the risk of surgical site infections. Ann Surg. 2012;256(3):538–43.

9. Dennett E, Omundsen M. Dealy to appendicectomy and associated morbidity: a retrospective review. ANZ J Surg. 2006;76:153–5.
10. Ditillo MF, Dziura JD, Rabinovici R. Is it safe to delay appendectomy in adults with acute appendicitis? Ann Surg. 2006;244(5):656–60.
11. Ingraham AM, Cohen ME, Bilimoria KY. Effect of delay to operation on outcomes in adults with acute appendicitis. Arch Surg. 2010;145:886–92.
12. Leppäniemi A, Jousela I. A traffic-light coding system to organize emergency surgery across surgical disciplines. Br J Surg. 2014;101(1):e134–40. doi:10.1002/bjs.9325.
13. Kim L, Tan ST. Economic impact of untimely surgical intervention for acute plastic surgery patients. NZMJ. 2008;121(1275):26–32.

2

Safety in selective surgical exploration in penetrating neck trauma

Frederico Teixeira, Carlos Augusto Metidieri Menegozzo*, Sérgio Dias do Couto Netto, Renato S. Poggeti, Francisco de Sales Collet e Silva, Dario Birolini, Celso de Oliveira Bernini and Edivaldo Massazo Utiyama

Abstract

Background: Selective management of penetrating neck injuries has been considered the standard of care with minimal risks to patient safety. In a previous non-randomized prospective study conducted at our center, selective management proved to be safe and reduced unnecessary exploratory cervicotomies. In the present study, the role of clinical examination and selective diagnostic tests were assessed by reviewing demographic and clinical data. A comparison of results between two groups (mandatory surgical exploration versus selective surgical exploration) was made to check the safety of selective management in terms of the rates of morbidity and mortality.

Methods: A retrospective analysis at the Emergency Department of the Hospital das Clínicas of the University of Sao Paulo was performed by a chart review of our trauma registry, identifying 161 penetrating neck trauma victims.

Results: Of the 161 patients, 81.6 % were stabbed and 18.4 % had gunshot injuries. Stratifying the wound entry points by neck zones, we observed that zone I was penetrated in 32.8 %, zone II in 44.1 % and zone III in 23.1 % of all the cases. Thirty one patients (19.2 %) had immediate surgical exploration, which had a mean length of stay of 6 days, a complication rate of 12.9 % and a mortality rate of 9.4 %. Of the 130 who underwent selective surgical exploration 34 (26.1 %) required operative procedures after careful physical examination and diagnostic testing based on clinical indications. The mean length of stay for the selective surgical exploration group was 2 days with a complication rate of 17.6 % with no mortality, and virtually all of them were related to associated injuries in distant body segment. No statistical significance was found comparing mortality and complication rates between the two groups. Selective approach avoided 59 % of unnecessary exploratory cervicotomies.

Conclusion: Careful evaluation of asymptomatic and stable patients with minor signs of injury can safely avoid unnecessary neck explorations with low rates of morbidity. This should be the standard management of such patients.

Keywords: Neck injury, Penetrating trauma, Cervical trauma, Surgical selective management

Background

One of the most important characteristics of the neck is the anatomical relationship between vital structures and their relative vulnerability to injuries. Penetrating neck injuries (PNI) can result in simultaneous lesions in the aerodigestive and respiratory tracts, vertebral column and calvarium, blood vessels and lymphatic ducts. For several years, especially due to the military experience in the World War II, penetrating neck injuries were treated with exploratory surgery and this was recognized as the optimal management [1, 2]. The rationale for this approach was based on morbidity and mortality associated with missed injuries, although resulted in a high rate of non-therapeutic cervicotomies [1, 3–5].

In the civilian population, the mandatory exploration policy was questioned in the past two decades with a number of prospective series in the literature reporting the usefulness of the selective management of penetrating neck injuries [3–6]. In a previous non-randomized prospective study including 53 patients with penetrating neck injuries admitted to our emergency departament, selective surgical approach safely reduced the rate of unnecessary exploratory cervicotomies [7].

* Correspondence: carlosmenegozzo@gmail.com
Departament of Surgery, Division of Surgical Clinic III, University of Sao Paulo School of Medicine, Sao Paulo, Brazil

On the other hand, many surgeons prefer selective surgical exploration based on mandatory use of diagnostic studies which can be expensive and not readily available, especially in most Latin American emergency departments [5, 8, 9]. Therefore, we performed a retrospective analysis of PNI management in an urban trauma center in Brazil. Our objective was to assess the safety of the selective approach. Our main outcomes included morbidity and mortality rates. Our secondary outcome was the avoidance of unnecessary cervicotomies.

Methods

A chart review of enetrating neck trauma patients was done in order to evaluate our experience. All patients who presented with penetrating neck injuries met the inclusion criteria. Exclusion criteria included superficial wounds, defined by injuries superficial to the plane of the platysma muscle, and death before admission. Demographic data, pre - hospital care, mechanism of injury, Revised Trauma Score (RTS) and Injury Severity Score (ISS) were obtained from the Emergency Department trauma registry.

All patients were initially assessed according to Advanced Trauma Life Support guidelines by the attending trauma surgical staff, led by an experienced trauma surgeon consultant. The site of injury was classified using anatomical landmarks: Zone I extending from the base of the neck to the cricoid cartilage; Zone II is the area between the cricoid and the inferior border of the mandible; and Zone III comprising the area between the angle of the mandible to the base of the skull [10]. First physical exam meant to divide these patients into two categories. The first category included those presenting with hard signsand symptoms [6, 9] of aerodigestive severe injuries such as bubbling, hoarseness, salivary fistula, expanding hematomas, profuse bleeding or hemodynamic instability; these patients underwent mandatory exploration. On the other hand, hemodynamically stable patients with soft signs and symptoms [6, 9] such as dysphagia, crepitation, stable hematoma, hemoptysis or hematemesis, were treated with the selective approach. Patients with suspected spinal cord injury had neurosurgical consultation, and the decision of surgical repair of these injuries was at the discretion of the neurosurgical team. Assympotmatic patients were physically evaluated, with local exploration, for the depth of the injury by the consultant surgeon. If a superficial wound was identified, simple suturing was performed, followed by hospital discharge.

Neck Computed Tomography was utilized in cases of suspected cervical fractures, spinal cord injuries or in the setting of concomitant severe facial or head injury. Esophagoscopy, laryngoscopy, bronchoscopy and swallow studies were performed based on trauma topography, presence of signs and symptoms suggestive of aerodigestive tract or subcutaneous emphysema signs on radiographic studies. Profuse bleeding from neck injury was initially managed with balloon tamponade [11]. Stable hematomas, audible bruits, palpable thrill or abnormal pulses in Zone II injuries were investigated using duplex scan. Angiographic studies were only performed in Zone I and III injuries with suspicious clinical findings, or uncertain duplex scan images of Zone II injuries.

All asymptomatic patients were observed for a minimum of 24 h. The surgical technique used was a vertical incision on the anterior border of the sternocleidomastoid muscle for Zone II and median sternotomy for Zone I injuries. Post auricular extension of the vertical incision was performed for distal vascular control in Zone III injuries. Occasionally bilateral vertical incisions were required for transfixating cervical lesions.

Statistical analysis and comparison was performed using chi-square and t-student tests using SPSS Statistics® software. A p value < 0.05 was considered statistically significant.

Results

During a five-year period, 181 patients were admitted with stab or gunshot injuries in the neck. Of those patients, 161 presented with neck wounds violating the platysma. Demographic information of the admitted patients is shown in Table 1. The time of arrival ranged from 15 min to 120 min, with a mean of 35 min. Of the gunshot injuries 17 (57 %) were considered transcervical. In 6 (3.4 %) stabbed patients the wound was created by mirrors, screw divers, razors and in one case by a circular saw. Surgical neck exploration was the treatment of choice for 65 (40 %) patients.

Thirty one patients admitted having hard signs of vascular or aerodigestive injuries were immediately taken to the operative room. The mechanism of injury was gunshot in 9 (29 %) and stabbing in 22 (71 %) cases.

In the mandatory neck exploration group, 8 (25.8 %) had Zone I injuries, 17 (54.8 %) Zone II injuries, and 6 (19.4 %) Zone III injuries. Of them, 7 (22.6 %) had major vascular injuries such as jugular, carotid and vertebral vessels, and 24 (77.4 %) had injuries on the trachea and larynx, esophagus or pharynx. The signs and symptoms which indicated immediate neck exploration are shown in Table 2.

Neck balloon tamponade was required in one patient, who presented with major vascular injury active bleeding in the oral cavity. One patient presented with profound shock and recalcitrant coagulopathy secondary to a carotid injury. Damage control with temporary arterial shunt was necessary in that case.

Table 1 Admission data of the 161 patients presenting with penetrating neck injuries

	Number of patients (%)
Gender	
Male	143 (88 %)
Female	18 (12 %)
Mean Age (years)	26
Pre-hospital care	
Land Unit	143 (89 %)
Aeromedic Unit	2 (1 %)
Other	16 (10 %)
Mechanism of Injury	
Gunshot Wound (GSW)	29 (18 %)
Stab Wound	
Knife	126 (78 %)
Other	6 (4 %)
Injury Location	
Zone I	53 (33 %
Zone II	71 (44 %)
Zone III	37 (23 %)
Management	
Selective Approach	130 (81 %)
Mandatory Surgery	31 (19 %)

Table 3 displays data about the patients of the Selective Approach Group. All of the stable patients who presented signs or symptoms of vascular injuries were investigated with duplex ultrasound for Zone II injuries and angiography for Zone I or Zone III injuries.

Fifty-four (41,5 %) patients had Zone II injuries and all of them underwent duplex ultrasound investigation. Angiography was performed in 16 (12.3 %) patients, with 6 Zone I and 9 had Zone III injuries. In only one case of Zone II injury, an angiography was performed due an inconclusive duplex ultrasound. Diagnosis of vascular injuries were made in 9 (13 %) stable patients by duplex ultrasound or angiography. All patients with minor vascular injuries, except one, were expectantly managed and no surgical exploration was necessary. In one patient a vertebral artery injury was identified. Selective

Table 2 Mandatory surgery group: clinical findings

	Number of patients (%)
Bleeding	20 (64 %)
Expanding Hematoma	7 (22 %)
Bubbling	2 (6 %)
Hard Aerodigestive Symptoms	1 (3 %)
Persistent hemorrhagic shock	1 (3 %)

Table 3 Selective approach group ($n = 130$)

	Number of patients (%)
Observation only	96 (74 %)
Surgical Exploration	34 (26 %)
Clinical Findings	
None	39 (30 %)
Bleeding	47 (36 %)
Disphagia or odinophagia	11 (8 %)
Stable Hematoma	10 (8 %)
Hoarseness	9 (7 %)
Hemoptysis	7 (5 %)
Emphysema	6 (5 %)
Stridor	1 (1 %)
Surgical Findings	
Pharingoesophageal Injury	10 (29 %)
Laringotracheal Injury	21 (62 %)
Combined Aerodigestive Injury	3 (9 %)

embolization of the artery was performed to control of the bleeding.

The patients with signs and symptoms of aerodigestive tract injuries were submitted to diagnostic investigation with esophagoscopy, laryngoscopy and bronchoscopy. In 34 patients, the diagnostic investigation with endoscopic tests indicated surgical exploration. Of them, 30 (88.2 %) were stabbed and 4 (11.8 %) had gunshot wounds. In the group of patients submitted to selective neck explorations, 7 (20.6 %) had Zone I injuries, 19 (55.9 %) had Zone II injuries and 8 (23.5 %) had Zone III injuries.

The trauma scores, morbidity and mortality of both groups are shown in Table 4. Mortality was observed only in the mandatory surgical exploration group. All 39 patients with no clinical findings were observed for at least 24 h and discharged without evidence of clinical

Table 4 Trauma scores and complications

	Selective approach ($n = 130$)	Mandatory surgery ($n = 31$)	
ISS (mean)	17	26	
RTS (mean)	7.62	5.83	
Complications			$p = 0.6$
Surgical site infection	2	2	
Haematoma	1	1	
Wound dehiscence	2	0	
Laryngeal recurrent injury	1	0	
Pharyngoesophageal fistulae	0	1	
Mortality	0	3	$P = 0.06$

compromise. A Selective management policy avoided non-therapeutic neck explorations in 59.6 % of the patients, as these patients had uncomplicated clinical courses with conservative management.

Discussion

The neck is a vulnerable area containing different vital organs of multiple physiological systems. Due to proximity of these anatomical structures, there is a high predisposition of multisystemic injuries with potentially life-threatening lesions of the laringotracheal and pharingoesophageal complexes, major blood vessels, spinal cord and cervical nerves. Mandatory surgical exploration was the mainstay form of treatment during past few decades, mostly because of this singular topographic characteristic. Moreover, reported cases of unrecognized neurovascular injuries, resulting from conservative treatment, prompted the widespread acceptance of mandatory surgical exploration for all injuries penetrating the platysma [12–18].

However, studies documenting the civilian experience in the management of penetrating neck injuries during the last 3 decades have shown high rates of non-therapeutic exploratory cervicotomies. As a consequence, Selective Approach of penetrating neck injuries based on clinical criteria and additional radiographic and endoscopic tests has emerged as an alternative management in several centers [19–31].

Neck injuries can represent a fair share of the trauma admissions in high-volume centers [4, 9], and the number of patients with neck trauma is rising in some countries, such as England [32]. Recent publications have highlighted the ongoing controversy about role of surgical exploration in the management of penetrating neck injuries [6, 24, 33–35].

Based on their cumulative experiences, busy trauma centers often adopt a policy of selective management for patients suffering PNI mainly based on clinical investigations and protocols [9, 20, 22, 24]. On the other hand, centers with limited number of admissions have a higher threshold for adjunctive investigation studies and favor the old policy of mandatory surgical exploration [36–38]. In fact, some studies promoted the mandatory exploration policy given the low morbidity and shorter length of stay [38]. This approach was stated as cost-effective and more accurate than imaging studies, especially endoscopic and contrast studies [39–41]. However, a publication from Nason et. al. showed no improvement in terms of hospital stay or morbidity in patients treated with mandatory exploration of penetrating neck injuries [5].

After analyzing a previous non-randomized prospective study validating the selective management of penetrating cervical injuries in our Trauma Service [7], we conducted a restrospective chart review of our patients who had PNI. Our goal was to obtain a realistic panorama of the assessment and management of patients admitted in a busy trauma center in Latin America with a larger cohort of patients.

The major indication for immediate surgery was active bleeding and expansive hematoma which comprises 87 % of surgical explorations in this group. In the selective management group 100 % of the injuries responsible for surgical explorations were in the aerodigestive tract. Adjunctive tests were indicated by judicious clinical examination based on the evolving concept that routine use of angiography and endoscopy in penetrating neck injuries patients rarely change the management [20, 22, 42, 43]. Demetriades et. al. found that the absence of clinical signs accurately excluded significant vascular and aerodigestive tract lesions [9]. Other studies show similar results regarding the safety of selective diagnostic testing [4, 23].

In this study, angiography was seldom indicated in the selective group and was almost restricted to Zones I and III injuries when clinical signs of vascular injuries were identified by detailed physical examination. Doppler examination is readily available and frequently performed at our institution making this noninvasive method of investigation useful when vascular injuries were suspected. An angiography was indicated in only one Zone II injury with an inconclusive duplex ultrasound result. Angiography was particular useful in a rare case of vertebral artery injury where therapeutic selective embolization was performed controlling the active bleeding. Since there is a reported complication in 0.2 % to 2 % of the catheter angiographies, some studies suggest the use of a safer, less costly and non-invasive diagnostic method such as duplex ultrasound, with similar accuracy [5, 9, 12]. Moreover, ultrasound is more widely available in trauma services.

Table 5 summarizes the accuracy of diagnostic studies in identifying lesions that required treatment, and includes data from other studies [4, 9, 44, 45]. The main

Table 5 Diagnostic accuracy in identifying lesions that required treatment

	PPV	NPV
Doppler	20 % [44], 100 % [9] Teixeira F et al. 12 %	100 % [9, 44], Teixeira F et al. 100 %
Angiography	80 % [4], 73 % [9], 18 % [44] Teixeira F et al. 12 %	100 % [4, 9, 44], Teixeira F et al. 100 %
Endoscopic (aeordigestive)	20 % [4, 9, 42], 37,5 % [45], Teixeira F et al. 100 %	100 % [4, 9, 42, 45], Teixeira F et al. 100 %

PPV positive predictive value, *NPV* negative predictive value

difference between our results and the published literature lies in the positive predictive value (PPV) of endoscopic studies. This is mainly because our approach was to surgically explore lesions detected by these studies, both to confirm it´s extent and also to repair or drain the injury site. Nevertheless, we recognize reports of nonoperative management of small aerodigestive lesions [4, 9, 42]. With vascular injuries, interestingly there was just one patient that required intervention after diagnostic evaluation. As such, when analyzing test accuracy for identifying lesions that require some form of intervention, one will note that doppler and angiography show low PPV and high NPV, which confirms their value in excluding significant lesions. Although high NPV has been previously shown, our low PPV differs from the published literature [4, 9, 44]. We consider this to be possibly related to selection bias and lack of standardization in test reports, and might not reflect the real PPV of these tests.

We do recognize that more recent publications advocate the use of Computerized Tomography Angiography (CTA) for the evaluation of penetrating neck injuries, showing good accuracy for vascular and aerodigestive lesions [6, 22]. Although not available in a great number of institutions and posing the risks inherent to the use of contrast, this modality offers timely, safe and accurate evaluation of major aspects of neck injuries.

Our retrospective analysis involved the management of patients prior to the adoption of that diagnostic tool as a routine practice in these patients in our service. As mentioned above, studies have showed that doppler ultrasound and endoscopic studies are accurate [5, 9, 12, 24, 42, 45] and maybe more available in some hospitals than CTA. Also, Thoma et al. published a prospective study in which complementary diagnostic studies were used based on physical examination findings and no CTA was performed, showing good results [4]. Hence, we believe that the present study could be used also for centers with limited resources, and that our results can help guiding management in these hospitals. Based in our results and the published data, we present an algorithm for management of PNI patients (Fig. 1).

When comparing results between mandatory and selective exploratory groups, postoperative morbidity and mortality were not significantly different between the groups. We found a complication rate of 4.5 % and 12.9 % in patients of selective approach and mandatory exploration groups, respectively. Other studies found lower rates of complication for surgically managed patients [5, 14, 39]. Mortality was observed only in mandatory surgery group (9.6 %), which could be partially explained by the patients´ higher ISS and RTS values at admission in that group. Solimann et. al. found similar results, while other groups report a lower mortality rate [4, 9, 31]. The mean time of hospitalization was lower in the selective approach group.

An important finding from our study is that almost 60 % of the patients were not submitted to non-therapeutic neck explorations, and no missed injuries were observed at follow up of selective managed patients. This is consistent with other studies showing avoidance of unnecessary cervicotomies in 30–89 % [4, 5, 37–40]. Low failure rates of selective managed patients have been reported, ranging from

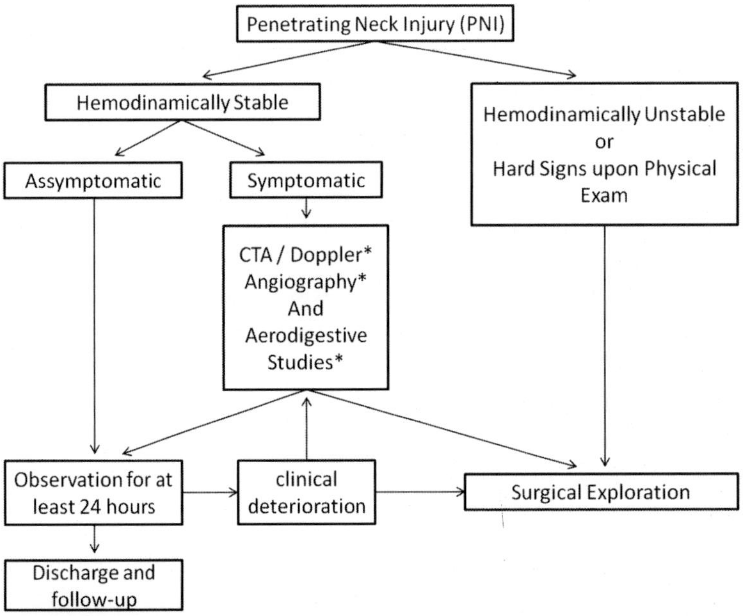

Fig. 1 Management Algorithm. *diagnosic studies should be used according to available resources and experience in each center

0 to 3 % [4, 9, 28, 31]. Also in concordance with these results, none of the patients selectively managed with observation died or had to undergo surgery.

Our study is limited by all aspects inherent to a retrospective analysis. Since patients were managed based on individualized criteria, not every patient underwent full diagnostic work-up. Therefore, it is reasonable to recognize that clinically non-relevant injuries may have been missed. Also, there was lack of uniformity concerning the operative technique description and diagnostic tests reports which could limit the interpretation of the results.

Conclusion

Management of patients with penetrating neck injuries is still challenging. Major signs and symptoms of vascular or aerodigestive injuries should prompt emergent surgical exploration. Our results further support previous evidence that selective management based in physical evaluation and diagnostic studies is safe and feasible in stable patients. These patients should be managed according to staff experience and resource availability. A selective approach is feasable and safely decreases the incidence of non-therapeutic cervicotomies and their complications.

Abbreviations

CTA, computerized tomography angiography; HCFMUSP, hospital das Clinicas of the University of Sao Paulo School of Medicine; ISS, injury severity score; NPV, begative predictive value; PNI, penetrating neck injury; PPV, positive predictive value; RTS, revised trauma score

Acknowledgements

We would like to thank Edna Frasson de Souza Montero for helping with the final revision of the article, and Lécio de Carvalho, Marilene Cardoso, and Peter Qi for grammatical revision and standardisation of language.

Funding

There are no funding sources to be declared.

Authors' contribution

FT, CAMM, SDN, RSP and FCS made substantial contributions to conception and design, or acquisition of data, or analysis and interpretation of data; DB, COB and EMU were involved in drafting the manuscript or revising it critically for important intellectual content; DB, COB and EMU gave final approval of the version to be published. All authors read and approved the final manuscript.

Competing interests

The authors declare that they have no competing interests.

References

1. Biffl WL, Moore EE, Rehse DH, Offner PJ, Franciose RJ, Burch JM. Selective management of penetrating neck trauma based on cervical level of injury. Am J Surg. 1997;174:678–82.
2. Fox CJ, Gillespie DL, Weber MA, Cox MW, Hawksworth JS, Cryer CM, Rich NM, O'Donnell SD. Delayed evaluation of combat-related penetrating neck trauma. J Vasc Surg. 2006;44:86–93.
3. Burgess CA, Dale OT, Almeyda R, Corbridge RJ. An evidence based review of the assessment and management of penetrating neck trauma. Clin Otolaryngol. 2012;37:44–52.
4. Thoma M, Navsaria PH, Edu S, Nicol AJ. Analysis of 203 patients with penetrating neck injuries. World J Surg. 2008;32(12):2716–23.
5. Nason RW, Assuras GN, Gray PR, Lipschitz J, Burns CM. Penetrating neck injuries: analysis of experience from a Canadian trauma centre. Can J Surg. 2001;44(2):122–6.
6. Sperry JL, Moore EE, Coimbra R, Croce M, Davis JW, Karmy-Jones R, et al. Western Trauma association critical decisions in trauma: penetrating neck trauma. J Trauma Acute Care Surg. 2013;75(6):936–40.
7. Lourencao JL, Nahas SC, Margarido NF, Rodrigues Junior AJ, Birolini D. Penetrating Trauma to the Neck: prospective study of 53 cases. Rev Hosp Clin Fac Med Sao Paulo. 1998;53(5):234–41.
8. Demetriades D, Charalambides D, Lakhoo M. Physical examination and selective conservative management in patients with penetrating injuries of the neck. Br J Surg. 1993;80:1534–6.
9. Demetriades D, Theodorou D, Cornwell E, Berne TV, Asensio J, Belzberg H, Velmahos G, Weaver F, Yellin A. Evaluation of penetrating injuries of the neck: prospective study of 223 patients. World J Surg. 1997;21(1):41–7. discussion 47–8.
10. Roon AJ, Christensen N. Evaluation and treatment of penetrating cervical injuries. J Trauma. 1979;19:391–7.
11. Gilroy D, Lakhoo M, Charalambides D, Demetriades D. Control of life-threatening haemorrhage from the neck: a new indication for balloon tamponade. Injury. 1992;23(8):557–9.
12. Bagheri SC, Khan HA, Bell RB. Penetrating neck injuries. Oral Maxillofac Surg Clin North Am. 2008;20(3):393-414
13. Bigger IA, Lippert KM. Arteriovenous fistula involving common carotid artery and internal jugular vein. Surgery. 1937;2:555.
14. Blair VP. A note on the treatment of secondary hemorrhage from branches of the common carotid artery. Ann Surg. 1921;74:313.
15. Fogelman MJ, Stewart RD. Penetrating wounds of the neck. Am J Surg. 1956;91:581–93.
16. McInnis WD, Cruz AB, Aust JB. Penetrating injuries to the neck. Am J Surg. 1975;130:416–20.
17. Mooro A. A case of arteriovenous aneurysm of the neck. Lancet. 1923;2:1186.
18. Markey JC, Hines JL, Nance FC. Penetrating neck wounds: a review of 218 cases. Am J Surg. 1975;130:416–20.
19. Insull P, Adams D, Segar A, Ng A, Civil I. Is exploration mandatory in penetrating zone II neck injuries. ANZ J Surg. 2007;77:261–4.
20. Inaba K, Munera F, McKenney M, Rivas L, Moya M, Bahouth H, Cohn S. Prospective evaluation of screening multislice helical computed tomographic angiography in the initial evaluation of penetrating neck injuries. J Trauma. 2006;61:144–9.
21. Schroeder JW, Baskaran V, Aygun N. Imaging of traumatic arterial injuries in the neck with an emphasis on CTA. Emerg Radiol. 2010;17:109–22.
22. Inaba K, Branco BC, Menaker J, Scalea TM, Crane S, DuBose JJ, Tung L, Reddy S, Demetriades D. Evaluation of multidetector computed tomography for penetrating neck injury: a prospective multicenter study. J Trauma Acute Care Surg. 2012;72:576–83. discussion 583Y574; quiz 803Y804.
23. Sekharan J, Dennis JW, Veldenz HC, Miranda F, Frykberg ER. Continued experience with physical examination alone for evaluation and management of penetrating zone 2 neck injuries: results of 145 cases. J Vasc Surg. 2000;32:483–9.
24. Tisherman SA, Bokhari F, Collier B, Cumming J, Ebert J, Holevar M, Kurek S, Leon S, Rhee P. Clinical practice guideline: penetrating zone II neck trauma. J Trauma. 2008;64(5):1392–405.
25. O'Brien PJ, Cox MW. A modern approach to cervical vascular trauma. Perspect Vasc Surg Endovasc Ther. 2011;23(2):90–7.
26. Weigelt JA, Thal ER, Snyder 3rd WH, Fry RE, Meier DE, Kilman WJ. Diagnosis of penetrating cervical esophageal injuries. Am J Surg. 1987;154(6):619–22.
27. Wood J, Fabian TC, Mangiante EC. Penetrating neck injuries: recommendations for selective management. J Trauma. 1989;29(5):602–5.

28. Ngakane H, Muckart DJ, Luvuno FM. Penetrating visceral injuries of the neck: results of a conservative management policy. Br J Surg. 1990;77(8):908–10.
29. Srinivasan R, Haywood T, Horwitz B, Buckman RF, Fisher RS, Krevsky B. Role of flexible endoscopy in the evaluation of possible esophageal trauma after penetrating injuries. Am J Gastroenterol. 2000;95(7):1725–9.
30. Offiah C, Hall E. Imaging assessment of penetrating injury of the neck and face. Insights Imaging. 2012;3(5):419–31.
31. Madsen AS, Laing GL, Bruce JL, Oosthuizen GV, Clarke DL. An audit of penetrating neck injuries in a South African Trauma service. Injury. 2016;47(1):64–9.
32. Harris R, Olding C, Lacey C, Bentley R, Schulte KM, Lewis D, Kandasamy N, Oakley R. Changing incidence and management of penetrationg neck injuries in the South East London Trauma Centre. Ann R Coll Surg Engl. 2012;94:240–4.
33. Mohammed GS, Pillay WR, Barker P, Robbs JV. The role of clinical examination in excluding vascular injury in haemodynamically stable patients with gunshot wounds to the neck. A prospective study of 59 patients. Eur J Vasc Endovasc Surg. 2004;28:425–30.
34. Eddy VA. Is routine angiography mandatory for penetrating injury to zone 1 of the neck? Zone 1 penetrating neck injury study group. J Trauma. 2000;48:208–13.
35. Ferguson E, Dennis JW, Vu JH, Frykberg ER. Redefining the role of arterial imaging in the management of penetrating zone 3 neck injuries. Vascular. 2005;13:158–63.
36. Bishara RA, Pasch AR, Douglas DD, Schuler JJ, Lim LT, Flanigan DP. The necessity of mandatory exploration of penetrating zone II neck injuries. Surgery. 1986;100:655–60.
37. Golueke PJ, Goldstein AS, Sclafani SJ, Mitchell WG, Shaftan GW. Routine versus selective exploration of penetrating neck injuries: a randomized prospective study. J Trauma. 1984;24:1010–4.
38. Pakarinen TK, Leppäniemi A, Sihvo E, Hiltunen KM, Salo J. Management of cervical stab wounds in low volume trauma centres: Systematic physical examination and low threshold for adjunctive studies, or surgical exploration. Injury. 2006;37:440–7.
39. Apffelstaedt JP, Mtiller R. Results of mandatory exploration for penetrating neck trauma. World J Surg. 1994;18:917–20.
40. Meyer JP, Barrett JA, Schuler JJ, Flanigan P. Mandatory vs selective exploration for penetrating neck trauma. Arch Surg. 1987;122(5):592–7.
41. Noyes LD, McSwain NE, Markowitz IP. Panendoscopy with arteriography versus mandatory exploration of penetrating wounds of the neck. Ann Surg. 1986;204(1):21–31.
42. Soliman A, Ahmad SM, Roy D. The role of aerodigestive tract endoscopy in penetrating neck trauma. Laryngoscope. 2014;124 Suppl 7:S1–9.
43. Van Waes OJ, Cheriex KC, Navsaria PH, van Riet PA, Nicol AJ, Vermeulen J. Management of penetrating neck injuries. Br J Surg. 2012;99 Suppl 1:149–54.
44. Demetriades D, Theodorou D, Cornwell 3rd E, Weaver F, Yellin A, Velmahos G, Berne TV. Penetrating injuries of the neck in patients in stable condition. Physical examination, angiography, or color flow doppler imaging. Arch Surg. 1995;130(9):971–5.
45. Zaidi SMH, Ahmad R. Penetrating neck trauma: a case for conservative approach. Am J Otolaryngol. 2011;32:591–6.

3

Elevated white blood cell count, decreased hematocrit and presence of macrohematuria correlate with abdominal organ injury in pediatric blunt trauma patients

Yehuda Hershkovitz[1], Sergei Naveh[1], Boris Kessel[2], Zahar Shapira[1], Ariel Halevy[1] and Igor Jeroukhimov[1*]

Abstract

Introduction: Computerized tomography (CT) has become an important diagnostic modality in trauma patients. Pediatric patients are particularly susceptible to ionized radiation making liberal CT use in this age group unacceptable. We aimed to identify parameters that might predict abnormal findings on abdominal CT leading to patient management changes.

Methods: Data on blunt trauma patients up to 15 years of age admitted to Assaf Harofeh Medical Center from January 2007 to October 2014 was retrospectively collected. All patients with abdominal CT scan as part of initial assessment were included. Medical and surgical data were extracted from the medial charts. Patients were divided into two groups. Group I: patients whose management was changed solely based on abdominal CT findings and Group II: patients with normal abdominal CT. The groups were compared by all the data parameters.

Results: Overall, 182 patients were included in the study. The groups were comparable by age and mechanism of injury. Management changes based on CT findings were found in 68 (37.4 %) patients. White blood cell count >14000, abnormally low hematocrit level and macrohematuria were associated with a diagnosis of intra-abdominal injury requiring patient management changes ($p < 0.05$). Group I patients had longer LOS. Fifteen patients (22 %) required active intervention based solely on CT findings. Physical examination, arterial blood gases and initial radiology examinations results did not correlate with abdominal CT findings.

Conclusions: Elevated WBC, decreased hematocrit and presence of macrohematuria strongly correlate with abdominal CT findings and lead to changes in patient management.

Keywords: Abdominal trauma, Pediatric trauma management, CT in blunt trauma

Introduction

The potential risk of radiation damage caused by CT scan dictates careful use of this imaging modality [1]. While in the management of a stable adult patient with blunt abdominal trauma the indications for a CT scan are established [2], its use in the pediatric population is still a matter of debate. It has been shown that the mechanism of injury as a sole indication for obtaining a CT scan in pediatric trauma victims does not clearly predict significant findings affecting patient management [3, 4].

The indications for abdominal imaging after blunt trauma are usually based on physical examination and mechanism of injury suggestive of intra-abdominal injury [5]. However, the clinical evaluation of children with potential abdominal trauma may be limited and often unreliable, especially in multisystem injuries [6].

Although abdominal CT is considered the best imaging modality for diagnosing intra-abdominal injury (IAI), less than 15 % of pediatric patients sustaining blunt trauma are found to have IAI on CT [5].

* Correspondence: igorjer65@gmail.com
[1]Division of Surgery, Assaf Harofeh Medical Center, Zerifin 70300, affiliated to the Sackler Faculty of Medicine, Tel Aviv University, Tel Aviv, Israel
Full list of author information is available at the end of the article

Increasing awareness of the hazards that exposure to radiation carries, especially in pediatric population, and given the scarcity of traumatic CT findings leading to intervention in these patients, led us to clarify factors that may help in the use of CT on a more selective basis.

The purpose of this study was to define objective clinical parameters on initial evaluation of children with blunt abdominal trauma that predict traumatic findings on abdominal CT scan which would influence the management plan.

Methods

A retrospective observational cross sectional study was performed at Assaf Harofeh Medical Center. The study was approved by the Institutional Review Board.

Charts of pediatric blunt trauma patients admitted from January 1, 2007 to September 30, 2014 that underwent abdominal CT as a part of initial evaluation were reviewed. All blunt trauma patients up to 15 years old with Abbreviated Injury Scale (AIS) severity score indicating abdominal injury were eligible for the study. Patients with decreased level of consciousness (GCS < 12) and patients who did not undergo abdominal CT were not included. Data regarding patient demographics, mechanism of injury, initial physical examination findings, Glasgow Coma Scale (GCS) on admission, laboratory data, radiologic interpretation of chest and pelvic roentgenograms, focused assessment with sonography in trauma (FAST) results, CT scan findings and required surgical procedures and length of hospital stay (LOS) were extracted from the medical charts.

Our institutional policy dictates overnight observation for every pediatric patient who has a CT scan as a part of trauma management.

Change in patient management was defined as an alteration in management based directly on the CT findings.

An abnormal CT was defined as a scan exhibiting any traumatic abnormality either apparent or occult (finding of free fluid in the peritoneal cavity).

The patients were divided into two groups. Group I included patients whose management was changed due to abdominal CT findings. This group included either patients admitted to the Intensive Care Unit (ICU) or patients hospitalized longer than 24 h as a result of the findings on abdominal CT. All the patients undergoing acute interventions including laparotomy, angiography/embolization or ERCP necessarily fell into this Group. Group II included patients whose management was not affected by abdominal CT findings.

Findings on physical examination were classified as normal or abnormal. Abdominal examination was considered abnormal if abrasions, contusions, seat-belt sign, abdominal distension, or tenderness on palpation were noted. Positive findings on the examination of extremities included presence of abrasions, lacerations, deformity/fracture, or tenderness on palpation. Laboratory tests obtained only on arrival were included. Laboratory results were classified as normal and abnormal (according to the patient's age). White blood cell (WBC) count up to 11,000 was considered normal, mildly elevated ranging from 11000 to 14000 and markedly elevated above 14000. Chest and pelvis roentgenogram were screened for trauma-related pathology. FAST was considered positive if intraperitoneal fluid was demonstrated.

Statistical analysis

In order to compare quantitative (continuous) variables between the two independent groups, the two sample *t*-test was applied as well as the non-parametric Mann–Whitney test. The association between the two categorical variables was assessed using either the Chi-square test or Fisher's exact test. All statistical tests applied were two-tailed. A p value less than 0.05 was considered statistically significant. Statistical analysis was performed using the Statistical Package for the Social Sciences (SPSS) software.

Results

Overall, 397 pediatric patients with abdominal trauma were admitted to our Medical Center during the study period. One hundred and eighty-two patients entered the study. The rest of the patients either had GCS lower than 12 (40 patients) or did not undergo abdominal CT (175 patients).

The mechanism of injury, demographics, GCS and Injury Severity Score (ISS) are summarized in Table 1. There was no difference in the patient characteristics between the two groups, with the exception of the ISS which was higher in Group I.

A positive physical examination did not predict clinically relevant findings on CT (Table 2). This relates to the analysis of positive findings on physical examination irrespective of body region.

CT revealed abdominal organs injury in 68 (37.4 %) patients (Table 3). Solid organs were injured in most cases (spleen 31, liver 19, kidney 17). Management altered by CT scan involved the need for active intervention in 15 out of 68 patients (22.1 %) [10 (14.7 %) patients underwent laparotomy, 2 (2.9 %) required an angiographic arterial embolization (for splenic and liver injury) and 3 patients (4.4 %) had an ERCP for suspected pancreatic duct injury]. Observation only sufficed in all other patients. Three out of 10 laparotomies (30 %) were performed in patients whose only finding on CT was free peritoneal fluid. Small bowel laceration was found in 2 cases and 1 had a mesenteric tear.

Table 1 Patient characteristics

		Group I 68 patients	Group II 114 patients	P value
Age		9.1 ± 4.1	8.7 ± 3.9	>0.05
Gender (male / female)		54 / 14	81 / 33	>0.05
Mechanism of injury	PHBC**	20.6 %	30.7 %	>0.05
	MVA passenger***	5.9 %	10.5 %	
	Fall	20.6 %	18.4 %	
	Assault	20.6 %	18.4 %	
	Bike	27.9 %	19.3 %	
	BHC****	4.4 %	2.6 %	
ISS*	1–8	13.2 %	78.9 %	<0.05
	9–14	17.6 %	11.4 %	
	15–24	51.5 %	4.4 %	
	>25	17.6 %	5.3 %	

*ISS, Injury Severity Score; ** PHBC; Pedestrian hit by car. *** MVA – Motor Vehicle Accident. **** BHC – Bicycle Hit by Car
*ISS, ** PHBC, *** MVA, **** BHC. *ISS*, Injury Severity Score; *PHBC*; Pedestrian hit by car; *MVA*, Motor vehicle accident; *BHC*, Bicycle hit by car

Overall LOS for Group I patients was 7.3 ± 6 days compared to 1.8 ± 2 days in Group II ($p < .005$). Forty-three Group II patients had non abdominal pathology (orthopedic, neurosurgical or urologic) that required admission for more than 24 h.

The presence of macrohematuria correlated with a change in management based on CT findings ($p < 0.05$). All 5 patients with macrohematuria were admitted. Four of them had renal injury and 1 patient had a liver laceration and pelvic fractures.

Laboratory tests were performed according to the decision of the surgeon on call, thus some tests results are missing in some of the patients. Detailed data is described in Fig. 1.

Markedly elevated WBC (>14000) and abnormally low hematocrit were significantly different between the groups ($p < 0.05$). Both correlated with abnormal CT findings requiring changes in patient management.

Abnormal pH, base excess and microhematuria did not predict positive CT findings ($p > 0.05$).

None of the initial imaging modalities (chest and pelvic X-rays, and FAST) were associated with intra-abdominal injury on CT.

Discussion

The role of CT is well established in the management of adult blunt trauma patients [2]. Hemodynamically stable patients with an abnormal physical examination, patients with altered levels of consciousness and patients whose mechanism of injury suspicious for internal organ injury undergo further evaluation with CT [7]. However, in the pediatric population, recent studies have shown that using CT scan, based solely on the mechanism of injury, is not justified [3, 4].

The pediatric patient is considered 10 times more susceptible to radiation in terms of estimated cancer incidence [1]. There is an understandable tendency to define predictive rules for the identification of intra-abdominal injuries in order to limit the use of CT [8–15].

We continue to define the role of CT in the management of pediatric trauma patients. A liberal policy to perform abdominal CT in every case of suspected abdominal trauma has been changed to a more conservative approach in our Institution. The goal of this study was to define readily available clinical parameters predicting a positive CT influencing treatment plan. We focused on physical examination, laboratory tests and initial imaging findings.

Table 2 Physical examination findings

	Group I	Group II	p
Head	33.8 %	25.4 %	>0.05
Neck	1.5 %	4.4 %	>0.05
Chest	14.7 %	9.6 %	>0.05
Abdomen	29.4 %	41.2 %	>0.05
Back	10.3 %	12.3 %	>0.05
Upper limbs	19.1 %	14.9 %	>0.05
Lower limbs	22.1 %	34.2 %	>0.05

Table 3 Group I CT findings

Injured organ	Number	Percent
Solid organ injury (liver, kidney or spleen)	52	76.4 %
Pancreas	7	10.3 %
Retroperitoneal hematoma	3	4.4 %
Moderate amount of free fluid	3	4.4 %
Bowel	2	2.9 %
Urinary bladder	1	1.5 %

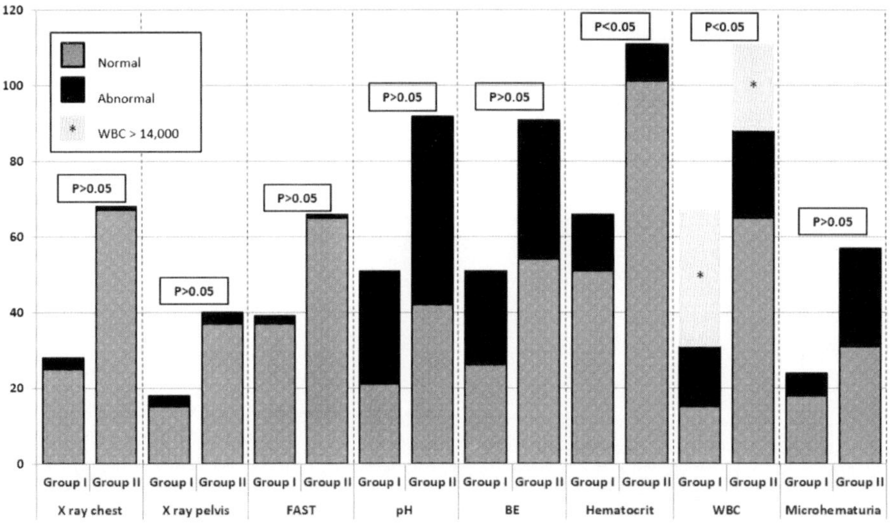

Fig. 1 Laboratory tests and imaging study results

The mechanism of injury was already evaluated in our previous work [4], where it was singled out in order to define its sole role in prediction of abdominal CT findings. Therefore it was not used in the current study as a variable, but rather as a patient characteristic in the two study groups.

Despite some data supporting the association of positive physical findings with intra-abdominal injury [8–10, 12, 13], our work has shown no such relation. Because of the small numbers in our study, analysis of the positive physical findings by regions was found statistically insignificant. There was an inconsistency in the documentation of the physical examination, nevertheless it seems logical to assume that at least positive findings would have been documented. Though in other works [8–10, 12, 16] positive findings on the physical examination of abdomen, chest and long bones fractures were predictive of intra-abdominal injury, our results show a lack of influence of the physical findings on the chance to discover traumatic pathology on the CT.

None of the initial imaging modalities (chest and pelvic X-rays and FAST) were associated with intra-abdominal injury on CT in our study. Beck [17] has reported that an abnormal pelvic roentgenogram predicts a positive CT scan. However, Kessel et al. [18] have questioned the usefulness of routine pelvic x-ray in stable multiple trauma patients, as in patients undergoing CT it did not change the therapeutic policy [18]. Streck et al. [12] found an abnormal chest X-ray to be associated with intra-abdominal injury, but the pelvic or femur roentgenogramm bore no such association [12].

The use of FAST in the management of pediatric trauma patients is debated in the literature. Soundappan et al. [19] and Soudack et al. [20] reported high sensitivity of the test (81 % and 92.5 % accordingly). However, Scaife et al. [21] found the sensitivity to be 50 %, which seems unacceptably low. It was concluded in this study that true positive FAST exams are uncommon and would rarely direct management. The limited role of FAST in stable pediatric patients has been shown by other authors [22, 23].

In our study, 105 patients underwent FAST (Table 2). Three (2.9 %) were positive, and of them 2 had findings on the following CT that led to a change in treatment plan.

In general, there is a low prevalence of laboratory test abnormalities in moderately injured pediatric patients (5.7 %) [24]. Rovalis et al. [25] showed that patients with a severe head injury had significantly higher WBC counts [25]. Schnüriger et al. [26] evaluated the relationship between a hollow viscus injury and WBC counts and concluded that the diagnostic value of serial WBC tests in predicting a hollow viscus injury is very limited. Holmes et al. [8] evaluated clinical and laboratory parameters for the identification of intra-abdominal injuries in pediatric blunt trauma patients. They have found the WBC to be higher in patients with intra-abdominal injuries, but the authors could not identify a clinically useful cutoff that would distinguish between the groups. In our study, a WBC > 14000 strongly correlated with positive abdominal CT findings.

The utility of the hematocrit for screening for unsuspected IAI remains unproven [8]. We found that a low hematocrit level is a significant predicting factor for IAI. Base excess is considered a predictor of mortality and severity of injury in trauma patients. In pediatric trauma patients though, it has been shown to be a weak prognostic factor [27]. In our study, a negative base excess level was not associated with abnormal CT findings.

The presence of macrohematuria is invariably associated with intra-abdominal injury in children [8, 9, 11–13, 24]. In this respect, our study does not differ from previous studies.

The data concerning free peritoneal fluid in pediatric blunt trauma is inconsistent. Holmes et al. [28] found isolated intraperitoneal fluid in 8 % of pediatric blunt trauma patients undergoing abdominal CT, and IAIs subsequently identified in 17 % of these patients. The likelihood of intra-abdominal injury increased with increasing amounts of fluid. In another study, 16 % of patients with intra-abdominal free fluid required laparotomy [29]. On the other hand, Christiano found free intra-abdominal fluid on 14 % of CTs performed for pediatric blunt abdominal injury [30], but only 3 % of them developed peritonitis and required surgery. Although the majority of patients will be eventually discharged without any intervention, the amount of patients requiring is not negligible, and therefore careful follow up with serial examination is necessary in selected cases. In our study, free intraperitoneal fluid was found in 38 (20.8 %) patients without any identifiable cause on CT. Three of them (8 %) eventually required surgery. Two had more than a minimal amount of fluid on the CT, and 1 patient developed signs of peritoneal irritation during the observation. Small bowel and mesentery laceration were found on laparotomy.

Our institutional policy dictates overnight observation for every pediatric patient who has undergone an abdominal CT, even if it was normal. One of the reasons is the known propensity of the CT to miss hollow viscus and pancreatic injuries [13].

The major limitations of this study include its retrospective nature and the relatively small amount of patients. Many of the patients did not have all the examinations because they were probably deemed unnecessary at the time of evaluation. Prospective studies including a large number of patients are needed for further evaluation of the role of CT in the pediatric trauma population.

Conclusion

Our data shows that an elevated WBC, a decreased hematocrit level and the presence of macrohematuria strongly implies abdominal CT findings leading to changes in management. The main influence resulting from CT was a change in the level of care (prolonged observation). It may also guide the need for active intervention in selected patients.

Study presentation

This study was presented at the "Best of the Best" session during the Third World Society of Emergency Surgery Congress (WSES) that took place in Jerusalem, Israel in July 2015.

Competing interests
The authors declare that they have no commercial associations, financial disclosures, or other competing interests with regard to this article. There are no sources of funding.

Authors' contributions

YH participated in the analysis and interpretation of the data; and drafting of the manuscript. SN participated in the acquisition of data; and drafting of the manuscript. BK, participated in the acquisition of data; and revising the article critically for important intellectual content. ZS participated in the analysis and interpretation of the data; and drafting of the manuscript. AH participated in the conception and design of the study; and revising the article critically for important intellectual content. IJ participated in the conception and design of the study; and revising the article critically for important intellectual content. All authors read and approved the final manuscript.

Author details
[1]Division of Surgery, Assaf Harofeh Medical Center, Zerifin 70300, affiliated to the Sackler Faculty of Medicine, Tel Aviv University, Tel Aviv, Israel. [2]Trauma Unit, Hillel Yaffe Medical Center, Hadera 38100, Israel.

References

1. Brenner D, Elliston C, Hall E, Berdon W. Estimated risks of radiation-induced fatal cancer from pediatric CT. AJR Am J Roentgenol. 2001;176(2):289–96.
2. Deunk J, Brink M, Dekker HM, Kool DR, Blickman JG, van Vugt AB, et al. Predictors for the selection of patients for abdominal CT after blunt trauma: a proposal for a diagnostic algorithm. Ann Surg. 2010;251(3):512–20.
3. Moore HB, Faulk LW, Moore EE, Pierraci F, Cothren Burlew C, Holscher CM, et al. Mechanism of injury alone is not justified as the sole indication for computed tomographic imaging in blunt pediatric trauma. J Trauma Acute Care Surg. 2013;75(6):995–1001.
4. Hershkovitz Y, Zoarets I, Stepansky A, Kozer E, Shapira Z, Klin B, et al. Computed tomography is not justified in every pediatric blunt trauma patient with a suspicious mechanism of injury. Am J Emerg Med. 2014;32(7):697–9.
5. Sivit CJ. Imaging children with abdominal trauma. AJR Am J Roentgenol. 2009;192(5):1179–89.
6. Saladino R, Lund D, Fleisher G. The spectrum of liver and spleen injuries in children: failure of the pediatric trauma score and clinical signs to predict isolated injuries. Ann Emerg Med. 1991;20(6):636–40.
7. Salim A, Sangthong B, Martin M, Brown C, Plurad D, Demetriades D. Whole body imaging in blunt multisystem trauma patients without obvious signs of injury: results of a prospective study. Arch Surg. 2006;141(5):468–73. discussion 73–5.
8. Holmes JF, Sokolove PE, Land C, Kuppermann N. Identification of intra-abdominal injuries in children hospitalized following blunt torso trauma. Acad Emerg Med. 1999;6(8):799–806.
9. Holmes JF, Sokolove PE, Brant WE, Palchak MJ, Vance CW, Owings JT, et al. Identification of children with intra-abdominal injuries after blunt trauma. Ann Emerg Med. 2002;39(5):500–9.
10. Cotton BA, Beckert BW, Smith MK, Burd RS. The utility of clinical and laboratory data for predicting intraabdominal injury among children. J Trauma. 2004;56(5):1068–74. discussion 74–5.
11. Holmes JF, Mao A, Awasthi S, McGahan JP, Wisner DH, Kuppermann N. Validation of a prediction rule for the identification of children with intra-abdominal injuries after blunt torso trauma. Ann Emerg Med. 2009;54(4):528–33.
12. Streck Jr CJ, Jewett BM, Wahlquist AH, Gutierrez PS, Russell WS. Evaluation for intra-abdominal injury in children after blunt torso trauma: can we reduce unnecessary abdominal computed tomography by utilizing a clinical prediction model? J Trauma Acute Care Surg. 2012;73(2):371–6. discussion 76.
13. Hynick NH, Brennan M, Schmit P, Noseworthy S, Yanchar NL. Identification of blunt abdominal injuries in children. J Trauma Acute Care Surg. 2014;76(1):95–100.
14. Karam O, Sanchez O, Chardot C, La Scala G. Blunt abdominal trauma in children: a score to predict the absence of organ injury. J Pediatr. 2009;154(6):912–7.

15. Holmes JF, Lillis K, Monroe D, Borgialli D, Kerrey BT, Mahajan P, et al. Identifying children at very low risk of clinically important blunt abdominal injuries. Ann Emerg Med. 2013;62(2):107–16. e2.
16. Miller D, Garza J, Tuggle D, Mantor C, Puffinbarger N. Physical examination as a reliable tool to predict intra-abdominal injuries in brain-injured children. Am J Surg. 2006;192(6):738–42.
17. Beck D, Marley R, Salvator A, Muakkassa F. Prospective study of the clinical predictors of a positive abdominal computed tomography in blunt trauma patients. J Trauma. 2004;57(2):296–300.
18. Kessel B, Sevi R, Jeroukhimov I, Kalganov A, Khashan T, Ashkenazi I, et al. Is routine portable pelvic X-ray in stable multiple trauma patients always justified in a high technology era? Injury. 2007;38(5):559–63.
19. Soundappan SV, Holland AJ, Cass DT, Lam A. Diagnostic accuracy of surgeon-performed focused abdominal sonography (FAST) in blunt paediatric trauma. Injury. 2005;36(8):970–5.
20. Soudack M, Epelman M, Maor R, Hayari L, Shoshani G, Heyman-Reiss A, et al. Experience with focused abdominal sonography for trauma (FAST) in 313 pediatric patients. J Clin Ultrasound. 2004;32(2):53–61.
21. Scaife ER, Rollins MD, Barnhart DC, Downey EC, Black RE, Meyers RL, et al. The role of focused abdominal sonography for trauma (FAST) in pediatric trauma evaluation. J Pediatr Surg. 2013;48(6):1377–83.
22. Coley BD, Mutabagani KH, Martin LC, Zumberge N, Cooney DR, Caniano DA, et al. Focused abdominal sonography for trauma (FAST) in children with blunt abdominal trauma. J Trauma. 2000;48(5):902–6.
23. Holmes JF, Brant WE, Bond WF, Sokolove PE, Kuppermann N. Emergency department ultrasonography in the evaluation of hypotensive and normotensive children with blunt abdominal trauma. J Pediatr Surg. 2001;36(7):968–73.
24. Isaacman DJ, Scarfone RJ, Kost SI, Gochman RF, Davis HW, Bernardo LM, et al. Utility of routine laboratory testing for detecting intra-abdominal injury in the pediatric trauma patient. Pediatrics. 1993;92(5):691–4.
25. Rovlias A, Kotsou S. The blood leukocyte count and its prognostic significance in severe head injury. Surg Neurol. 2001;55(4):190–6.
26. Schnuriger B, Inaba K, Barmparas G, Eberle BM, Lustenberger T, Lam L, et al. Serial white blood cell counts in trauma: do they predict a hollow viscus injury? J Trauma. 2010;69(2):302–7.
27. Levi Y, Jeroukhimov I, Peleg K, Rozenfeld M, Shavit I, Kozer E. Base excess as a predictor for injury severity in pediatric trauma patients. J Emerg Med. 2013;45(4):496–501.
28. Holmes JF, London KL, Brant WE, Kuppermann N. Isolated intraperitoneal fluid on abdominal computed tomography in children with blunt trauma. Acad Emerg Med. 2000;7(4):335–41.
29. Venkatesh KR, McQuay Jr N. Outcomes of management in stable children with intra-abdominal free fluid without solid organ injury after blunt abdominal injury. J Trauma. 2007;62(1):216–20.
30. Christiano JG, Tummers M, Kennedy A. Clinical significance of isolated intraperitoneal fluid on computed tomography in pediatric blunt abdominal trauma. J Pediatr Surg. 2009;44(6):1242–8.

Occult fractures of the proximal femur: imaging diagnosis and management of 82 cases in a regional trauma center

Bogdan Deleanu[1,2], Radu Prejbeanu[1,2], Eleftherios Tsiridis[6], Dinu Vermesan[1,2], Dan Crisan[1*], Horia Haragus[1], Vlad Predescu[4,5] and Florin Birsasteanu[2,3]

Abstract

Background: Occult hip fractures are often difficult to identify in busy trauma units. We aimed to present our institutions experience in the diagnosis and treatment of occult fractures around the hip and to help define a clinical and radiological management algorithm.

Method: We conducted a seven-year retrospective hospital medical record analysis. The electronic database was searched for ICD-10 CM codes S72.0 and S72.1 used for proximal femoral fractures upon patient discharge. We identified 34 (4.83 %) femoral neck fractures and 48 (4.42 %) trochanteric fractures labeled as occult.

Results: The majority of the cases were diagnosed by primary MRI scan (57.4 %) and 12 were diagnosed by emergency CT scan (14.6 %). For the remaining cases the final diagnosis was confirmed by 72 h CT scan in 9 patients (representing 39 % of the false negative cases) or by MRI in the rest of 14 patients. MRI was best at detecting incomplete pertrochanteric fracture patterns (13.45 % of total) and incomplete fractures of the greater trochanter (3.65 % of total) respectively. It also detected the majority of Garden I femoral neck fractures (20.7 % of total). CT scanning accurately detected 100 % of Garden 2 fractures (2.44 %) and 25 % (3.65 %) of the complete pertrochanteric fractures (false negative 25 %).

Conclusion: Occult fractures should be suspected in all patients with traumatic onset of hip pain that is inconsistent with normal radiographic findings. MRI is the golden standard but not as readily available not as cheap and not quite as quick to perform as as a CT scan. The latter which in turn can provide falsely negative results in the first 24 h. Improved imaging protocols could expedite management and improve treatment.

Keywords: Occult, Hip, Fracture, X-ray, MRI, CT scan

Background

The estimated prevalence of occult hip fractures varies between 2 and 10 % of the total hip fractures [1–7].

Occult are defined, those fractures that cannot be detected by radiographic standard examination until several weeks after injury [8]. Their importance resides in their "occult" status, meaning that they are not identifiable by routine emergency X-rays. In the Emergency Room (ER) most of the times only a pelvic or hip AP view is obtained, with some services requiring a complete trauma X-Ray set with lateral, inlet, outlet and Judet oblique views. The necessity of these explorations is however disputed as the presence of a concomitant pelvic fracture either radiographically visible or occult and a occult proximal femur fracture has been excluded by previous studies [9]. Radiographically unapparent fractures can be easily mislabeled as hip soft tissue trauma and treated conservatively, with no restriction on weightbearing.

Definitive diagnosis of occult fractures of the proximal femur is without exception an imaging one. MRI is the imaging method of choice, better tolerated by patients providing a faster diagnosis of occult fractures of the hip, it is therefore recommended that the MRI is performed in an emergency setting whenever it is available

* Correspondence: crisan.dan@gmail.com
[1]I-st Clinic of Orthopedics and Trauma, Pius Brinzeu Emergency Clinical County Hospital, 10 I. Bulbuca Blvd, 300737 Timisoara, Romania
Full list of author information is available at the end of the article

[2, 4, 5, 10]. But not all services can provide emergency access to MR scanning, while CT scanning is more widespread and cheaper to perform. There is still no consensus over the use of CT in detecting occult hip fractures and it has been demonstrated that even modern 64 slice machines can yield false negative results [11].

We aimed to present our institutions experience in the diagnosis and treatment of occult fractures around the hip and to help defining a clinical and radiological management algorithm.

Method

We conducted a seven-year retrospective search on the hospital medical record (Hipocrate, RCS Software, Bucharest, Romania) between 2005-2012. The electronic database of a regional trauma center was searched for ICD-10 codes S72.0 (intracapsular) and S72.1 (extracapsular) used for proximal femoral fractures upon patient discharge. We identified 769 femoral neck and 926 pertrochanteric fractures that were treated in our clinic during this period. Out of these, 34 (4.83 %) femoral neck fractures and 48 (4.42 %) pertrochanteric fractures were labeled as occult. The fracture distribution by fracture subtype can be seen in Fig. 1.

Emergency AP radiographs routinely investigate hip trauma with the hips in neutral rotation. These are almost always sufficient for establishing a diagnosis and a management strategy for the case. For cases with suspected occult fracture further imaging was carried out either with an MRI (General Electric Signa Horizon LX 1 Tesla) or a CT scan (Philips Brilliance MX 16 slice). No contrast was used in either method. For the cases with an inconclusive emergency CT and eloquent hip symptoms such as pain in the Scarpa triangle, in the greater trochanter region, on weight-bearing or during passive movement of the hip joint, an MRI scan was performed during the following 24 h or a second CT scan at 72 h for establishing the diagnosis.

Five patients were self-discharged from the ER without allowing us to establish final diagnosis. All five patients were reexamined in the next 1-3 days by a senior orthopedic surgeon due to ongoing hip symptoms and an outpatient MRI scan was performed. Most patients with hip fractures are elderly patients and the occult fractures group fitted this demographic distribution with 80 patients that were aged 60 and over, out of which 67 were aged 70 or over and only two young patients who were aged less than 60 years. The patients that decided to leave the ER were all over 75 years of age and did so upon consultations with their families. Thirty-eight patients had at least one neurological condition such as Parkinson's disease, cortical atrophy or stroke history, which ranged in severity from mild to serious. The majority of diagnosed cases were treated surgically whilst conservative management was reserved for the incomplete and totally undisplaced occult fractures according to the literature [12, 13].

Suspicion of an occult hip fracture should arise when there is a inconsistency between the trauma history and physical examination on one hand and the imaging results on the other. For example a young patient with high-energy hip trauma that has a negative X-ray but presents with a nonweightbearing painful hip should be further investigated. The patient may be able to bear weight but also present significant hip pain spontaneous and/or on palpation mobilization and this should also prompt for further imaging studies. Elderly patients with occult hip fractures almost always have sustained a trivial trauma and present non or partial weightbearing with pain in the anterior portion of the hip.

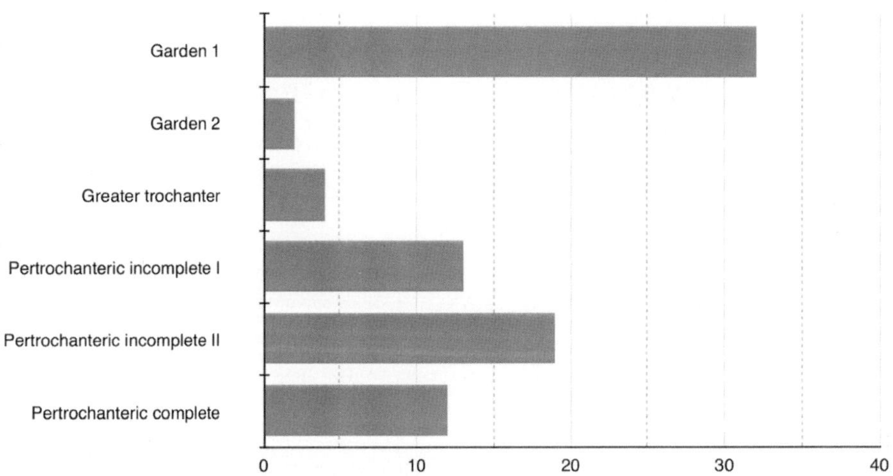

Fig. 1 Distribution of the occult fractures in fracture types. Pertrochanteric incomplete I represents <50 % of the bicortical distance fractured. Pertrochanteric incomplete II represents >50 % of the bicortical distance fractured

All data were recorded electronically using Microsoft Office Excel spread sheets (Microsoft Corporation, Redmond, US-WA) and the statistical analysis was performed using XLStat (Addinsoft SARL New York, US-NY). Approval for this study was obtained from our Hospital's institutional review board (IRB) and informed consent was obtained from each patient.

Results

From a total of 82 identified occult fractures 47 were diagnosed by MRI (57,4 % 95 % CI: 27,4 %–90,9 %) and 12 were diagnosed by emergency CT (14,6 % 95 % CI: 6,0 %-21,9 %). For the remaining 23 cases the final occult fracture diagnosis was confirmed by 72 h CT scan in 9 cases (11 % 95 % CI: 3,7 % – 9,5 % representing 39 % of the false negative cases) or by MRI in the rest of 14 cases (17 % 95 % CI: 3 % – 33,6 %, representing 61 % of the false negative cases) (Fig. 2).

MRI was best ($p = 0.048$) at detecting incomplete pertrochanteric fracture patterns in 84,6 % of the cases (13,45 % of total 95%CI: 12,1 % – 20,7 %) and incomplete fractures of the greater trochanter 75 % (3,65 %) and detected the majority (53 %) of Garden I femoral neck fractures (20,7 % of total). CT scanning accurately detected 100 % of Garden 2 fractures (2,44 % of total) and 25 % of the complete pertrochanteric fractures (3,65 % of total) but with more false negative results (23 false negative results based on acute scan; 28 % of total).

For femoral neck fractures in the elderly (Fig. 3a, b and c), the treatment of choice was hip hemiarthroplasty with a bipolar head and an uncemented stem (Taperlock, Biomet, Warsaw). Three parallel neck screws were used for 2 young patients with good bone stock. Pertrochanteric fractures (Fig. 3d, e and f) were routinely treated by intramedullary nailing (Gamma, Stryker, New Jersey) or extramedullary fixation with a sliding hip screw. Both techniques allowed immediate weight-bearing and early mobilization. Femoral neck fractures concomitant or iatrogenic were not detected in the patients undergoing nailing.

Out of the 82 cases investigated 34 were managed conservatively. Non-operative treatment consisted of bed rest initially and nonweightbearing on the affected leg no sooner than 3 weeks from the trauma. No attempt to manipulate the fracture was made since these were all nondisplaced fractures. No immobilization or skeletal traction was used. Progressive weightbearing was initiated at 6 weeks, starting with 10 %-20 % of total weight and increasing at a rate of 10 %-15 % per week under the direct supervision of a physical therapist. Radiographic evaluation was performed weekly for the first 4 weeks and monthly for the subsequent 3 months.

The relatively high rate of nonoperative treatment (34 cases, 46 % of total) was the result of a number of factors namely: incomplete fractures of the greater trochanter (4 cases, 4,9 %) and incomplete pertrochanteric fractures (13 cases, 15,8 %) In those cases the risk to benefit ratio would not justify the surgical intervention and the consensus of the trauma meeting of our units was in favor of conservative management. Furthermore associated comorbidities (7 cases, 8,5 %) were another rationale to selecting conservative treatment and finally the patient choice (10 cases, 12,2 %).

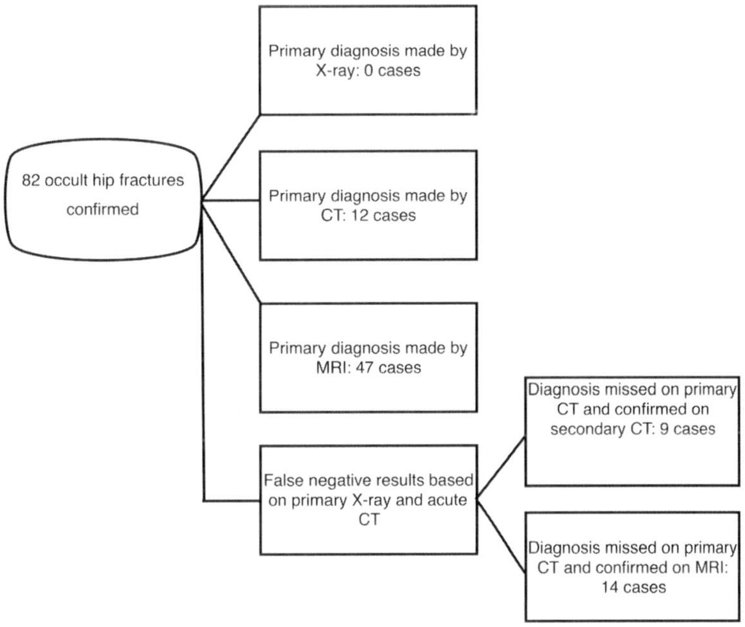

Fig. 2 Case stratification showing the diagnostic algorithm used and the number of fractures diagnosed primarily and secondarily by MRI and CT scan

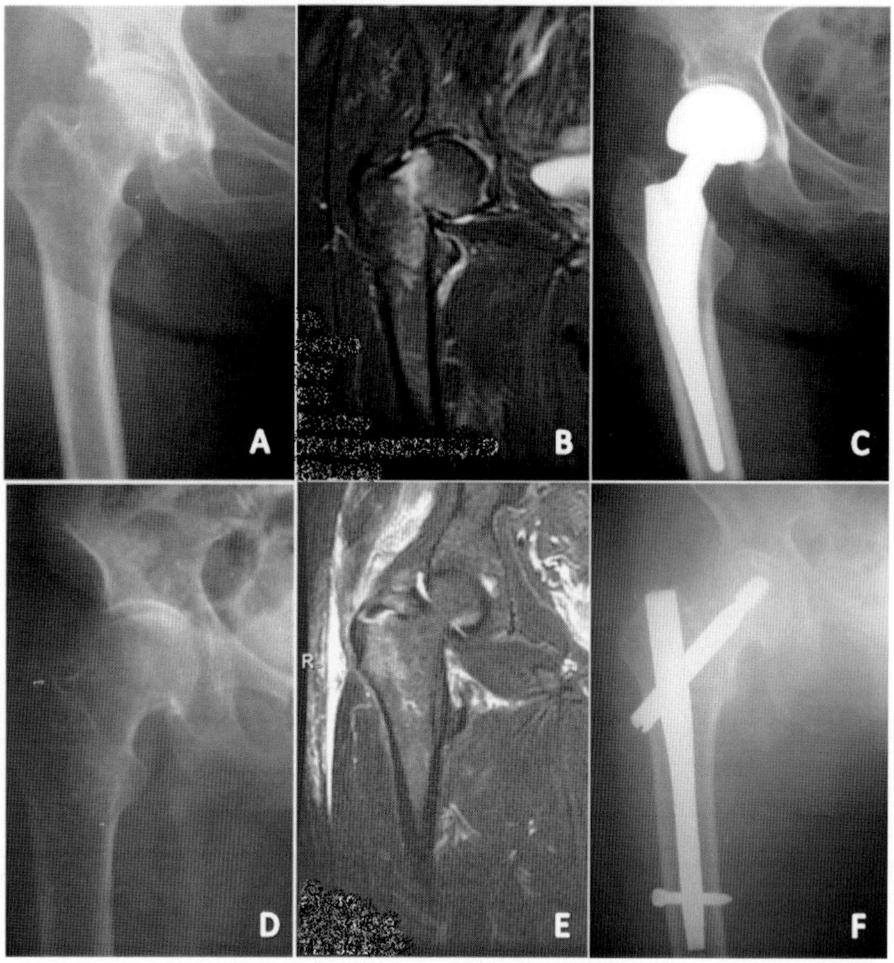

Fig. 3 **a** X-Ray of occult femoral neck fracture of the right hip. **b** MRI of the same case showing a Garden II femoral neck fracture. **c** Postoperative X-ray showing a uncemented bipolar hip. **d** X-Ray of occult pertrochanteric fracture of the right hip. **e** MRI of the same case showing a incomplete pertrochanteric fracture (>50 %). **f** Postoperative X-ray showing osteosynthesis with a Gamma 3 nail (Stryker, NJ)

Discussion

In the current study we present an imaging diagnosis protocol we have developed over the last 10 years using the best imaging modality available in an efficient manner and integrated this data with the selection of established treatment methods.

A hip MRI was preferred if available in the first 24 h. For all the 47 cases investigated by a primary MRI a positive occult hip fracture diagnosis was obtained. An emergency CT scan was performed in 35 cases when the MRI was not available during the first 24 h. This led to a true positive diagnosis in 12 cases. For the remaining 23 patients with negative x-rays and negative emergency CT, but with persistent hip pain, the diagnosis was obtained next day by an MRI scan in 14 cases, or a CT scan in 9 cases 72 h later.

If clinical suspicion of a missed fracture arises with inconclusive radiological results [14] different imaging studies should be employed to investigate the primary cause of hip pain [3]. Further radiographic investigation of the hip is usually not carried out with standardized (oblique, Judet, inlet, outlet) [4] or experimental views [15] or particular digital image processing techniques [16].

Both orthopedic surgeons and radiologists alike consider MRI to be the gold standard in the detection of occult fractures [3, 6, 17–22],with T(1)-weighted coronal MRI having 100 % sensitivity while for T(2)-weighted imaging there was 84.0 % sensitivity [23]. Pandey et al. conducted an ER based study evaluating patients with traumatic hip pain and negative X-rays by MRI. They identified 22 fractures out of 33 suspected cases, but did not provide a total number of hip fractures for the period [21]. Dominguez et al. found 4.4 % of patients with hip trauma and negative X-rays had a hip or pelvic fracture identified by MRI, representing 9.9 % of the total number of hip fractures [4].

CT scanning has been employed for the detection of occult hip fractures [24] with 93 % sensitivity and 95 % specificity. A 72 h delay is advised for further improving sensitivity [25]. In a study by Dunker et al. of 193 hips in elderly patients with negative or inconclusive radiographs, CT scans performed within 24 h after low hip trauma detected 41 femoral neck and 68 pertrochanteric fractures [26]. Jordan et al. in a recent paper recognized the main advantage of CT in its availability (usually 24/7 in a trauma center) and its smaller cost compared to MRI, in conformity with other authors, restating the role of CT in investigating occult hip fractures [2, 5]. A comparative study by Lubovsky et al. concluded that MRI was more accurate and provided less misdiagnosis than CT on a relatively small group of 13 patients [19] while a paper by Hakkarinen reports 4 patients out of 24 occult hip fractures that had a negative 64 slice CT scan and a positive MRI, concluding that while CT scanning is a useful tool in detecting occult hip fractures (18 fractures out of 24 were identified by CT only) false negative results are possible even with 64 slice CT while no fractures were missed by MRI [11]. One of the main shortcomings of computer tomography is the emission of X-rays and the rather high dose of weight dependent ionizing radiation that the patient would receive that it is doubled if a repeat 72 h CT is necessary [27].

Another imaging investigation described in literature is bone scintigraphy using technetium Tc 99 m polyphosphate, with a sensitivity of 98 % [28]. It is dependent on the timing of the examination, with a lower sensitivity and specificity than MRI. It is also less reliable in very old patients and those with circulatory disturbances [12]. Furthermore, the time necessary for a MRI acquisition is much shorter, with trauma protocols taking less than fifteen minutes to perform [1]. Alternative modalities have been evaluated for their value in diagnosing proximal femur fractures. Sonography was found to have 100 % sensibility and 65 % specificity compared to MRI. It could therefore be proposed as a screening tool for occult hip fractures in the absence of readily available MRI [29]. Auscultatory percussion technique is another useful method to assess patients who present with posttraumatic hip pain and normal radiographs [30].

Limitations include the retrospective design of our study and the use of a 16 slice CT scanner, not the most efficient for diagnosing occult hip fractures [11]. The investigation was however performed by a senior radiologist and the evaluation was done together with a senior orthopedic surgeon limiting the bias and false negative results.

Conclusions

In conclusion, any patient with a suspected hip fracture (meaning a patient with significant posttraumatic hip pain, spontaneous, on palpation, mobilization or gait) and negative X-rays should receive further imaging exploration in the first 24 h. If MRI is readily available it should be preferred as it has better accuracy in detecting occult hip fractures. If for whatever reason an MRI cannot be performed in the first 24 h, an emergency CT scan should be used instead. This is often easier to accomplish, as CT is available round the clock in trauma centers and from our experience sufficient for establishing a diagnosis for the majority of patients. However in the case of a negative 24 h CT the patient should be further investigated. Again the MRI should be the investigation of choice, and if not available followed by a repeat CT after 72 h.

Abbreviations

AP: Antero-posterior; ER: Emergency room; CT: Computer tomography; ICD-10: International Statistical Classification of Diseases and Related Health Problems 10th Revision; MRI: Magnetic resonance imaging; X-ray: Radiography.

Competing interests

The authors declare that they have no competing interests.

Authors' contributions

Bogdan Deleanu is the main surgeon, having treated most of the cases involved in the study. He is also responsible for the main idea regarding the the conception and design of the study.
Radu Prejbeanu is treating surgeon for some of the cases involved. He also refined the concept of the study.
Dan Crisan is secondary surgeon and responsible for the design of the study, drafting the article, the acquisition, analysis and interpretation of data.
Horia Haragus is secondary surgeon and analysis and interpretation of data and paper review.
Dinu Vermesan primary surgeon and critical reviewer.
Florin Birsasteanu was involved in the conception of the study improving it with important intellectual content.
Vlad Predescu provided critical review of the article.
Eleftherios Tsiridis provided valuable insights during the initial and ulterior review process and final approval of the version to be submitted.
All authors read and approved the final manuscript.

Authors' information

None.

Acknowledgements

Funding

No funding was received for the design, during the completion phase or for the publication of the manuscript.

Author details

[1]I-st Clinic of Orthopedics and Trauma, Pius Brinzeu Emergency Clinical County Hospital, 10 I. Bulbuca Blvd, 300737 Timisoara, Romania. [2]Victor Babes University of Medicine and Pharmacy, 2 Eftimie Murgu Square, 300041 Timişoara, Romania. [3]Department of Radiology, Pius Brinzeu Emergency Clinical County Hospital, 10 I. Bulbuca Blvd, 300737 Timisoara, Romania. [4]St. Pantelimon Clinical Emergency Hospital, 340 - 342 Pantelimon Road, Sector 2, 033092 Bucharest, Romania. [5]Carol Davila University of Medicine and Pharmacy, 8 Eroii Sanitari Blvd, 050474 Bucharest, Romania. [6]Aristotle University Medical School, 54124 Thessaloniki, Greece.

References

1. Lim A. Occult hip fractures in elderly patients: is CT enough? General Medicine: Open Access. 2013;1(1):1–2.
2. Gill SK, Smith J, Fox R, Chesser TJS. Investigation of occult hip fractures: the use of CT and MRI. Scientific World Journal. 2013;2013:1–4.

3. Cannon J, Silvestri S, Munro M. Imaging choices in occult hip fracture. J Emerg Med. 2009;37:144–52.
4. Dominguez S, Liu P, Roberts C, Mandell M, Richman PB. Prevalence of traumatic hip and pelvic fractures in patients with suspected hip fracture and negative initial standard radiographs–a study of emergency department patients. Acad Emerg Med. 2005;12:366–9.
5. Jordan RW, Dickenson E, Baraza N, Srinivasan K. Who is more accurate in the diagnosis of neck of femur fractures, radiologists or orthopaedic trainees? Skeletal Radiol. 2012;42:173–6.
6. National Clinical Guideline Centre (UK). The Management of Hip Fracture in Adults. London: Royal College of Physicians (UK); 2011.
7. Lee K-H, Kim H-M, Kim Y-S, Jeong C, Moon C-W, Lee S-U, et al. Isolated fractures of the greater trochanter with occult intertrochanteric extension. Arch Orthop Trauma Surg. 2010;130:1275–80.
8. O'Grady SD. Mosby, 2009. Mosby's dictionary of medicine, nursing & health professions. Mosby Elsevier. Nurse Educ Pract. 2010;10:0. ISBN:978-0-323-04937-5.
9. Lakshmanan P, Sharma A, Lyons K, Peehal JP. Are occult fractures of the hip and pelvic ring mutually exclusive? J Bone Joint Surg Br. 2007;89:1344–6.
10. Agency for Healthcare Research and Quality [http://www.guideline.gov/content.aspx?id=47668].
11. Hakkarinen DK, Banh KV, Hendey GW. Magnetic resonance imaging identifies occult hip fractures missed by 64-slice computed tomography. J Emerg Med. 2012;43:303–7.
12. Rubin G, Malka I, Rozen N. Should we operate on occult hip fractures? Isr Med Assoc J. 2010;12:316–7.
13. Rizzo PF, Gould ES, Lyden JP, Asnis SE. Diagnosis of occult fractures about the hip. Magnetic resonance imaging compared with bone-scanning. J Bone Joint Surg Am. 1993;75:395–401.
14. Helland EB, Tollefsen I, Reksten G. Radiographic diagnosis of the occult hip fracture: experience in 16 patients. Acta Orthop. 2000;71:639–41.
15. Harding J, Chesser TJS, Bradley M. The bristol hip view: its role in the diagnosis and surgical planning and occult fracture diagnosis for proximal femoral fractures. Scientific World Journal. 2013;2013:703783–4.
16. Botser IB, Herman A, Nathaniel R, Rappaport D, Chechik A. Digital image enhancement improves diagnosis of nondisplaced proximal femur fractures. Clin Orthop Relat Res. 2009;467:246–53.
17. Frihagen F, Nordsletten L, Tariq R, Madsen JE. MRI diagnosis of occult hip fractures. Acta Orthop. 2005;76:524–30.
18. Hossain M, Barwick C, Sinha AK, Andrew JG. Is magnetic resonance imaging (MRI) necessary to exclude occult hip fracture? Injury. 2007;38:1204–8.
19. Lubovsky O, Liebergall M, Mattan Y, Weil Y, Mosheiff R. Early diagnosis of occult hip fractures MRI versus CT scan. Injury. 2005;36:788–92.
20. Nachtrab O, Cassar-Pullicino VN, Lalam R, Tins B, Tyrrell PNM, Singh J. Role of MRI in hip fractures, including stress fractures, occult fractures, avulsion fractures. Eur J Radiol. 2012;81:3813–23.
21. Grad WB, Desy NM. Bilateral occult hip fracture. CJEM. 2012;14(6):372–7.
22. Lee YP, Griffith JF, Antonio GE, Tang N, Leung KS. Early magnetic resonance imaging of radiographically occult osteoporotic fractures of the femoral neck. Hong Kong Med J. 2004;10:271–5.
23. Iwata T, Nozawa S, Dohjima T, Yamamoto T, Ishimaru D, Tsugita M, et al. The value of T1-weighted coronal MRI scans in diagnosing occult fracture of the hip. J Bone Joint Surg Br. 2012;94:969–73.
24. Collin D, Dunker D, Göthlin JH, Geijer M. Observer variation for radiography, computed tomography, and magnetic resonance imaging of occult hip fractures. Acta Radiol. 2011;52:871–4.
25. Gangopadhyay S, Akra GA, Nanu AM. Occult hip fractures in the elderly: a protocol for management. Eur J Orthop Surg Traumatol. 2006;17:153–6.
26. Dunker D, Collin D, Göthlin JH, Geijer M. High clinical utility of computed tomography compared to radiography in elderly patients with occult hip fracture after low-energy trauma. Emerg Radiol. 2012;19:135–9.
27. Israel GM, Cicchiello L, Brink J, Huda W. Patient size and radiation exposure in thoracic, pelvic, and abdominal CT examinations performed with automatic exposure control. AJR Am J Roentgenol. 2010;195:1342–6.
28. Brunner LC, Eshilian-Oates L, Kuo TY. Hip fractures in adults. Am Fam Physician. 2003;67:537–42.
29. Safran O, Goldman V, Applbaum Y, Milgrom C, Bloom R, Peyser A, et al. Posttraumatic painful hip: sonography as a screening test for occult hip fractures. J Ultrasound Med. 2009;28:1447–52.
30. File P, Wood JP, Kreplick LW. Diagnosis of hip fracture by the auscultatory percussion technique. Am J Emerg Med. 1998;16:173–6.

5

Emergency General Surgery: evolution of a subspecialty by stealth

L. Pearce*, S. R. Smith, E. Parkin, C. Hall, J. Kennedy and A. Macdonald

Abstract

Background: Emergency surgical patients account for around half of all NHS surgical workload and 80 % of surgical deaths. Few trainees opt to CCT in General Surgery, and there is no recognised subspecialty training program in Emergency General Surgery (EGS). Despite this lack of training and relevant assessment by examination, there appears to be an increasing number of EGS posts advertised. This study aims to provide information about potential future employment opportunities for surgical trainees.

Methods: All consultant surgeon posts, advertised in the British Medical Journal between January 2009 and December 2014 were included. Data collected included specialty, region and institute of advertised post. For the purposes of statistical analysis, data was divided into two separate year bands: 2009–2011 and 2012–2014. Statistical analysis was by Chi-squared test; $p < 0.01$ was considered statistically significant. An online tool was also used to determine experience and attitudes towards EGS amongst Consultant members of the ASGBI and all UK trainees in national training number (NTN) posts.

Results: Over the six-year study period, there were 1240 consultant job adverts in a general surgical specialty. Nine hundred and 75 were substantive posts; the region with the most jobs was London and the South East ($n = 278$). There were 55 jobs advertised in EGS, either with (20) or without (35) another subspecialty. The number of EGS adverts increased significantly in 2012–14 compared to 2009–11 ($p = 0.008$). 229 (28 %) Consultants and 309 (22 %) trainees responded to the survey. 16 % of consultants work in NHS institutions with Emergency General Surgeons. Only 21 % of trainees believe EGS will be delivered by EGS consultants in the future whilst 8.2 % of trainees stated EGS as their career plan. Less than half of all UK consultant surgeons see EGS as a subspecialty.

Conclusions: This data demonstrates increasing societal need for EGS consultants over the last six years and the emergence of Emergency Surgery as a new subspecialty. In order to meet the EGS needs of the NHS, general surgical training and the examination system need to be revised.

Background

Centralisation of services within the UK's National Health Service (NHS) has led to increasing subspecialisation within general surgery over the last ten years. Whilst this may be considered beneficial for elective care, numbers of surgeons with the diverse skill set required for the Emergency General Surgery (EGS) workload (50 % of all surgical workload, 80 % of surgical deaths) is reducing. More recently, through the publication of key documents and statements [1–5], there has been an increase in focus on Emergency General Surgical patients and the acute care surgical services that institutions are able to provide to manage them. However, for subspecialists, general surgical emergencies (often outside of their trained subspecialty) continue to be a major part of their consultant practice [6].

Standards have been set for the provision of emergency surgical care in the UK [2]. Senior prompt decision making has been shown to improve emergency surgical patient experience and outcomes [7, 8]. Consultant leadership is essential to ensure the safety of patients managed by the relatively new concept of ambulatory emergency care services within surgery [9].

Several different models of acute surgical service provision have been implemented by NHS institutions across the UK. Some larger centres provide simultaneous

* Correspondence: lpearce@doctors.org.uk
Clinical Research Fellow, Department of General Surgery, Central Manchester University Hospitals Foundation Trust, Oxford Road, Manchester M13 9WL, UK

upper gastrointestinal, lower gastrointestinal and hepatobiliary daytime and 'out of hours' acute service. However, this model of care reduces subspecialist availability for elective work (rewarded by NHS tariffs) and is not possible in hospitals with small numbers of subspecialty consultants.

Many centres have appointed Consultant Emergency General Surgeons to provide a consultant led and consultant delivered acute care surgical service for emergency patients. As such, the term 'Emergency General Surgeon' is now one with which we are becoming increasing familiar in the UK. However, EGS remains an unrecognised UK training subspecialty without a separate higher surgical training programme [10] or modular competency based assessment.

Aims

This study aims to ascertain UK Consultant and Trainees experiences and attitudes towards Emergency General Surgery and to provide information about potential future employment opportunities for trainees.

Methods

An online survey tool was used (www.surveymonkey.net) to determine UK experience and attitudes towards Emergency General Surgery (EGS). Two separate online links were sent to consultant members of the ASGBI and all UK trainees in national training number (NTN) posts.

A review of all consultant general surgeon posts advertised in the British Medical Journal (BMJ) between 1st January 2009 and 31st December 2014 (72 months) was undertaken. Posts in general surgical specialities were included. Advertisements for plastic surgery, orthopaedic, cardiothoracic, urology, otorhinolaryngology, academic posts, senior lecturer and locum agency posts were excluded.

Job adverts were categorised as follows:

- Academic
- Breast
- Breast and general surgery
- Colorectal
- Colorectal and general surgery
- EGS/EGS and general surgery
- EGS and another subspecialty
- Endocrine
- Endocrine and general surgery
- General only
- Hepatobiliary
- Hepatobiliary and general surgery
- Remote and rural surgery
- Transplant
- Trauma
- Upper gastrointestinal
- Upper gastrointestinal and general surgery
- Vascular
- Vascular & general surgery
- Other

Data was also collected on the region, term and basis of appointment (locum or substantive, full or part time) and specialty advertised.

All analyses were performed using Stata, version 11.2 (College Station, TX, USA). We divided the data up into two discrete year bands – 2009–11 & 2012–14 – and explored how job adverts had changed over time using the Chi-squared test. $P < 0.01$ was considered statistically significant.

Results

Whilst 44 % of consultants surveyed view EGS as a subspecialty, a minority of consultant surgeons surveyed (16 %) currently work in institutions with EGS consultants. More recently appointed consultants less often felt ready for independent EGS duty than those appointed previously (10–20 years in post; 80 % ready compared with 2–5 years in post; 62 % ready). More than half (52 %) of consultants in post for less than five years would have felt 'better' prepared' for EGS with a dedicated period of EGS training, compared with 13 % of those in post for less than twenty years ($p = 0.022$). Nearly all trainees (92.4 %) felt more intensive training in emergency surgery would be beneficial to their general surgical training i.e. 6-month post in acute surgery. Seventy per cent of Consultant surgeons envisage a future model of EGS cover utilising EGS surgeons compared with 21 % of trainees.

There were 1240 consultant jobs in a general surgical specialty advertised in the BMJ over the 6-year study period. Nine hundred and 75 were substantive posts. Eighty nine per cent of all posts ($n = 1104$) were advertised on a full time basis with less than full time considered in ten percent of posts ($n = 124$). Only one percent of all posts were advertised on a purely part time basis (80 % breast subspecialty).

The region with the most jobs was London and the South East ($n = 278$) (see Table 1). The total number of posts was 645 in 2009–11 and 595 in 2012–14. Table 2 displays job adverts according to subspecialty, comparing 2009–11 with 2012–14.

In total, there were 55 jobs advertised in EGS, either with (20) or without (35) another subspecialty. The number of EGS adverts increased significantly in 2012–14 compared to 2009–11 ($p = 0.008$). London and the South East were the highest recruiters to EGS posts (10 % of all consultant surgeon posts advertised in the region). There was a borderline decrease in the number of breast & general jobs advertised ($p = 0.021$). Numbers

Table 1 Regional consultant surgeon job advertisements in the British Medical Journal 2009–2014

Region	Number of posts advertised
North West	155
North East	13
North & Yorkshire	136
West Midlands	98
East Midlands	73
Eastern	95
London	115
South West	106
South East	163
Scotland	191
Wales	52
N. Ireland	43
Total	1240

of vascular & general jobs and purely general jobs did not change significantly over time.

Discussion

It is an exciting time for Emergency General Surgery in the UK and changes should be embraced. Our study has highlighted the disparity between public and societal need, and the career aspirations of UK higher surgical trainees.

We have demonstrated evidence of an expanding national acute surgical workforce in the form of Emergency General Surgeons. Apart from a borderline decrease in the number of breast & general jobs, recruitment to other subspecialties has not changed significantly over the past 6 years.

International models of care and the provision of training

Focus upon elective subspecialisation, and subsequent centralisation of services, has resulted in near extinction of the traditional "general surgeon" who regularly operated on multiple organ systems. There is worldwide debate surrounding the provision of acute care surgical services [11], appropriate models of emergency surgical care provision and related issues of decreased training time, operative exposure and ever increasing "super-sub-specialisation" [12].

In recent years, international surgical colleges have published standards for emergency surgical care [2, 13, 14], but there remains abundant multifactorial heterogeneity between institutional models facilitating acute care surgical service provision [11]. The development of the specialty of Acute Care Surgery (ACS), Trauma and

Table 2 Consultant surgeon job advertisements in the British Medical Journal 2009–2014

Specialty	2009–2011	2012–2014	Overall
Academic	1	1	2
Breast	104	94	198
Breast & general	34	16	50
Colorectal	94	98	192
Colorectal & general	69	52	121
EGS/EGS & general	11	24	35
EGS & other specialty	8	12	20
Endocrine	2	2	4
Endocrine & general	1	2	3
General only	79	91	170
HPB	24	18	42
HPB & general	1	3	4
Remote & rural	4	0	4
Transplant	18	24	42
Trauma	2	2	4
UGI	61	44	105
UGI & general	50	52	102
Vascular	70	55	125
Vascular & general	10	4	14
Other	2	1	3
Total	645	595	1240

Critical Care in the USA has provided dedicated acute care subspecialty training for surgical residents. Whilst the training models are varied as dictated by widespread geographical variability in case mix (and particular trauma services) there is a minimum standard required within the curriculum for Acute Care Surgeons as detailed by the American Association for the Surgery of Trauma.

The Netherlands, Germany, Sweden and the UK are yet to develop nationally and establish a dedicated acute care surgical service [15]. Despite no UK national agreement on an appropriate acute model of care and a dedicated subspecialty emergency surgical training programme in the UK, our results show an increase in EGS appointments in the last 3 years. Similar appointments are being made in other European countries [16].

Recent changes in UK Training

Surgical training has also become increasingly subspecialised. In 2013, vascular higher surgical training was uncoupled from general surgical training. Consequently, future vascular surgeons will not be adequately trained to provide acute emergency general surgical care at consultant level. Furthermore, few trainees opt to pursue a Completion Certificate of Training (CCT) in general surgery and EGS (or ACS) is not a recognised subspecialty. Our study demonstrates significant increase in numbers of emergency general surgical consultant posts but lack of expansion of UK consultant subspecialty posts in the last 3 years. Trainees are therefore facing unpredictable employment opportunities at the end of higher surgical subspecialty training in the UK.

Training in EGS

EGS is often perceived to be associated with unpredictable out of hours operating, 'disruption' to elective services and adverse outcomes by trainee participation in cases [7]. However, there is clear evident public and societal need for emergency general surgeons, which has been acknowledged by NHS organisations and Consultant surgeons. Despite this, UK higher surgical training programmes have not, in the most part, sought to address potential short falls in emergency general surgical training, and competencies or encouraged trainees to pursue a career in EGS. Numbers of index emergency procedures (i.e. laparotomies) at CCT fall short of the detailed clinical competencies, case mix and volume of cases required for CCT in other subspecialties. Emergency general surgical training remains acquired during out of hours service provision (limited by European Working Time Directive) on an ad hoc basis, is not standardised and a workforce gap has been created.

Future of EGS

Hospitals in the UK and beyond are appointing more emergency general surgeons, but their exact role within an organisation and their level of surgical competence has not been clearly defined. Individuals appointed to these roles should be trained to make appropriate clinical decisions in the management of emergency general surgical patients and be able to perform complex emergency procedures. They will also need to enable trainees to acquire the necessary skill set for independent emergency surgical practice.

The increase in EGS posts demonstrated in our study highlights potential employment opportunities for future higher surgical trainees and supports the need for a dedicated modular or higher surgical training programme in EGS. As not all emergency surgical skills can be developed in the elective setting, a dedicated period of emergency surgical training and assessment during higher surgical training could be beneficial by facilitating exposure to an array of complex and common emergency cases within the constraints of EWTD.

Conclusion

It is likely that EGS provision in the UK NHS will continue to undergo significant change over the next decade. EGS is emerging as a subspecialty in its own right and trainees should consider future employment opportunities when declaring chosen subspecialty training. The Higher Surgical Training programme and examination system in general surgery should be modified to address these changes to ensure emergency surgical patients in the NHS receive expeditious, high quality care.

Competing interests

The authors declare that they have no competing interests.

Authors' contributions

LP was involved in design of the study, data collection for posts and survey data, data analysis and writing of the manuscript. SS was involved in egs post data collection and writing of the manuscript. EP collected egs post data and performed data analysis. CH collected survey data and performed data analysis and proof reading of manuscript. JK collected EGS post data. AM was involved in design of the study. All authors read and approved the final manuscript.

References

1. RCSEng. The higher risk surgical patient; towards improved care for a forgotten group. England: Royal College of Surgeons; 2011. http://www.rcseng.ac.uk.
2. RCSEng. Emergency surgery: standards for unscheduled care. England: Royal College of Surgeons; 2011. http://www.rcseng.ac.uk.
3. Concerns about UK emergency surgery death rates. Lancet 384, 1238 (2014).
4. Barrow E, Anderson ID, Varley S, Pichel AC, Peden CJ, Saunders DI, et al. Current UK practice in emergency laparotomy. Ann R Coll Surg Engl. 2013; 95:599–603.
5. Saunders DI, Murray D, Pichel AC, Varley S, Peden CJ. Variations in mortality after emergency laparotomy: the first report of the UK Emergency Laparotomy Network. Br J Anaesth. 2012;109:368–75.

6. Garner JP, Prytherch D, Senapati A, O'Leary D, Thompson MR. Sub-specialization in general surgery: the problem of providing a safe emergency general surgical service. Colorectal Dis. 2006;8:273–7.
7. Kasotakis G, Lakha A, Sarkar B, Kunitake H, Kissane-Lee N, Dechert T, et al. Trainee participation is associated with adverse outcomes in emergency general surgery: an analysis of the National Surgical Quality Improvement Program database. Ann Surg. 2014;260:483–90. discussion 490–3.
8. Suen K, Hayes IP, Thomson BN, Shedda S. Effect of the introduction of an emergency general surgery service on outcomes from appendicectomy. Br J Surg. 2014;101:e141–6.
9. Tribouloy JP. Ambulatory emergency surgery. Presse Med. 2014;43:301–4.
10. Training, J.C.o.S. Guidelines for the award of a CCT in general surgery. 2014. http://www.jcst.org.
11. Bhagvan S, Civil I. Acute care surgery: can New Zealand afford to wait? N Z Med J. 2009;122:71–6.
12. Soreide K. Trauma and the acute care surgery model–should it embrace or replace general surgery? Scand J Trauma Resusc Emerg Med. 2009;17:4.
13. Model of Care for Acute Surgery; National Clinical Programme in Surgery. Royal College of Surgeons of Ireland. 2013. www.rcsie.ie.
14. Emergency Surgery Position Paper. Royal australasian college of surgeons. 2015. http://www.surgeons.org.
15. International comparisons o fselected service lines in seven health systems. Annex 7 - review of service lines: Emergency Surgery. Evidence report October 27th 2014. http://www.gov.uk.
16. Poole GH, Glyn T, Srinivasa S, Hill AG. Modular acute system for general surgery: hand over the operation, not the patient. ANZ J Surg. 2012;82:156–60.

One year experience of swine dermal non-crosslinked collagen prostheses for abdominal wall repairs in elective and emergency surgery

Giulia Montori[1*], Federico Coccolini[1], Roberto Manfredi[1], Marco Ceresoli[1], Luca Campanati[1], Stefano Magnone[1], Michele Pisano[1], Elia Poiasina[1], Gabriela Nita[1], Fausto Catena[2] and Luca Ansaloni[1]

Abstract

Introduction: The approach to the abdominal wall surgical repair is dramatically changed in the last years. This study evaluates our institutional outcomes about the usage of biological meshes for abdominal wall repair in different setting: in elective surgery, in emergency surgery and in abdominal wall repair following open abdomen (OA) procedure.

Methods: A database was prospectively conducted (January–December 2014) and data were reviewed for patients who underwent to an abdominal wall reconstruction with swine dermal non-cross linked collagens prostheses either in elective or emergency setting, and following OA/laparostomy procedure. Demographic data, co-morbidities, indications for surgery, intra-operative details, post-operative complications and outcome (peri-operative, 3, 6, 9-months) were analyzed.

Results: A total of 30 cases were reported: 9 in elective surgery (Group 1), 4 in emergency surgery (Group 2) and 17 with abdominal wall closure following OA management (Group 3). Two meshes were removed: 1 in the Group 1 and 1 in the Group 3. During follow-up only one patient in the Group 3 had a recurrence of the incisional hernia. Mortality rate was 11.1 % at 3 months in Group 1, 0 % in the Group 2, and 29.4 % in peri-operative period in the Group 3.

Conclusions: The use of non-cross linked biological meshes can be safe and versatile in different situations from elective to emergency surgery, and also for the reconstruction of the abdominal wall after OA procedure, with an acceptable recurrence and mortality rate.

Keywords: Biological mesh, Ventral hernia, Abdominal wall repair, Swine dermal collagen, Open abdomen, Laparostomy, Emergency surgery

Background

Abdominal wall hernia is one of the most common conditions encountered by general surgeons. Procedures to repair abdominal wall defects are more than 990.000 each year in USA, with an estimated 567.000 of them performed in emergency [1, 2]. Similar data are reported in other Western countries [3]. In most cases emergency hernia repair are performed in adults over 65 years old [2]. These age-related increasing rates of emergency hernia repair are associated with increased morbidity and mortality risks [2]. In these particular situations the use of biological materials can be safer than synthetic meshes [4]. Actually in the late 1990s, biologic materials for hernia repair were introduced as a possible biocompatible material to support "in vivo" tissue regeneration to restore the physiological function of the abdominal wall [4, 5]. Although these biomaterials enacted a new conceptual approach in abdominal wall reconstruction [5, 6], the main reported problems related with the use of biological meshes are: wound infections, seromas, fistula formation, recurrence of the defect (25–28 % in grade 3–4 of the Ventral Hernia Working Group (VHWG) classification [4]) and costs [7, 8]. Nevertheless definitive conclusions about the use of these biological

* Correspondence: giulia.montori@gmail.com
[1]Unit of General and Emergency Surgery, Papa Giovanni XXIII Hospital, P.zza OMS 1, 24128 Bergamo, Italy
Full list of author information is available at the end of the article

materials are difficult to drawn due to: lack of adequate follow-up, use either of different surgical techniques and/or different types of biological meshes and absence of high levels of evidence studies [7, 8]. However there are many advantages in using biological meshes compared to the synthetic prostheses: less prosthetic erosions and/or fistulization, less chronic pain, and minor risk of infection [9].

Porcine dermal prostheses are manufactured by collagenic tissue harvesting, followed by a variety of patented chemical treatments and delipidation processes [10]. Although natural cross-links exist in native collagen and function to stabilize the structure of the collagenic proteins, giving mechanical strength and protection from collagenase [10], however some prostheses undergo to an additional phase chemical cross-linking process to increase the collagen strength [10]. The addition of chemical cross-linking between the collagen chains seems to further reduce the bacterial and host collagenase enzymes activity, slowing the degradation process of the prostheses. For this reason the indications report in literature suggest a use of cross-linked mesh in more contaminated field [11]. However some authors reports that porcine biologic non-cross-linked mesh has been used to support the repair of abdomen wall with a hernia recurrence rates of 7 % in case of underlay position, while in the cross-linked porcine mesh group infection and explantation rates were relatively higher [9]. These data indicate that there is currently no ideal biologic mesh for complex hernia repair and the candidate for biologic mesh implantation has not been clearly defined yet. A Randomized Control Trial (SIMBIOSE study: use of biological mesh versus standard wound care in infected incisional ventral hernias) is ongoing to evaluate the efficacy of biologic mesh in infected field [12].

This study evaluates our institutional outcomes about the usage of biological meshes for abdominal wall repair in three different setting: in elective surgery, in emergency surgery and following open abdomen (OA)/laparostomy procedure.

Methods

An analysis was performed on a prospectively maintained database from January 1st, 2014 to December 31st, 2014 of all patients who underwent primary or recurrent hernia repair with the usage of swine dermal collagens prostheses at Papa Giovanni XXIII Hospital (Bergamo, Italy). Enclosed patients were divided into 3 groups: abdominal wall reconstruction in elective surgery (Group 1), in emergency surgery (Group 2) and following OA/laparostomy management (Group 3). In all patients were used 1.4 mm thick, non-cross linked swine dermal collagen prostheses, with different dimensions (8*14, 10*20, 25*18, 20*30) (Protexa™, Tecnoss, Giaveno, Italy), fixed to the fascia with resorbable PDS 1 or 0. In case of elective surgery and in clean field the antibiotic prophylaxis used was Cefazolin 2 g, in the dirty and contaminated field the antibiotic theraphy was accord to the WSES guideline for the management of the intra-abdominal infection (IAI) [13]. Patients data were collected and analyzed evaluating demographic characteristics, co-morbidities, surgical indications, intra-operative details, complications (according to the Dindo-Clavien classification [14]) and outcome (peri-operative, at 3, 6, 9 months). Incisional hernia was classified according to the VHWG classification [4]. In case of septic implant, the peritonitis severity was evaluated according to the Mannheim Peritonitis Index (MPI) at the first laparotomy and at every subsequent abdominal exploration if indicated [15]. The severity of the trauma was calculated according to the Injury Severity Score (ISS) [16]. Balthazar score was used to evaluate the severity of pancreatitis [17]. The OA was classified according to the Björck classification [18].

Results

Thirty patients undergoing abdominal wall reconstruction with indication for biologic mesh placement and with swine dermal non-crosslinked collagen prostheses implant were enrolled in the study period. Of these patients, 9 were in Group 1 (Table 1), 4 in Group 2 (Table 2), and 17 in Group 3 (Table 3). According to the Hernia Grading System [4] 5 of the 30 patients presents a clean surgical site but high comorbidities, 21 patients have a contaminated field, and four patients have a dirty surgical site.

Demographics characteristics

In Group 1, nine patients were enrolled: four of them were female. The mean age was 68.3 years (range 53–83). In all patients the surgical indication was incisional hernia repair. The use of the biological mesh was imposed due to the co-morbidities of the patients (grade 2 VHWG classification) and due to the presence of a previous wound infection and/or gastrointestinal tract resection (grade 3 VHWG classification). In six patients one or more comorbidities were present and listed as follows: immunodepression, a concomitant malignancy, abdominal aortic aneurism, diabetes, cardiopathy, bronchopneumopathy chronic obstructive. The others 3 patients have no comorbidity. However all these nine patients presented an intra-operative condition requiring the placement of a biological prosthesis: six patients underwent to colic anastomosis for colic resection, one patient had a prosthetic infection, and two patients had intra-abdominal infections (abscess from acute appendicitis and a ischemic small bowel).

In Group 2, four patients were enclosed (2 were female), with a mean age of 76.5 years (range 66–89). In this group the surgical indications were the following:

Table 1 Patients characteristics underwent to abdominal wall repair in elective surgery

Characteristics (*N* = 9)	Value	*N* (%)
Gender	Male	5 (55.6)
	Female	4 (44.4)
Age	Mean (SD), yrs	68.3 (±9.3)
	Median (range), yrs	68 (53–83)
Surgical indications	Incisional hernia	9 (100)
Comorbidities[a]	Immunodepression	4
	Abdominal aortic aneurism	1
	Diabetes	1
	Malignancy	3
	Cardiopathy	2
	BPCO	2
	None	3
Indications for the positioning of the prostheses	Colic anastomosis	6 (66.7)
	Previous prosthetic infection	1 (11.1)
	Intraabdominal infection	2 (22.2)
Prosthetic position	Onlay	0 (0)
	Inlay	0 (0)
	Retromuscolar	6 (66.7)
	Preperitoneal	0 (0)
	Intraperitoneal	3 (33.3)
Hospital stay	Mean (SD), dys	21 (±21)
	Median (range), dys	14 (7–70)
Mortality rates	At 1 month	0
	At 3 months	1 (11.1)
	At 6 months	0
	At 9 months	0

(*SD* standard deviation; *pts* patients, *yrs* years, *BPCO* bronchopneumopathy chronic obstructive)

[a]More than one patient has more than one comorbidity

Table 2 Patients characteristics underwent to abdominal wall repair in emergency surgery

Characteristics (*N* = 4)	Value	*N* (%)
Gender	Male	2 (50)
	Female	2 (50)
Age	Mean (SD), yrs	76.5 (±9.4)
	Median (range), yrs	75.5 (66–89)
Surgical indications	Complicated incisional hernia	1 (25)
	Diverticular perforation and incisional hernia	1 (25)
	Eventration and ileo anastomosis	1 (25)
	Recto-vaginal fistula and incisional hernia	1 (25)
Comorbidities[a]	Corticosteroid therapy	2
	Cardiovascular disease	2
	Inflammatory bowel disease	1
	Cerebrovascular disease	1
	None	2
Prothetic position	Onlay	1 (25)
	Inlay	1 (25)
	Retromuscolar	2 (50)
	Preperitoneal	0 (0)
	Intraperitoneal	0 (0)
Hospital stay	Mean (SD), dys	21.5 (±16.8)
	Median (range), dys	16.5 (7–45)
Mortality rates	At 1 month	0 (0)
	At 3 months	0 (0)
	At 6 months	0 (0)
	At 9 months	0 (0)

(*SD* standard deviation, *pts* patients, *dys* days, *yrs* years)

[a]More than one patient has more than one comorbidity

abdominal hernia complicated with an enterocutaneous fistula, a diverticular perforation with a large incisional hernia, an eventration complicating a previous surgery with a small bowel resection and anastomoses, and an incisional hernia with a recto-vaginal fistula in Crohn disease. Two patients presented more than one comorbidity: corticosteroid therapy, cardio-vascular disease, inflammatory bowel disease, and cerebrovascular disease. The other two patients had no previous diseases.

In Group 3, 17 patients were analyzed (9 patients were female). The mean age was 62.6 years (range 18–79). The main frequent comorbidities were: presence of cardiopathy and vasculopathy, the malignancy (gastric and colic cancer), and an immunosuppressed status. The others comorbidities present were the following: abdominal aortic aneurism, hemodialysis, and diabetes. Only three patients had no comorbidity. Seven patients (41.2 %) underwent to an OA procedure for intra-abdominal sepsis (anastomotic leak, appendicular peritonitis, biliary peritonitis), four patients (23.6 %) for intestinal ischemia, three patients (17.6 %) for trauma, two patients (11.8 %) after vascular surgery complications (duodenal perforation after exclusion of aortic aneurism), one patient (5.8 %) for severe acute pancreatitis. In 12 patients (70.6 %) the choice for the OA was to prevent the abdominal compartment syndrome; in 5 cases (29.4 %) the OA was performed to treat an increase of intra-abdominal pressure. In all patients the abdominal closure was planned at the first laparotomy and the decision of the biological prostheses usage was related to the intra-operative condition at the moment of the abdominal wall reconstruction. Eight patients (47 %) were from the Intensive Care Unit (ICU). For the three trauma patients the mean and median ISS were 38.3 (SD ± 14.3)

Table 3 Patients characteristics underwent to abdominal wall repair in open abdomen

Characteristics ($N = 17$)	Value	*N* (%)
Gender	Male	8 (47)
	Female	9 (53)
Age	Mean (SD), yrs	62.6 (±18.6)
	Median (range), yrs	72 (18–79)
Surgical indications to open abdomen	Intra-abdominal sepsis and/or post-operative complications	7 (41.2)
	Pancreatitis	1 (5.8)
	Trauma	3 (17.6)
	Vascular complications	2 (11.8)
	Intestinal ischemia	4 (23.6)
Comorbidities[a]	Corticosteroid therapy	2
	Cardiopathy and vasculopathy	9
	Malignancy	6
	Infectious diseases, immunodepression	5
	Abdominal aortic aneurism	4
	Hemodialisis	1
	Diabetes	1
	None	3
Provenience of the pts	ICU	8 (47)
	Ward	5 (29.5)
	Emergency department	4 (23.5)
ISS ($N = 3$)	ISS mean (SD)	38.3 (±14.3)
	ISS median (range)	35 (26–54)
Bathazar score ($N = 1$)	E	
MPI ($N = 14$)	MPI mean (SD)	26.6 (±8.8)
	MPI median (range)	26 (15–43)
	<21	4 (28.6)
	21–29	5 (35.7)
	>29	5 (35.7)
Bjorck classification at the first laparotomy	Ia	7 (41.4)
	Ib	4 (23.5)
	IIa	0 (0)
	IIb	6 (35.1)
	III	0 (0)
	IV	0 (0)
Bjorck classification at the closure	Ia	13 (76.6)
	Ib	0 (0)
	IIa	3 (17.6)
	IIb	0 (0)
	III	0 (0)
	IV	1 (5.8)

Table 3 Patients characteristics underwent to abdominal wall repair in open abdomen ***(Continued)***

Causes of OA	Prevention of ACS	12 (70.6)
	Treatment of ACS	5 (29.4)
Type of OA	NPWT	16 (94.2)
	Skin closure	1 (5.8)
Closure abdominal wall	Mean (SD), dys	6.1 (±3.5)
	Median (range), dys	6 (1–15)
Stoma	Yes	4 (23.5)
	- colostomy	2 (50)
	- ileostomy	1 (25)
	- urostomy	1 (25)
	No	13 (76.5)
Intestinal anastomosis	Yes	11 (64.7)
	No	6 (35.3)
Enterocutaneous fistula	Yes	1 (5.8)
	No	16 (94.2)
Fascia closure	Yes	9 (53)
	No	8 (47)
Prothetic position	Onlay	2 (11.8)
	Inlay	1 (5.8)
	Retromuscolar	9 (52.8)
	Preperitoneal	0 (0)
	Intraperitoneal	5 (29.6)
Hospital stay	ICU	
	Mean (SD), dys	23.9 (±18.2)
	Median (range), dys	20 (2–71)
	Ward	
	Mean (SD), dys	28.4 (±21.2)
	Median (range), dys	23 (0–70)
Mortality rates	Peri-operative	5 (29.4)
	At 3 months	0 (0)
	At 6 months	0 (0)
	At 9 months	0 (0)

(*NPWT* negative pressure wound therapy, *pts* patients, *dys* days, *yrs* years, *SD* standard deviation, *ISS* Injury Severity Score, *MPI* Mannheim Peritoneal Index, *OA* Open Abdomen)
[a]More than one patient has more than one comorbidity

and 35 (range 26–54) respectively. For the patient with pancreatitis the Balthazar score before surgery was E.

Intraoperative details

In Group 1, the mesh was placed intra-peritoneally in three patients and in the retromuscolar plane in six patients.

In Group 2, the mesh was placed inlay (as a bridge between the medial edges) and onlay (in the subcutaneous space) in one patient each, and in the retromuscolar plane in two patients.

In Group 3, in 14 patients (the three trauma patients were excluded) the mean MPI was 26.6 (range 15–43). Four patients had a MPI < 21, five patients had a MPI between 21 to 29 and five patients had a MPI up to 29. According to the Björck score the majority of the patients (7 patients) had a grade Ia at the first laparotomy. Four patients had a grade Ib, and six patients had a grade IIb. At the closure, the rate of grade Björck Ia was in 13 patients (3 patients had a Björck IIa, and 1 patient a Björck IV). In 16 patients the OA was managed with a negative pressure wound therapy (NPWT) technique, and in 1 case the skin closure technique was performed. At the definitive intervention, the fascial closure was performed in nine patients (53 %), in the others eight patients only the posterior fascia was closed. In all 17 patients the abdominal wall was reinforced with a biological mesh: in nine patients the mesh was placed in the retromuscolar plane (sublay), in five patients intraperitoneally, in two patients onlay, and in 1 pt it was placed inlay. The time to definitive abdominal closure after OA was 6.1 days, with a range of 1–15. In four patients (25 %) a stoma was performed, meanwhile 11 patients (70.6 %) had an intestinal resection and anastomoses during the abdomen revision.

Outcome

In two patients the mesh was removed: in the first case (Group 1) because the patient was re-operated for an intestinal ischemia, in the other patient (Group 3) for a duodenal fistula. In the last case the patient was left open and the wound was treated with a Vacuum Assisted Therapy (VAC).

In Group 1 the mean hospital stay was 21 days (range 7–70). The follow up at 3-months was completed for 9 patients: 2 patients has a grade I complication (wound infection), 1 patient had a grade IVb (re-operated for a small bowel ischemia), 1 patient died for a septic shock in a leucopenia, 4 patients were free from complications. One patient was lost at the follow-up. Four patients completed the follow-up at 6 months: 3 patients were free from complications, one patient died for a septic shock in leucopenia for the important lymphoproliferative disorder associated with recent chemotherapy regimen. One patient was lost at the follow-up. No patients completed the 9-months follow-up. One patient (11.1 %) died (septic shock in leucopenia).

In Group 2 the mean hospital stay was 21.5 days (range 7–45). One patient presented a grade I complication (wound infections), one patient presented a grade II complication (wound dehiscence) requires a vacuum-assisted closure technique. Two patients had no complications. One patient was lost to follow-up. The overall mortality was 0 %.

In the Group 3 the mean and median ICU stay was 23.9 days (range 2–71), and the mean ward stay was 28.4 days (range 0–70). In peri-operative time: 4 patients presented a grade I complication (wound infection), 1 patient presented a IIIb complications (a duodenal fistula due to a dehiscence of the duodenal perforation that required another surgical intervention and a VAC therapy to manage the fistula) and the patient is still hospitalized. Seven patients were free from complications. Five patients died (2 for aortic rupture, 2 for septic shock, and 1 for respiratory insufficiency and septic shock). Twelve patients completed the follow-up at 3 months: 1 patient presented a Grade II complication (incisional hernia non complicated), 1 patient require the pursuit of the VAC therapy to manage the duodenal fistula. Seven patients are free of complications. Three patients were lost to follow-up. No patients died at 3 months follow-up. Six patients completed the follow-up at 6 months: 1 patient presented a Grade II complication (incisional hernia non complicated). Two patients were healthy. Three patients were lost to follow-up. No patients died at 6 months follow-up. Two patients completed the follow-up at 9 months: 1 patient had no complications. One patient was lost to follow-up. No patients died at 9 months follow-up. The overall peri-operative mortality was 29.4 % (5 patients).

Discussion

Incisional hernia remains a common complication in abdominal surgery and occurs after elective laparotomy with an incidence from 2 to 20 % or more [7, 19, 20]. However, these rates can increase (as high as 50 %) after abdominal closure in emergency surgery and in the abdominal repair following OA procedure [21–23]. The approach to the abdominal wall surgical repair is dramatically changed in the last years due to the availability of new repair materials, like biologic prostheses. Although in last years many studies tried to find an agreement about specific technique and materials that should be applied to repair of complex ventral hernia, at present, no strong consensus has been found yet [4, 24]. However the use of biologic prostheses is actually accepted by the medical community for addressing abdominal wall defects, particularly in contaminated and potentially contaminated fields [11, 25]. Despite this, the numerous advantages of biologic materials have been proven [11, 26, 27].

The present study reports a one-year experience about the usage of biological prostheses in different fields from elective surgery to emergency surgery and OA procedure. We analyze our surgical indications to the usage of biological meshes to evaluate the outcomes and the feasibility in these fields.

In the first group we considered only the patients underwent to ventral hernia repair in elective surgery. In all patients the abdominal wall defect was associated with high risk of contamination or an already existing infection imposed the positioning of a biological prostheses.

The decision of the positioning of the prosthesis was based on the VHWG and the Italian Biological Prostheses work-group recommendations [4, 11], according to the degree of contamination potential or effective, and according to co-morbidities of the patient. In literature also others studies confirmed and supported these recommendations [7, 28, 29]. In our study, more than half of the patients of this group had more than one comorbidity (in particular immunosuppression and malignancy), that associated with a local wound infection or intra-abdominal infection have prevented the use of a synthetic mesh. In two third of patients the mesh was placed in the retromuscolar space, in line with the literature [9, 30]. The "sublay" position (posterior to the rectus muscle) has been the most used, in fact it allows for better tissue incorporation and lower chance of bacterial contamination, increases neo-angiogenesis and avoids the direct contact with intra-abdominal viscera [1, 9]. In this group only one patient died at three months for a septic shock, and in one case we had to remove the mesh because the patient was re-operated for an intestinal ischemia.

At the analysis of the second group (patients underwent to ventral hernia repair in emergency conditions) we found that the presence of wound infection or intra-abdominal infection are the main indication requiring a biological mesh positioning. This decision was also dictated by the important comorbidities present in half of patients. The other important point has been the age of patients (older than patients in others group, with a median age of 75.5 years). In last year the number of elderly patients (>65 years) underwent to ventral hernia repair in emergency setting is increasing [2]. A recent study reports that the risk of operative factors associated with the risk of surgical site infection were open procedures, incisional/ventral repairs, and hernia repairs with bowel obstruction/necrosis [2]. Into account of these data and according to the VHWG recommendations [4] we decided to repair the abdominal wall defect with a biological mesh, with favorable outcomes and with an acceptable hospital stay (median 16.5 days).

The third group was the largest group. The problem of abdomen closure after OA procedure remains the most critical point for these patients [21–23]. Data about long-terms outcome after repair of abdominal wall in OA procedure are still lacking and the durability of the different biologic meshes has not been clinically proved [26, 31]. Our surgical indications for an OA procedure requiring a biological prostheses positioning were the difficulty to close the abdominal wall (the anterior and the posterior fascia) or to reinforce the closure of the posterior fascia (when the anterior fascia was impossible to close). The main causes for a laparostomy were secondary peritonitis, intestinal ischemia and trauma. The conditions that required leaving the abdomen open remains the abdominal compartment syndrome (ACS) or the conditions that promote an intra-abdominal hypertension (IAH) (intestinal ischemia, acute severe pancreatitis, vascular complications), or in case of damage control surgery (trauma) [13, 26, 32–34]. Recently the approach to the intra-abdominal sepsis was changed and leaving the abdomen open in that condition has been proven to reduce mortality and post-operative complications [31, 35]. The primary goal remains the source control and a temporary abdominal closure was considered a valid instrument to manage severe abdominal sepsis [35]. In our series the traumatized patients undergone to OA had severe trauma (ISS > 25). In the two-third of cases we have proceed to OA management to prevent an ACS; in only one-third OA procedure was considered as treatment of the IAH or of the ACS. In patients with intra-abdominal sepsis the scoring system to estimate the severity and prognosis of secondary peritonitis we used was the MPI [15]. Literature reports that a MPI greater that 29 relates with high mortality rates (100 % vs 0–2.3 % in patients with MPI < 21) [15]. In our series one–third of patients have severe peritonitis (MPI > of 29), and these MPI values associated with the important comorbidities may be the responsible for the high peri-operative mortality rate (29.4 % at our analysis). In the present series the status of the OA has been evaluated at the first laparotomy and at the last one according to the Björck classification [18]. Data reported an increased number of patients presenting a Grade 1A (clean OA without adherence between bowel and abdominal wall or fixity) at the abdomen closure (from 41.4 %, at the first laparotomy, to 76.6 %, at the last laparotomy). These results showed the efficacy of the OA treatment in reducing the intra-abdominal contamination. Regarding to the technique used for temporary abdominal closure we used the NPWT in almost all cases. This strategy seems to be the best in preventing evisceration, actively remove any infected or toxic fluid from the peritoneal cavity, prevent the formation of entero-atmospheric fistulas, preserve the fascia and the abdominal wall domain, make reoperation easy and safe, and achieve early definitive closure [23, 26, 36]. Our goals were to close the abdomen wall as soon as possible (within 5–7 days) [26, 27, 37] to reduce the OA complications. A recent prospective controlled trial and a systematic review suggested that use of a dynamic fascial sutures combined with NPWT in the treatment of OA for intra-abdominal sepsis is safe and associated to a low rate of incisional hernias and entero-atmospheric fistula [22, 23]. However in our series almost all patients despite the NPWT alone, the closure of the abdominal wall happened in an average of 6.1 days, but in 53 % of cases the fascia was closed with a mesh in the retromuscolar space [9, 30]. The main complications after OA remain the enterocutenaous fistula and the long-term ventral hernia, in addition to the high rate of morbidity and mortality associated with the procedure [8, 26, 38]. A recent meta-analysis about OA and temporary abdominal closure techniques in non-trauma patients (4358 patients) reported a mortality rate near to 30 %, with an overall rate of fistula of 12.1 %, with a 14.6 % in series applying NPWT without fascial traction, and of 5.7 % after NPTW with fascial traction [38]. Others studies reported a high delayed facial closure rate ranging from 34 % and 73.6 % in septic patients, with lower rates in trauma patients due to the more frequent early abdominal closure [23]. In our study only one patient had a duodenal fistula and required the removal of the prostheses (being managed with a VAC therapy to control the spillage of duodenal contents [38]) and only one patient presented an incisional hernia without complications. These low rates of incisional hernia are probably due to the lack of a long-term follow-up. The other complications in present study were related wound infection or dehiscence that were managed with local wound dressing. Also in our data the rate of perioperative mortality remains high (29.4 %), similar with the data find in the literature (30 %), however this is probably due to the extremely compromised conditions of the patients and the paucity of cases [2, 38].

Despite the limitations present study showed that the use of non-cross-linked porcine dermal meshes in different surgical setting, particularly in elderly and septic patients is safe and effective, without worsening morbidity and mortality.

Conclusions

The present one-year prospective analysis shows that the use of swine dermal non cross-linked collagen prostheses for abdominal wall repair is safe and effective in general and emergency surgery, particularly in elderly and in immune-compromised patients. However more data are necessary. For this reason the development of big prospective studies are mandatory.

Competing interest

The authors declare that they have no competing interests.

Authors' contributions

GM and FeCo collected data and wrote the manuscript. LA did the statistical analysis and reviewed the manuscript. All authors read and approved the final manuscript.

Author details

[1]Unit of General and Emergency Surgery, Papa Giovanni XXIII Hospital, P.zza OMS 1, 24128 Bergamo, Italy. [2]General surgery department, Ospedale Maggiore, Parma, Italy.

References

1. Coccolini F, Poiasina E, Bertoli P, Gossetti F, Agresta F, Dassatti MR, et al. The Italian register of biological prostheses. Eur Surg Res. 2013;50(3–4):262–72.
2. Beadles CA, Meagher AD, Charles AG. Trends in emergent hernia repair in the United States. JAMA Surg. 2015;150:194–200.
3. Ansaloni L, Coccolini F, Fortuna D, Catena F, Di Saverio S, Belotti LM, et al. Assessment of 126,913 inguinal hernia repairs in the Emilia-Romagna region of Italy: analysis of 10 years. Hernia. 2014;18(2):261–7.
4. Ventral Hernia Working Group, Breuing K, Butler CE, Ferzoco S, Franz M, Hultman CS, et al. Incisional ventral hernias: review of the literature and recommendations regarding the grading and the technique of repair. Surgery. 2010;148(3):544.
5. Coccolini F, Catena F, Catena F, Poiasina E, Poletti E, Ansaloni L. Biomaterials in abdominal wall surgery: change your mind! Ann Surg. 2014; [Epub ahead of print].
6. Sipe JD. Tissue engineering and reparative medicine. Ann NY Acad Sci. 2002;961:1–9.
7. Kissane NA, Itani KMF. A decade of ventral incisional hernia repairs with biologic acellular dermal matrix: what have we learned? PRSJ. 2012;130;5S-2:194S–2.
8. Peralta R, Latifi R. Long-Term outcomes of abdominal wall reconstruction. What are the real numbers? World J Surg. 2012;36:534–8.
9. Diaz Jr JJ, Cullinane DC, Khwaja KA, Tyson GH, Ott M, Jerome R, et al. Eastern Association for the Surgery of Trauma: management of the open abdomen, part III-review of abdominal wall reconstruction. J Trauma Acute Care Surg. 2013;75(3):376–86.
10. Smart NJ, Bryan N, Hunt JA, Daniels IR. Porcine dermis implants in soft-tissue reconstruction: current status. Biologics Target and Therapy. 2014;8:83–90.
11. Coccolini F, Agresta F, Bassi A, Catena F, Crovella F, Ferrara R, et al. Italian Biological Prosthesis Work-Group (IBPWG): proposal for a decisional model in using biological prosthesis. World J Emerg Surg. 2012;7(1):34.
12. Biological Meshes in Infected Fields: a Randomized Controlled Trial (SIMBIOSE). https://clinicaltrials.gov/ct2/show/NCT01594450.
13. Sartelli M, Viale P, Catena F, Ansaloni L, Moore E, Malangoni M, et al. 2013 WSES guidelines for management of intra-abdominal infections. World J Emerg Surg. 2013;8(1):3.
14. Dindo D, Demartines N, Clavien PA. Classification of surgical complications: a new proposal with evaluation in a cohort of 6336 patients and results of a survey. Ann Surg. 2004;240(2):205–13.
15. Mishra SP, Tiwary SK, Mishra M, Gupta SK. An introduction of tertiary peritonitis. J Emerg Trauma Shock. 2014;7(2):121–3.
16. Baker SP, O'Neill B, Haddon Jr W, Long WB. The injury severity score: a method for describing patients with multiple injuries and evaluating emergency care. J Trauma. 1974;14(3):187–96.
17. Chatzicostas C, Roussomoustakaki M, Vardas E, Romanos J, Kouroumalis EA. Balthazar computed tomography severity index is superior to Ranson criteria and APACHE II and III scoring systems in predicting acute pancreatitis outcome. J Clin Gastroenterol. 2003;36(3):253–60.
18. Björck M, Bruhin A, Cheatham M, Hinck D, Kaplan M, Manca G, et al. Classification–important step to improve management of patients with an open abdomen. World J Surg. 2009;33(6):1154–7.
19. Le Huu NR, Mege D, Ouaïssi M, Sielezneff I, Sastre B. Incidence and prevention of ventral incisional hernia. J Visc Surg. 2012;149:e3–14.
20. Sbitany H, Know E, Chern H, Finlayson E, Varma MG, Hansen SL. Outcomes analysis of biological mesh use for abdominal wall reconstruction in clean-contaminated and contaminated ventral hernia repair. Ann Pl Surg. 2013; [Epub ahead of print].
21. Kaoutzanis C, Lichtle SW, Mouawad NJ, Welch KB, Lampman RM, Wahl WL, et al. Risk factors for postoperative wound infections and prolonged hospitalization after ventral/incisional hernia repair. Hernia. 2013;19(1):113–23.
22. Fortelny RH, Hofmann A, Gruber-Blum S, Petter-Puchner AH, Glaser KS. Delayed closure of open abdomen in septic patients is facilitated by combined negative pressure wound therapy and dynamic fascial suture. Surg Endosc. 2014;28(3):735–40.
23. Atema JJ, Gans SL, Boermeester MA. Systematic review and meta-analysis of the open abdomen and temporary abdominal closure techniques in Non-trauma patients. World J Surg. 2015;39(4):912–25.
24. Latifi R, Leppaniemi A. Compelx andominal wall defects and enterocutaneous fistulae in the era of biological mesh: did we make any real progress? World J Surg. 2012;36:495–6.

25. Lee L, Mata J, Landry T, Khwaja KA, Vassiliou MC, Fried GM, et al. A systematic review of synthetic and biologic materials for abdominal wall reinforcement in contaminated fields. Surg Endosc. 2014;28:2531–46.
26. Demetriades D, Salim A. Management of the open abdomen. Surg Clin North Am. 2014;94(1):131–53.
27. Godat L, Kobayashi L, Costantini T, Coimbra R. Abdominal damage control surgery and reconstruction: world society of emergency surgery position paper. World J Emerg Surg. 2013;8(1):53.
28. Nieuwenhuizen J, Eker HH, Timmermans L, Hop WC, Kleinrensink GJ, Jeekel J, et al. A double blind randomized controlled trial comparing primary closure with mesh augmentes closure to reduce incisional hernia incidence. BMC Surg. 2013;13:48.
29. Butler CE, Baumann DP, Janis JE, Rosen MJ. Abdominal wall reconstruction. Curr Probl Surg. 2013;50:557–86.
30. Muysoms F, Campanelli G, Champault GG, DeBeaux AC, Dietz UA, Jeekel J, et al. EuraHS: the development of an international online platform for registration and outcome measurement of ventral abdominal wall hernia repair. Hernia. 2012;16(3):239–50.
31. Regner JL, Kobayashi L, Coimbra R. Surgical strategies for management of open abdomen. World J Surg. 2012;36:497–510.
32. Kirkpatrick AW, Roberts DJ, De Waele J, Jaeschke R, Malbrain ML, De Keulenaer B, et al. Intra-abdominal hypertension and the abdominal compartment syndrome: updated consensus definitions and clinical practice guidelines from the World Society of the Abdominal Compartment Syndrome. Intensive Care Med. 2013;39(7):1190–206.
33. Sartelli M, Catena F, Ansaloni L, Coccolini F, Corbella D, Moore EE, et al. Complicated intra-abdominal infections worldwide: the definitive data of the CIAOW Study. World J Emerg Surg. 2014;9:37.
34. Navsaria P, Nicol A, Hudson D, Cockwill J, Smith J. Negative pressure wound therapy management of the "open abdomen" following trauma: a prospective study and systematic review. World J Emerg Surg. 2013;8(1):4.
35. Dutton WD, Diaz JJ, Miller RS. Critical care issues in managing complex open abdominal wound. J Int Care Med. 2012;27(3):161–71.
36. Olona C, Caro A, Duque E, Moreno F, Vadillo J, Rueda JC, et al. Comparative study of open abdomen treatment: ABThera™ vs. abdominal dressing™. Hernia. 2015;19(2):323–8.
37. Sugrue M, D'Amours SK, Kolkman KA. Temporary abdominal closure. Acta Clin Belg. 2007;62 Suppl 1:210–4.
38. Demetriades D. Total management of the open abdomen. Int Wound J. 2012;9 Suppl 1:17–24.

7

Geriatric Assessment as a qualification element for elective and emergency cholecystectomy in older patients

Jakub Kenig*, Piotr Wałęga, Urszula Olszewska, Aleksander Konturek and Wojciech Nowak

Abstract

Background: Older patients experience a higher incidence of postoperative complications after cholecystectomy compared with younger patients. However, most studies have not considered patient frailty, particularly regarding emergency cholecystectomy. The aim of this prospective study was to evaluate outcomes in frail older patients eligible for elective and emergency cholecystectomy.

Methods: Preoperative Geriatric Assessment (GA) was performed in consecutive patients aged 65+ years, operated for biliary disease. The GA evaluated the functional, cognitive, comorbidity, depressive, nutritional, and polypharmacy status and patients with two or more abnormal domains were considered frail. Outcomes of interest were 30-day postoperative mortality, morbidity, and length of hospital stay (LOS).

Results: A total of 126 patients (median age 74; range 65–93 years) were included. There was no difference between elective frail and non-frail patients regarding postoperative mortality (0 %) and morbidity (6 % vs. 5 %; $p = 0.76$). LOS was not significantly longer in the frail group (5.6 vs. 4 days; $p = 0.22$). In the emergency-admitted patients, almost all complications occurred in the frail population (mortality 5 % vs. 0 %; morbidity 36.7 % vs. 3.3 %, compared with non-frail patients, respectively; $p < 0.01$) and LOS was significantly longer (10.3 (frail) vs. 6 days (non-frail);$p = 0.03$). Frail status was a significant independent predictive factor for postoperative complications in the emergency population, only (odds ratio: 3.4 (1.2–9.7); $p = 0.02$).

Conclusions: Elective laparoscopic cholecystectomy is a safe and effective surgical technique also for older frail patients. In emergency settings, frail patients have significantly more complications and a longer LOS. However, the role of severity of frailty and the most reliable GA tools require further study.

Keywords: Geriatric assessment, Frailty, Surgery in older patients, Cholecystectomy

Background

Several studies, concerning surgical treatment of biliary disease, have shown that older patients more often have complicated gallstone disease, more emergency and open operations, higher postoperative morbidity and mortality rates, and a longer postoperative hospital stay compared with younger patients [1–6]. However, most studies have not considered the larger heterogeneity of co-morbidity and physical strength in this group of patients, which further contributes to the complexity of treatment. This relates especially to frail patients who have reduced physiologic reserve associated with increased susceptibility to disability because of age-related loss of physical, cognitive, social, and physiological functioning [7]. In these patients, standard preoperative medical history, physical examination, biochemistry, and imaging tests often do not provide the information needed for optimal and tailored treatment, leading to both under- and overtreatment [8]. On the other hand, a Geriatric Assessment (GA), can provide a comprehensive health appraisal to guide targeted geriatric interventions and appropriate treatment selection [7, 8]. This systemic approach was mostly investigated in surgical,

* Correspondence: jkenig@cm-uj.krakow.pl
3rd Department of General Surgery, Jagiellonian University Medical College, Pradnicka str. 35-37, 31-202 Kraków, Poland

oncologic patients [9] but not among patients with biliary diseases apart from one study by Lasithiotakis et al. [10]. Furthermore, the appropriate assessment can be even more complex in case of patients with acute cholecystitis. At present, such "patient-related" treatment guidelines do not exist, taking into consideration local pathological changes, patient clinical status and the subsequent treatment decisions [11]. Therefore, the aim of this prospective study was to evaluate postoperative outcomes in frail older patients eligible for elective and emergency cholecystectomy. To our knowledge, this is the first prospective study to assess the outcome of frail older patients undergoing emergency cholecystectomy.

Methods

Study population

Between June 2014 and December 2015, we prospectively enrolled consecutive patients over 65 years of age with symptomatic gallstone disease, acute cholecystitis requiring elective or emergency surgery, respectively. The study was conducted at a tertiary referral hospital. The ethics committee approved this study and informed consent was obtained from all patients or their caregivers.

Inclusion criteria for the elective patients were symptomatic and sonographically detected cholelithiasis. Inclusion criteria for the emergency patients were acute cholecystitis according to the 2013 Tokyo Guidelines [12]. Patients with pancreatitis at the time of surgery were excluded. Three patients who were unable to give consent or answer the GA questions were excluded and two additional patients were excluded because of incomplete data.

Study protocol

All patients were assessed using the GA, which was performed on the day of admission by trained physicians or, for emergency patients, by trained physicians or nurses. The GA comprised the validated instruments presented in the Table 1, with the range and the literature-based cut-off scores [13–20].

The results of each test were recorded and each test was also scored on a dichotomous scale, based on whether an impairment in any of the parameters was present.

All operations were performed by residents under the direct supervision of a consultant (who also served as the first assistant) or by the consultants themselves. Laparoscopic cholecystectomy was performed using a standard three- or four-port technique and all emergency patients were treated surgically within 24 h after admission. Severity grading for the acute cholecystitis patients was according to the 2013 Tokyo Guidelines [12].

Frailty model

A cumulative deficit model of frailty was used. The equally weighted deficits, as a measure of accumulated vulnerability, included ADL/IADL, Geriatric Depression Score, BOMC/CDT, the Mini-Nutritional Assessment, CCS, and the Polypharmacy Assessment. The functional (ADL/IADL) and cognitive domains (BOMC/CDT) were considered abnormal if one of the assessment tools showed literature-based impairment. The detection of deficits in two or more GA domains indicated an increased risk of disability or death and was used as the cut-off score for the GA set and also as the definition of frailty.

Outcome measures

The primary outcome, complications, was defined as any event occurring within 30 days of surgery that required treatment not routinely applied in the post-operative period. The severity of predefined complications was classified according to the Clavien–Dindo scale [21]. Grade I and II complications were classified as minor morbidity, and Grade III and IV complications as major morbidity. Postoperative mortality was defined as death within 30 days after surgery. LOS was calculated as the period from the admission day until discharge from hospital.

Table 1 Glossary of the tests used in the geriatric assessment with the range and the literature-based cut-off scores

TEST		NUMBER OF ITEMS	RANGE	CUT-OFF SCORE
ADL [13]	Functional status	6	0–6	<5
IADL [14]		8	0–8	≤7
BOMC Test [15]	Cognitive assessment	6	0–28	>10
CDT-test [16]		7	0–7	>3
Charlson Comorbidity Scale [17]	Comorbidity	19	0–37	>3
Geriatric Depression Scale [18]	Depression	15	0–15	>5
MNA full [19]	Nutritional assessment	18	0–30	<24
Polypharmacy [20]	Polypharmacy	1	0-∞	≥5 drugs/day

ADL Activities of daily living, *IADL* Instrumental Activities of Daily Living, *BOMC* Blessed Orientation-Memory-Concentration Test, *CDT* Clock Drawing Test, *CCS* Charlson Comorbidity Scale, *GDS* Geriatric Depression Scale, *MNA* Mini Nutritional Assessment

Statistical analysis

The data were analyzed using Statistica 10.0 software (StatSoft, Krakow, Poland). Categorical variables are described as percentages of the total population, while continuous variables are reported as the median and range. Pearson's chi-square or Fisher's exact test was used to compare categorical variables and the unpaired Student's t-test was used for comparisons.

Univariate and multivariate analysis was conducted to investigate the association between the GA set and 30-day postoperative morbidity (including a comparison of "any" with "no" complications and "major" with "no/minor" complications), adjusted for age and sex. Because of the small number of fatal events, postoperative mortality was not analyzed separately but as part of the "major morbidity" category. Statistical significance was defined as two-sided $p \leq 0.05$.

Results

The study sample comprised 66 elective patients (48 female and 18 male) and 60 emergency-admitted patients (34 female and 26 male). The median age was significantly lower among elective patients: 71 vs. 76 years of age; $p < 0.01$. Patients' baseline characteristics are shown in Table 2.

Table 2 Patients' baseline characteristics

Factor	Elective patients	Emergency patients
Number (female/male ratio) *[n]*	66 (48/18)	60 (34/26)
• 65–74 / 75–84 / 85+ *[n]*	40/20/6	25/27/8
Median age *[years (range)]*	71 (65–86)	76 (65–93)
ECOG-PS [44] *[n]*:		
• 0	19	5
• 1	34	24
• 2	12	12
• 3	1	16
• 4	0	3
ASA [45] *[n]*:		
• 1	8	1
• 2	48	25
• 3	10	30
• 4	0	4

ECOG-PS Eastern Cooperative Oncology Group performance status, *ASA* American Society of Anesthesiologists

Laparoscopic cholecystectomy was successfully performed in 57 (86 %) elective and 42 (70 %) emergency patients. The conversion to open cholecystectomy was performed in two patients (3 %) in the elective group and in five patients (8.3 %) in the emergency group. Seven (10.6 %) and 13 (21.7 %) patients had primary open cholecystectomy in the elective and emergency group, respectively, due to severe pulmonary and/or cardiac comorbidities after consultation with the anesthesiologists, numerous laparotomies in the upper abdomen. The mean operation time was 79 min (range, 30–180 min). Emergency frail patients had a non-significantly longer operation time compared with emergency fit patients (85 vs. 71 min; $p = 0.14$). There was no difference between frail and fit patients operated electively (77 vs. 76 min; $p = 0.87$).

The severity of acute cholecystitis in emergency admitted patients according to the revised 2013 Tokyo Guidelines was as follows: Grade I: two patients (3.3 %); Grade II: 39 patients (65 %); and Grade III: 19 patients (31.7 %).

Descriptive analysis of the GA components and frailty frequency

The Table 3 presents the results of the GA instruments with literature-based cut-off scores and the proportion of patients who had abnormal results in the test.

Table 4 shows the results of the cumulative deficit model of the GA. The frequency of frailty was significantly higher among emergency patients compared with elective patients (34 vs. 46 patients, respectively; $p < 0.01$). The cumulative number of abnormal domains among frail patients was between two and five (elective patients) and between two and six (emergency patients). Additionally, significantly more frail emergency patients had Grade III (severe) acute cholecystitis according to the 2013 Tokyo Guidelines (17 vs. three patients, (frail emergency patients vs. fit emergency patients, respectively); $p < 0.01$).

Outcomes

The discharge status was to home in all elective cases and to skilled nursing facilities in 8.3 % ($n = 5$) of emergency patients. There were no readmissions and there was no mortality among the elective patients. In the emergency group, the 30-day mortality was 5 % ($n = 3$) with patients dying on the 1st, 3rd, and 10th postoperative day because of progressive circulatory insufficiency. The 30-day morbidity was 10.6 % (including 6.1 % major morbidities) and 36.7 % (including 10 % major morbidities), in the elective vs. the emergency group of patients, respectively. Comparing the incidence of both 30-day postoperative overall and major complications between frail and non-frail patients, there was no statistically significant difference (6 % vs. 5 %, $p = 0.76$) in the elective group. All four occurrences of major complications (postoperative bleeding, bile leakage, abscess formation) in the elective group were observed among patients with chronic severe inflammatory processes and were connected to the surgical technique. In comparison, in the emergency group, almost all mortality and major complications were observed in the frail populations (36.7 vs. 3.3 %; $p < 0.01$) - Table 5.

Table 3 Elements of the Geriatric Assessment with the proportion of patients with abnormal test results

TEST	ELECTIVE PATIENTS *[n] (%)*	EMERGENCY PATIENTS *[n] (%)*
ADL (cut-off score <5)		
• Dependent	0 (0 %)	10 (17 %)
IADL (cut-off score ≤7)		
• Dependent	2 (3 %)	19 (32 %)
MNA full (cut-off score <24)		
• Malnutrition	10 (15 %)	24 (40 %)
BOMC (cut-off score >10)		
• Impaired	4 (6 %)	19 (32 %)
CDT-test (cut-off score >3)		
• Impaired	25 (38 %)	25 (42 %)
GDS (cut-off score >5)		
• Depressed	13 (20 %)	19 (32 %)
CCS (cut-off score ≥3)		
• ≥3	9 (14 %)	27 (45 %)
Polypharmacy		
• >5 drugs/day	21 (32 %)	29 (48 %)

ADL Activities of Daily Living, *IADL* Instrumental Activities of Daily Living, *MNA* Mini Nutritional Assessment, *BOMC* Blessed Orientation-Memory-Concentration, *CDT-test* Test, Clock Drawing Test ; *CCS* Charlson Comorbidity Scale, *GDS* Geriatric Depression Scale, $p > 5$ Polypharmacy >5 drugs/day

Comparing the LOS of frail and non-frail patients, the frail group had non-significantly longer mean hospital stay (5.6 vs. 4 days; $p = 0.22$) in the elective group. In the emergency group, the LOS was significantly longer among frail patients (10.3 vs. 6 days, frail emergency patients vs. non-frail emergency patients, respectively; $p = 0.03$).

Cumulative effect of GA in determining surgical outcome

The results of the univariate and multivariate logistic regression analysis showed that age and sex did not increase the surgical risk either in the elective or the emergency group. The frailty status was not predictive of all and major postoperative complications in the elective group. In turn, frailty was an independent risk factor for all complications in the emergency group. It was not possible to build a model for the major complications in the emergency group because of an insufficient number of patients in this subgroup (major complications were observed only among frail patients). The results of the multivariate logistic regression are presented in Table 6.

Table 4 Validated assessment tools used in the Geriatric Assessment, with frailty frequency

GERIATRIC ASSESSMENT	ELECTIVE PATIENTS	EMERGENCY PATIENTS
ADL/IADL + MNA + BOMC/CDT + CCS + GDS + Polypharmacy (>5 drugs/day)	34 (51.5 %)	46 (76.7 %)

ADL Activities of daily living, *IADL* Instrumental Activities of Daily Living, *MNA* Mini Nutritional Assessment, *BOMC* Blessed Orientation-Memory-Concentration, Test, *CDT* Clock Drawing Test, *CCS* Charlson Comorbidity Scale, *GDS* Geriatric Depression Scale

Discussion

In this study, almost half of the elective and two thirds of the emergency older patients were frail. However, the procedure was performed safely with no 30-day postoperative mortality and a low number of major complications, for both frail and non-frail elective patients. In contrast, we encountered poorer outcomes in emergency operated patients. All of the cases of mortality and major comorbidity occurred in frail emergency patients, which was confirmed by regression analysis. Frail status was not a risk factor for overall and major postoperative complications in the elective group but was a significant independent predictive factor for postoperative complications in the emergency population. Similarly, the LOS was not significantly longer in the elective frail group of patients and was significantly longer in the emergency frail population.

Published studies show that elective laparoscopic cholecystectomy is a feasible and safe procedure in older patients, including in a group of octogenarians. The authors report no or single cases of mortality and usually a higher, but acceptable, rate of postoperative complications when compared with a younger population [1–6, 22, 23]. However, the authors of a meta-analysis of laparoscopic versus open cholecystectomy in older patients, including studies up to June 2013, concluded that further high-quality evidence is necessary to draw definitive conclusions, although the best available evidence supports the selective use of laparoscopy [24]. Older patients with acute cholecystitis have more frequent primary open cholecystectomies, a higher conversion rate and, in most studies, a worse postoperative outcome [25–28]. We obtained similar results with no mortality in the elective population, a low postoperative complication rate, and most of the procedures were performed using minimally invasive techniques. Similar to other studies, older patients with acute cholecystitis had a higher rate of mortality, morbidity, primary open cholecystectomies, and conversions in our study. However, the frailty factor was not considered in these studies and advanced age alone is not necessarily synonymous with vulnerability to adverse health outcomes.

Another problem with the frailty concept is the choice of the best assessment model, which is still debatable. Three of them are most frequently cited in the current literature: the multi-domain GA, the cumulative deficit score (CDS), and the frailty phenotype model [7]. Most

Table 5 Severity of all postoperative complications according to the Clavien–Dindo classification among frail and non-frail elective and emergency patients

Clavien-Dindo classification	Number of complications			
	Elective patients		Emergency patients	
	Frail	Non-frail	Frail	Non-frail
Grade I	1	1	1	1
Grade II	2	1	10	2
Grade IIIa	0	0	1	0
Grade IIIb	2	2	2	0
Grade IVa	0	0	5	0
Grade IVb	0	0	0	0
Grade V	0	0	3	0

trials evaluating the multi-domain GA in surgical patients have analyzed the relationship between individual elements of the GA and the outcomes, showing a statistically significant predictive possibility of postoperative complications [29–32]. In our study, domains as a single risk factor were not relevant in the elective patients, both in the univariate and multivariate regression analysis. In turn, in the emergency group some domains (I-ADL, CDT, CCI, Polypharmacy) turned out to be the risk factor of postoperative outcome, however, only in the univariate analysis (data not included in the paper).

Robinson et al. and Kim KI et al. showed that a cumulative deficit frailty score was independently associated with postoperative mortality [33, 34]. Similarly, in our previous study, this model turned out to be also predictive of 30-day postoperative morbidity in oncologic patients with solid cancer eligible for abdominal surgery. However, the number of incorporated GA domains had a great influence on the prevalence of frailty and on adequate surgical risk assessment [35]. Another problem is the cut-off of two abnormal domains, which was used as a frailty definition in our study. We extrapolated the guidelines of Geriatric Assessment used by the SIOG in the older oncologic patients [36]. However, there is still no "golden standard" regarding the number of impaired domains that should be considered as a frailty marker.

Kristjansson et al., Kwang-il et al., Tan et al., and Makary et al. used a frailty phenotype model and observed that impairments were also independently associated with adverse in-hospital events, prolonged LOS, and post-discharge institutionalization [37–40].

However, none of these studies analyzed exclusively patients eligible for cholecystectomy. Lasithiotakis et al. performed the only study including a frailty assessment in 57 older patients eligible for elective laparoscopic cholecystectomy. In contrast to our results, they observed that the GA might predict 30-day postoperative complications and a prolonged stay. This and our study have common features: similar median age, a cumulative model used to assess frailty (with five out of six similar domains and the same cut-offs), almost the same number of patients identified as frail (56.1 vs. 51.5 %), and a similar method of reporting outcomes [10]. However, our study has a few important differences. The study by Lasithiotakis et al. included only patients with uncomplicated biliary disease whereas our study included consecutive patients also presenting with severe chronic cholecystitis (intraoperative finding in patients admitted electively) and these patients experienced the major postoperative complications. Unfortunately, our study period included the highest number of bile leakages ever experienced in our institution, in both the fit and frail groups. Moreover, our study included also the Geriatric Depression Scale in the frailty assessment, which is a proven predictor of postoperative adverse outcome [41].

Although, we are in favor of the use of the cumulative deficit model, it still remains unclear which measure of frailty should be used in surgical patients. All of the frailty models evaluate the same concept but from a different perspective and further research is needed to determine the best approach.

It is also important to note the severity of acute cholecystitis in our case series. Previous studies have shown that perioperative outcomes are influenced by the severity of gallbladder disease rather than chronological age [42]. In our emergency population, only 3 % of patients had a Grade I score and more than one third had Grade III acute cholecystitis according to the 2013 Tokyo Guidelines, which is one of the highest reported results. Moreover, the timing of the surgery plays an important role [43] but this factor was not significant in regression and correlation analysis (data not presented) in our study.

Table 6 Results of the multivariate logistic regression of the cumulative number of impairments in the Geriatric Assessment set on postoperative outcome (adjusted by age, sex)

GERIATRIC ASSESSMENT	ELECTIVE PATIENTS OR (95 % CI)		EMERGENCY PATIENTS OR (95 % CI)	
	ALL	MAJOR	ALL	MAJOR
ADL/IADL + MNA + BOMC/CDT + CCS + GDS + Polypharmacy (>5 drugs/day)	1.2 (0.5-2.7) $p = 0.63$	0.89 (0.3-2.6) $p = 0.84$	3.4 (1.2-9.7) $p = 0.02$	-[a]

All variables were considered dichotomous; *OR* odds ratio, *95% CI* 95% confidence interval, The statistically significant values appear in bold font; [a]There were no cases of major complications in the non-frail group. *ADL* Activities of Daily Living, *IADL* Instrumental Activities of Daily Living, *MNA* Mini Nutritional Assessment, *BOMC* Blessed Orientation-Memory-Concentration ,Test, *CDT* Clock.Drawing Test, *CCS* Charlson Comorbidity Scale, *GDS* Geriatric Depression Scale

We believe that the severity of the surgical insult is of great importance in frail patients. In our study, in patients eligible for elective cholecystectomy, this factor did not appear to be strong enough to influence the reduced physiologic reserve and outcomes in frail patients and this could be a result of further heterogeneity within this population. The identification of frailty alone appears to be insufficient in patients undergoing surgery and it should be supported by its magnitude. The number of abnormal deficits in the cumulative model of frailty could be one such factor. Additionally, meticulous surgical technique in experienced hands is of paramount importance for this particular group. Therefore, the influence of the surgeon, the surgical technique, and the reaction of the patient's body to the stress connected with the operative procedure in the context of frailty require further study.

Conclusion

Elective laparoscopic cholecystectomy is a safe and effective surgical technique also for older frail patients. In emergency settings, frail patients have significantly more complications and a longer LOS compared with the fit population. However, the role of severity of frailty and the most reliable GA tools require further study.

Abbreviations

ADL, activities of daily living; ASA score, the American Society of Anesthesiologist's score; BOMC, the blessed orientation-memory-concentration test; CCS, the charlson comorbidity scale; CDS, the cumulative deficit score; CDT, the clock drawing test (CDT); ECOG-PS, the performance status eastern cooperative oncology group performance status; GA, geriatric assessment; GDS, the geriatric depression scale; IADL, instrumental activities of daily living; LOS, length of hospital stay; MNA, the mini nutritional assessment

Acknowledgments

We thank all of the nurses in the Surgical Department for their help during the study period.

Funding

This research received no specific grant from any funding agency, commercial or not-for-profit sectors.

Authors' contributions

JK - Study conception and design, Acquisition of data, Analysis and interpretation of data. Drafting of manuscript; PW - Acquisition of data, Drafting of manuscript; UO - Acquisition of data, Drafting of manuscript; AK - Acquisition of data, Drafting of manuscript; WN - Drafting of manuscript, Critical revision of manuscript All authors read and approved the final manuscript.

Competing interests

The authors declare that they have no competing interests.

References

1. Pessaux P, Tuech J-J, Derouet N, Rouge C, Regenet N, Arnaud J-P. Laparoscopic cholecystectomy in the elderly. Surg Endosc. 2000;14:1067–69.
2. Brunt LM, Quasebarth MA, Dunnegan DL, Soper NJ. Outcomes analysis of laparoscopic cholecystectomy in the extremely elderly. Surg Endosc. 2001;15:700–5.
3. Weber D. Laparoscopic surgery, an excellent approach in elderly patients. Arch Surg. 2003;138:1083–88.
4. Uecker J, Adams M, Skipper K, Dunn E. Cholecystitis in the octogenarian: is laparoscopic cholecystectomy the best approach? Am Surg. 2001;67:637–40.
5. Nielsen LBJ, Harboe MK, Bardram L. Cholecystectomy for the elderly: no hesitation for otherwise healthy patients. Surg Endosc. 2014;28:171–77.
6. Agrusa A, Romano G, Frazzetta G, Chianetta D, Sorce V, Di Buono G, Gulotta G. Role and outcomes of laparoscopic cholecystectomy in the elderly. Int J Surg. 2014;12:37–9.
7. Morley JE, Vellas B, van Kan GA, Anker SD, Bauer JM, Bernabei R, Cesari M, Chumlea WC, Doehner W, Evans J, Fried LP, Guralnik JM, Katz PR, Malmstrom TK, McCarter RJ, Gutierrez Robledo LM, Rockwood K, von Haehling S, Vandewoude MF, Walston J. Frailty consensus: a call to action. J Am Med Dir Assoc. 2013;14(6):392–7.
8. Rubenstein LZ, Stuck AE, Siu AL, Wieland D. Impacts of geriatric evaluation and management programs on defined outcomes: overview of the evidence. J Am Geriatr Soc. 1991;39:8–16.
9. Puts MTE, Hardt J, Monette J, Girre V, Springall E, Alibhai SM. Use of geriatric assessment for older adults in the oncology setting: a systematic review. J Natl Cancer Inst. 2012;104(15):1134–64.
10. Lasithiotakis K, Petrakis J, Venianaki M, Georgiades G, Koutsomanolis D, Andreou A, Zoras O, Chalkiadakis G. Frailty predicts outcome of elective laparoscopic cholecystectomy in geriatric patients. Surg Endosc. 2013;27:1144–50.
11. Campanile FC, Catena F, Coccolini F, Lotti M, Piazzalunga D, Pisano M, Ansaloni L. The need for new "patient-related" guidelines for the treatment of acute cholecystitis. World J Emerg Surg. 2011;6:44–6.
12. Takada T, Strasberg SM, Solomkin JS, Pitt HA, Gomi H, Yoshida M, Mayumi T, Miura F, Gouma DJ, Garden OJ, Büchler MW, Kiriyama S, Yokoe M, Kimura Y, Tsuyuguchi T, Itoi T, Gabata T, Higuchi R, Okamoto K, Hata J, Murata A, Kusachi S, Windsor JA, Supe AN, Lee S, Chen XP, Yamashita Y, Hirata K, Inui K, Sumiyama Y. Tokyo guidelines revision committee. TG13: updated Tokyo guidelines for the management of acute cholangitis and cholecystitis. J Hepatobiliary Pancreat Sci. 2013;20(1):1–7.
13. Katz S, Akpom CA. A measure of primary sociobiological function. Int J Health Serv. 1976;6:493–507.
14. Lawton MP, Brody EM. Assessment of older people: self-maintaining and instrumental activities of daily living. Gerontologist. 1969;9:179–86.
15. Tomlinson BE, Roth M. The association between quantitative measures of dementia and senile change in cerebral grey matter of elderly subjects. Br J Psychiat. 1968;114:797–811.
16. Watson YI, Arfken CL, Birge SL. Clock completion: an objective screening test for dementia. J Am Geriatr Soc. 1993;41:1235–40.
17. Charlson ME, Pompei P, Ales KL, MacKenzie CR. A new method of classifying prognostic comorbidity in longitudinal studies: development and validation. J Chronic Dis. 1987;40:373–83.
18. Brink TL, Yesavage JA, Lum O, Heersema P, Adey MB, Rose TL. Screening test for geriatric depression. Clin Gerontol. 1982;1:37–44.
19. Guigoz Y, Vellas B, Garry PJ. Mini nutritional assessment: a practical assessment tool for grading the nutritional state of elderly patients. Facts Res Gerontol. 1994;2:15–59.
20. Curtis LH, Ostbye T, Sendersky V, Hutchison S, Dans PE, Wright A, Woosley RL, Shulman KA. Inappropriate prescribing for elderly Americans in a large outpatient population. Arch Intern Med. 2004;164:1621–25.
21. Dindo D, Demartines N, Clavien PA. Classification of surgical complications. A New proposal with evaluation in a cohort of 6336 patients and results of a survey. Ann Surg. 2004;240:205–13.
22. Chung JY, Chang WY, Lin TW, Lu JR, Yang MW, Lin CC, Chang CJ, Chou AH. An analysis of surgical outcomes in patients aged 80 years and older. Acta Anaesthesiol Taiwan. 2014;52(4):153–8.
23. Fukami Y, Kurumiya Y, Mizuno K, Sekoguchi E, Kobayashi S. Cholecystectomy in octogenarians: be careful. Update Surg. 2014;66(4):265–68.
24. Antoniou SA, Antoniou GA, Koch OO, Pointer R, Granderath FA. Meta-analysis of laparoscopic vs open cholecystectomy in elderly patients. World J Gastroenterol. 2014;20(46):17626–34.

25. Teixeira JP, Ribeiro C, Pinho A, Graca L, Moreira LM, Maia JC. Laparoscopic cholecystectomy in acute cholecystitis in the elderly. Hepatogastroenterology. 2014;61(129):18–21.
26. Chang WT, Yu FJ, Hsieh MY, Huang MC, Lee KT, Chen JS. Laparoscopic cholecystectomy in aged patients. Hepatogastroenterology. 2009;56(93): 950–55.
27. Polychronidis A, Botaitis S, Tsaroucha A, Tripsianis G, Bounovas A, Pitiakoudis M, Simopoulos C. Laparoscopic cholecystectomy in elderly patients. J Gastrointestin Liver Dis. 2008;17(3):309–13.
28. Lee S, Na B-G, Yoo Y-S, Mun S-P, Choi N-K. Clinical outcome for laparoscopic cholecystectomy in extremely elderly patients. Ann Surg Treat Res. 2015; 88(3):145–51.
29. Audisio R. And PACE study participants. Shall we operate? preoperative assessment in elderly cancer patients (PACE) can help. A SIOG surgical task force prospective study. Crit Rev Oncol Hematol. 2008;65:156–63.
30. Kothari A, Phillips S, Bretl T, Block K, Weigel T. Components of geriatric assessment predict thoracic surgery outcomes. J Surg Res. 2011;166:5–13.
31. Kristjansson SR, Jordhøy MS, Nesbakken A, Skovlunde BA, Johannessen H, Wyller TB. Which elements of a comprehensive geriatric assessment (CGA) predict post-operative complications and early mortality after colorectal cancer surgery? J Geriatr Oncol. 2010;1:57–65.
32. Fukuse T, Satoda N, Hijiya K, Fujinaga T. Importance of a comprehensive geriatric assessment in prediction of complications following thoracic surgery in elderly patients. Chest. 2005;127:886–91.
33. Robinson TN, Eiseman B, Wallace JI, Church SD, McFann KK, Pfister SM, Sharp TJ, Moss M. Redefining geriatric preoperative assessment using frailty, disability and co-morbidity. Ann Surg. 2009;250:449–55.
34. Kim KI, Park KH, Koo KH, Han HS, Kim CH. Comprehensive geriatric assessment can predict postoperative morbidity and mortality in elderly patients undergoing elective surgery. Arch Geront Geriat. 2013;56:507–12.
35. Kenig J, Olszewska U, Zychiewicz B, Barczynski M. Mituś-Kenig M (2015) Cumulative deficit model of geriatric assessment to predict the postoperative outcomes of older patient with solid abdominal cancer. J Geriatr Oncol. 2015;6(5):370–9.
36. Wildiers H, Heeren P, Puts M, Topinkova E, Janssen-Heijnen M, Extermann M, Falandry C, Artz A, Brain E, Colloca G, Flamaing J, Karnakis T, Kenis C, Audisio R, Mohile S, Repetto L, Van Leeuwen B, Milisen K, Hurria A. International society of geriatric oncology consensus on geriatric assessment in older patients with cancer. Clin Oncol. 2014;32:2595–603.
37. Kristjansson SR, Nesbakken A, Jordhoy MS, Skovlund E, Audisio RA, Johannessen HO, Bakka A, Wyller TB. Comprehensive geriatric assessment can predict complications in elderly patients after elective surgery for colorectal cancer: a prospective observational cohort study. Crit Rev Oncol Hematol. 2010;76:208–17.
38. Tan KY, Kawamura YJ, Tokomitsu A, Tang T. Assessment for frailty is useful for predicting morbidity in elderly patients undergoing colorectal cancer resection whose comorbidities are already optimized. Am J Surg. 2012;204:139–43.
39. Makary MA, Segev DL, Pronovost PJ, Syin D, Bandeen-Roche K, Patel P, Takenaga R, Devgan L, Holzmueller CG, Tian J, Fried LP. Frailty as a predictor of surgical outcomes in older patients. J Am Coll Surg. 2010;210:901–8.
40. Kristjansson SR, Rønninga B, Hurria A, Skovlundd E, Jordhøye MS, Nesbakkeng A, Wyller TB. A comparison of two pre-operative frailty measures in older surgical cancer patients. J Geriatr Oncol. 2012;3:1–7.
41. Leung JM, Sands LP, Mullen EA, Wang Y, Vaurio L. Are preoperative depressive symptoms associated with postoperative delirium in geriatric surgical patients? J Gerontol A Biol Sci Med Sci. 2005;60(12):1563–68.
42. Rao A, Polanco A, Qiu S, Kim J, Chin EH, Divino CM, Nguyen SQ. Safety of outpatient laparoscopic cholecystectomy in the elderly: analysis of 15248 patients using the NSQIP database. J Am Coll Surg. 2013;217(6):1038–43.
43. Kuwabara K, Matsuda S, Fushimi K, Ishuukawa KB, Horiguchi H, Fujimori K. Relationships of age, cholecystectomy approach and timing with the surgical and functional outcomes of elderly patients with cholecystitis. Int J Surg. 2011;9(5):392–99.
44. Oken MM, Creech RH, Tormey DC, Horton J, Davis TE, McFadden ET, Carbone PP. Toxicity and response criteria of the eastern cooperative oncology group. Am J Clin Oncol. 1982;5:649–55.
45. American Society of Anesthesiologists. New classification of physical status. Anesthesiology. 1963;24:111.

8

Critically ill patients with acute cholecystitis are at increased risk for extensive gallbladder inflammation

Marios Papadakis†, Peter C. Ambe*† and Hubert Zirngibl

Abstract

Background: Acute cholecystitis is a common diagnosis and surgery is the standard of care for young and fit patients. However, due to high risk of postoperative morbidity and mortality, surgical management of critically ill patients remains a controversy. It is not clear, whether the increased risk of perioperative complications associated with the management of critically ill patients with acute cholecystitis is secondary to reduced physiologic reserve per se or to the severity of gallbladder inflammation.

Methods: A retrospective analysis of prospectively collected data of patients undergoing laparoscopic cholecystectomy for acute cholecystitis in a university hospital over a three-year-period was performed. The ASA scores at the time of presentation were used to categorize patients into two groups. The study group consisted of critically ill patients with ASA 3 and 4, while the control group was made up of fit patients with ASA 1 and 2. Both groups were compared with regard to perioperative data, postoperative outcome and extent of gallbladder inflammation on histopathology.

Results: Two hundred and seventeen cases of acute cholecystitis with complete charts were available for analysis. The study group included 67 critically ill patients with ASA 3 and 4, while the control group included 150 fit patients with ASA 1 and 2. Both groups were comparable with regard to perioperative data. Histopathology confirmed severe cholecystitis in a significant number of cases in the study group compared to the control group (37 % vs. 18 %, $p = 0.03$). Significantly higher rates of morbidity and mortality were recorded in the study group ($p < 0.05$). Equally, significantly more patients from the study group were managed in the ICU (40 % vs. 8 %, $p = 0.001$).

Conclusion: Critically ill patients presenting with acute cholecystitis are at increased risk for extensive gallbladder inflammation. The increased risk of morbidity and mortality seen in such patients might partly be secondary to severe acute cholecystitis.

Keywords: Acute cholecystitis, Critically ill patients, Laparoscopic cholecystectomy

Background

Acute cholecystitis (AC) is usually an indication for surgery. Current evidence suggests early cholecystectomy to be superior to interval or delayed cholecystectomy with regard to outcome and cost of treatment [1–8]. However, the heterogeneity of patients with acute cholecystitis (AC) makes it almost impossible to standardize treatment. Thus, while healthier and "fit for surgery" candidates are generally surgically managed, controversy exists in the management of elderly and critically ill patients [9–17]. Medical management with antibiotics, fasting, antiemetic and pain medication as well as percutaneous gallbladder aspiration or drainage have been employed as alternative treatment options [12, 16, 18–21]. These options have either been used as a definite means of treatment or as a bridge to surgery after cooling down the acute inflammation.

Patients with reduced physiologic reserves, that is critically ill and elderly patients, have been shown to be at increased risk for postoperative morbidity following gallbladder surgery for acute cholecystitis. However, it is not

* Correspondence: peter.ambe@helios-kliniken.de
†Equal contributors
Helios Klinikum Wuppertal, Department of Surgery II, Witten – Herdecke University, Heusner Str. 40, 42283 Wuppertal, Germany

clear whether or not this increased risk of postoperative morbidity is secondary to reduced physiologic reserve per se or to the extent of gallbladder inflammation. The aim of this study therefore was to investigate whether or not critically ill patients with acute cholecystitis are at increased risk for extensive gallbladder inflammation.

Patients and methods

Following the approval of the ethic committee of the Witten – Herdecke University, a retrospective analysis of a prospectively maintained database of patients undergoing surgery for acute cholecystitis was performed. A written consent was obtained from each patient included. The data of all consecutive patients with AC scheduled for surgery from January 2012 until December 2014 were extracted by two independent investigators.

Patients were admitted following presentation in the emergency department or following referral from the department of internal medicine. Acute cholecystitis was suspected in patients presenting with pain to the right upper quadrant. The diagnosis was confirmed following findings from abdominal ultrasound sonography and blood chemistry as outlined in the Tokyo Guidelines [22, 23].

As part of our institutional standards, all patients with AC were put on i.v. antibiotics usually Tazobactam. Surgery was scheduled as soon as possible depending on the presence or absence of comorbidities needing special consultation and correction. The time interval between admission and surgery was calculated for each patient.

Laparoscopic cholecystectomy (LC) is a standard procedure in our department. In all cases LC was performed using four trocars. Surgery began with the placement of an 11 mm trocar just above the umbilicus after a mini-laparotomy. Occasionally, a Veress needle was used to create pneumoperitoneum. The maximum intraabdominal pressure was set at 12 mmHg. Surgery proceeded with the placement of a 12 mm trocar in the epigastrium slightly to the left of middle line and two 5 mm trocars in the right upper abdomen under visual control. The leading surgeon was either an attending surgeon with expertise in laparoscopic surgery, a fellow or a senior resident under supervision. Single shot antibiotic was administered before incision depending on the time interval between the last antibiotic application and begin of surgery. The gallbladder was removed via the supraumbilical mini-laparotomy using an endobag. Histopathology was performed in all cases.

The data of each patient was put into the database after discharge from the hospital. Demographic data including sex, age, body mass index (BMI) and medical comorbidity score as defined by the American Society of Anesthesiologists (ASA) at the time of surgery were retrieved for each patient. Preoperative data including; white blood count (WBC), c - reactive protein (CRP), platelet count and findings from abdominal ultrasound sonography were recorded for each patient. Perioperative data including surgical procedure, the course of surgery and the duration of surgery (time from incision to suture) were registered in each case. Postoperative data including; complications, management in the intensive care unit and the length of stay (LOS) were recorded for each case. The final histopathology records were consulted for the extent of gallbladder inflammation. The following terminologies were used to define the extent of gallbladder inflammation:

- edematous choleystitis was diagnosed in cases with gallbladder wall edema with interstitial fluid, dilated capillaries and lymphatics.
- necrotizing cholecystitis was diagnosed following the presence of scattered superficial necrosis of the gallbladder wall
- gangrenous cholecystitis was characterized by loss of mucosal lining and vascular architecture with profuse inflammation changes secondary influx of inflammatory cells [24].

The terminologies used to describe the extent of gallbladder inflammation on histopathology in this series are primarily german and correspond grossly with English terminologies used elsewhere [25]. Edematous cholecystitis was considered „uncomplicated while empyematous, necrotizing and gangrenous cholecystitis were referred to as „complicated cholecystitis".

In this study, a critically ill patient was defined as any patient with reduced physiologic reserve presenting with acute cholecystitis. Although the ASA score relies mostly on chronic conditions, it does account to some degree for the acute illness. Thus critically ill patients were defined as those with relevant chronic conditions presenting with AC [26]. The study group therefore consisted of patients with ASA 3 and 4, while the control group was made up of patients with ASA 1 and 2.

The Statistical Package for Social Science (SPSS®), IBM, version 22 was employed to analyze the collected data. Continuous variables were described using absolute case numbers and percentages. Since the data were not normally distributed, central tendencies were described using median values with the corresponding interquartile ranges with a 95 % confidence interval. Statistical significances were calculated using chi square test with the level of significance placed at $p < 0.05$.

Both groups would be compared with regard to perioperative findings and postoperative outcomes. Primary outcome was the extent of gallbladder inflammation on histopathology. Secondary outcomes included the duration of surgery, the rate of conversion, postoperative morbidity as defined by Clevian and Dindo [27], the need of ICU management and the LOS.

Results

Within the period of investigation, 1024 cholecystectomies were performed in our department. The indication for surgery was AC in 405 cases. After excluding cases with negative pathology (cases with chronic cholecystitis presenting with acute biliary colics) and incomplete data (ASA, BMI and gallbladder wall thickness per ultrasound sonography), 217 cases of AC were included for analysis, Fig. 1. The demographic features of the cases included are summarized in Table 1. The study group was significantly older compared to the control group, $p = 0.02$.

Cardiovascular disorders including high blood pressure, ischemic heart disease, hypertensive heart disease, atrial fibrillation and peripheral artery disease constituted the leading concomitant disorders in the study and were recorded in 55 cases (82 %). Type 2 diabetes was present in 27 cases (40 %). Chronic obstructive pulmonary disease was present in 18 cases (26.8 %) while chronic kidney disease was seen in 16 cases (23 %).

The perioperative characteristics in this study are presented in Table 2. There was no significant difference amongst both groups with regard to perioperative findings. Early cholecystectomy was performed within 72 h of symptom onset in over 80 % (54/67) of the study group and in about 91 % (137/150) of the control group. Delayed cholecystectomy, that is surgery after 72 h of symptom onset was performed in 19.4 % (13 cases) of the study group and in 8.7 % (13 cases) of the control group. This difference was statistically significant, $p = 0.02$.

Conversion from laparoscopic to open surgery was necessary in 14 cases (6.5 %). While conversion was necessary in just three cases (4.5 %) in the study group, 11 cases (7.3 %) were converted in the control group. This difference was not statistically significant, $p = 0.42$. All converted cases were monitored in the ICU.

Table 1 Demographic characteristics

Characteristics	Study group	Control group	*p*-value
Number of cases	67	150	/
Sex: female	28 (42.4 %)	66 (44.0 %)	0.44
male	38 (57.6 %)	84 (56.0 %)	
Median Age (yrs)	76.0	59.0	0.02
Interquartile range	19.0	25.0	
Median BMI (kg/m^2)	27.1	27.4	0.88
Interquartile range	6.5	5.7	

The study group was significantly older compared to the control group. *Yrs* years, *BMI* body mass index

Complications were recorded in 25 (11.5 %) cases in the entire study population. These included 14 (20.9 %) cases in the study group and 11 (7.3 %) cases in the control group. This difference was statistically significant, $p = 0.004$). The postoperative outcomes of both groups are summarized in Table 3, while the complications recorded in both groups are presented in Table 4.

ICU management was necessary in 40.9 % of cases in the study group, while only 8 % of cases in the control group required ICU admission. This difference was statistically significant, $p = 0.001$.

Uncomplicated cholecystitis was diagnosed in 63.6 % (42/67) of study group and in 82.0 % (123/150) of the control group following histopathology. Significantly ($p = 0.03$) more complicated gallbladder inflammation was evident in the study group (25/76 : 37.3 %) compared to the control group (27/150 : 18 %), Table 5. Three cases of mortality (1.4 %) were recorded in this series including two cases (1.3 %) in the study group and one case (1.5 %)

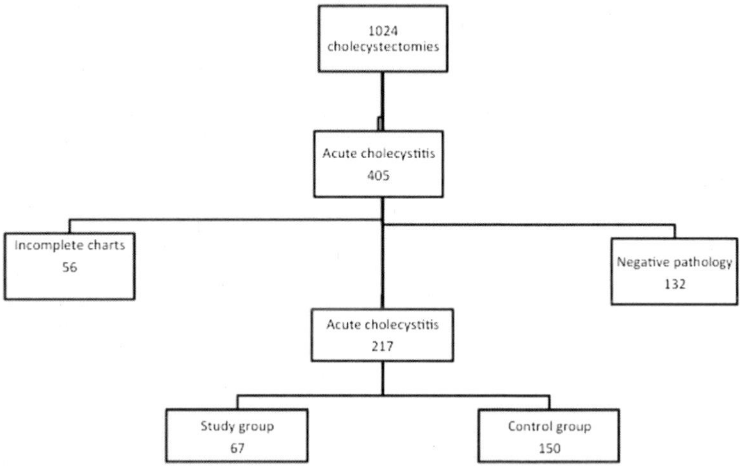

Fig. 1 Distribution of the study population. The study group consisted of 67 critically ill patients while the control group was made up of 150 healthier patients

Table 2 Perioperative data

Features	Study group	Control group	*p*-value
Median gallbladder wall thickness	6.0	5.0	0.26
Interquartile range	11.0	4.0	
WBC/ul	12.6	10.8	0.50
Interquartile range	8.5	6.8	
CRP	10.5	3.7	0.14
Interquartile range (mg/dl)	20.5	12.9	
Median time to surgery	24.0	24.0	0.10
Interquartile range (h)	60.0	42.0	
Median duration of surgery	98.0	87.0	0.28
Interquartile range (min)	63.0	58.0	
Conversion to open surgery	3/66 (4.5 %)	11/150 (7.3 %)	0.43

Both groups were comparable in terms of perioperative data
h hours, *min* minutes, *CRP* c – reactive protein, *WBC* white blood count

in the control group. This difference was not statistically significant, $p = 0.172$.

Discussion

This study was designed to investigate whether or not critically ill patients with acute cholecystitis could be at risk for extensive gallbladder inflammation. The charts of 217 patients undergoing laparoscopic cholecystitis for acute cholecystitis within a three-year-period in a university hospital were retrospectively reviewed. Patients with relevant chronic conditions (ASA scores > 2) presenting with AC were classified as critically ill. The study group consisted of 67 critically ill patients with ASA > 2, while the control group was made up of 150 fit patients with ASA ≤ 2. Although the study group was significantly older than the control group, both groups were comparable with regard to perioperative data. The rates of morbidity and mortality were significantly higher in the study group. Equally, significantly more patients from the study group required ICU management following surgery. Histopathology confirmed extensive gallbladder inflammation in the form of gangrenous, necrotizing and empyematous cholecystitis in a significant number of cases from the study group.

Table 3 Postoperative data

Features	Study group	Control group	P - value
ICU admission	27/67 (40.3 %)	12/150 (8.0 %)	0.001
Morbidity rate	14/67 (20.9 %)	11/150 (7.3 %)	0.004
Median length of stay	6.0	4.0	0.001
Interquartile range (d)	6.0	3.0	

The need for ICU management, the rate of morbidity and the median length of postoperative hospital stay were significantly higher in the study group.
d: days

Table 4 Complications

Complications	Study group	Control group
Grade I	4	4
Grade II	2	0
Grade III	5	6
Grade IV	1	0
Grade V	2	1

Postoperative complications according to the classification by Dindo et al. [27]
Study group:
I: delayed bowel movement 2x, superfacial wound bleeding 1x, wound dehiscence 1x
II: Pneumonia 2x
III: Bile leak 2 x, bilioma drainage 1x, bleeding 1x, subphrenic hematoma 1x
IV: Acute renal failure (Dialysis)
V: Mortality 1x (pulmonary embolism), 1 x pulmonary failure
Control group:
I: wound dehiscence 2x, wound infection 1x, small bilioma 1x
III: Subphrenic abscess 3x, Hematoma 1x, bile duct injury 2x
V: Mortality 1x (myocardial infarction)

Although acute cholecystitis is a common illness, the great divergence in the clinical course and possible concomitant medical conditions make it extremely difficult to standardize management. While early surgery is generally accepted as the standard of care for young and fit patients, the management of critically ill patients has been vague and is still a cause of controversy due to high rates of morbidity and mortality associated with the surgical management of such patients [4, 5, 9, 12, 13, 16, 20, 28].

Besides reduced physiologic reserve, many confounding factors like age, sex, timing of surgery as well as surgical expertise have been shown to influence postoperative outcome [1, 7, 29–33]. Current data suggests that the extent of gallbladder inflammation may equally affect postoperative outcomes as is the case with gangrenous and empyematous cholecystitis [34–37]. However, it is not known whether or not the high rates of complications associated with surgery for acute cholecystitis in critically ill patients is due to reduced physiologic reserve per se or to the extent of gallbladder inflammation. In this study, complicated cholecystitis (gangrenous, necrotizing and empyematous) was present in over 37 % of the study population compared to just 18 % of the control group.

Timing of surgical intervention has been a matter of debate for a long time. However, current evidence suggests a better outcome in patients managed within 72 h of symptom onset [1, 4, 38]. Although no statistically significant difference was seen amongst both groups with respect to the median time interval from diagnosis to surgery, surgery was performed later on patients with ASA scores > 2 as demonstrated by the interquartile range of 60 h in the study group. Indeed, delay cholecystectomy was performed in significantly more patients from the study group compared to the control group. This finding was not surprising since some of

Table 5 Histopathology

Histopathology	Study group	Control group	P -value
Uncomplicated acute cholecystitis	42/67 (62.6 %)	123/150 (82.0 %)	0.42
Empyematous cholecystitis	5/67 (7.5 %)	4/140 (2.7 %)	
Gangrenous cholecystitis	14/67 (20.9%)	14/150 (9.3 %)	0.02
Necrotizing cholecystitis	5/67 (7.5 %)	9/150 (6.0 %)	

Uncomplicated cholecystitis was seen in a vast majority of cases in both groups. Complicated cholecystitis was diagnosed in significantly more patients from the study group, $p = 0.02$

these patients required a correction of comorbid conditions prior to surgery.

There was no difference amongst both groups with regard to the rate of conversion. The rates of complications and mortality were significantly higher in the study group. Equally, the need for postoperative ICU management was significantly higher in the study groups. Although these findings are in accordance with current literature [39, 40], only 40 % of the study groups required ICU management in this series. This however is of little clinical implication, since the indication for ICU management varies amongst institutions.

With the exception of age, both groups were comparable in terms of baseline characteristics. This was also true for perioperative features in both groups. Therefore, the results recorded in this study cannot be blamed on these factors. Equally, surgical expertise was not an issue since both groups were managed by experienced surgeons. The results seen in this study therefore must be blamed either on reduced physiologic reserve per se or on the extent of gallbladder inflammation. However, since postoperative complications were recorded in a significant number of cases in patients with extensive gallbladder inflammation, the extent of inflammation rather than reduced physiologic reserve should be blamed for these complications.

The extent of gallbladder inflammation seems to depend on the duration of symptoms. Unequivocal evidence supporting the superiority of early cholecystectomy has become available over the last years [4, 5, 7, 8, 28, 41]. Delaying surgical intervention might be associated with worsening of inflammation. This seems to be the case with the study groups. The optimal time frame for surgery was most probably missed because of the need of specialist consultations and correction of comorbidities prior to surgery. Within this period, an initially uncomplicated cholecystitis probably got worse, resulting to a complicated form (gangrenous, empyematous or necrotizing cholecystitis).

In our department, same admission laparoscopic cholecystectomy represents the standard of care for patients with acute cholecystitis. Medical treatment is performed in a very small number of extremely morbid patients. Interventional methods like percutaneous cholecystostomy is not performed in our department. Therefore, it remains unclear, if and how the outcomes seen in this study would have been altered by medical and interventional treatment options.

Taken together, our results suggest that patients with reduced physiologic reserve presenting with acute cholecystitis are at increased risk for extensive gallbladder inflammation. The time spent on specialist consultation and for the correction of comorbidities prior to surgery forces such patients out of the optimal time frame for surgery. Delaying surgery in order to correct comorbidities may exacerbate the extent of inflammation, thereby leading to an increased risk of postoperative morbidity and the need of ICU management.

Our results argue for a timely management of critically ill patients with AC. First, surgery is best performed within 72 h of symptom onset. Second, medical treatment should be offered to patients who due to comorbidities cannot be managed within the safe time frame for surgery. However, the heterogeneity in the presentation and disease course in patients presenting with acute cholecystitis makes the clinical decision-making extremely difficult. This is especially true for patients who fail to recover on medical treatment and therefore have to undergo surgical management at the most unsuitable time. Therefore, the clinical decision-making must be individualized.

Although all patients included in this study were consecutive recruited and there was no risk of selection bias, the study design represents a major limitation of this study. Furthermore, it remains speculative, whether or not the outcomes recorded in this series might have been altered by medical or intervention treatment options. Thus, the trend reported in this series warrants further investigation.

Conclusion

Critically ill patients presenting with acute cholecystitis are at increased risk for extensive gallbladder inflammation. The increased risk of morbidity and mortality seen in such patients might in part to be secondary to severe acute cholecystitis.

Consent

Written informed consent was obtained from each patient for the publication of this study and any accompanying images.

Abbreviation

AC: acute cholecystitis; ASA: American Society of Anesthesiologists; BMI: body mass index; CRP: C-reactive protein; ICU: intensive care unit; LC: laparoscopic cholecystectomy; LOS: length of stay; SPSS: statistical package for social sciences; WBC: white blood count.

Competing interest

The authors declare no conflict of interest.

Authors' contribution

PA concepted the study. PA and HZ designed the study. PA and MP collected the data. PA analyzed the data. PA, MP and HZ interpreted the results. PA drafted the manuscript. All the authors critically reviewed the manuscript and approved the final version.

References

1. Ambe P, Weber SA, Christ H, Wassenberg D. Cholecystectomy for acute cholecystitis. How time-critical are the so called "golden 72 hours"? Or better "golden 24 hours" and "silver 25–72 hour"? A case control study. World J emergency surgery : WJES. 2014;9(1):60.
2. Degrate L, Ciravegna AL, Luperto M, Guaglio M, Garancini M, Maternini M, et al. Acute cholecystitis: The golden 72-h period is not a strict limit to perform early cholecystectomy. Results from 316 consecutive patients. Langenbecks Arch Surg. 2013;398(8):1129–36.
3. Gurusamy K, Samraj K, Gluud C, Wilson E, Davidson BR. Meta-analysis of randomized controlled trials on the safety and effectiveness of early versus delayed laparoscopic cholecystectomy for acute cholecystitis. Br J Surg. 2010;97(2):141–50.
4. Gutt CN, Encke J, Köninger J, Harnoss JC, Weigand K, Kipfmüller K, et al. Acute cholecystitis: Early versus delayed cholecystectomy, a multicenter randomized trial (ACDC Study, NCT00447304). Ann Surg. 2013;258(3):385–91.
5. Kolla SB, Aggarwal S, Kumar A, Kumar R, Chumber S, Parshad R, et al. Early versus delayed laparoscopic cholecystectomy for acute cholecystitis: a prospective randomized trial. Surg Endosc. 2004;18(9):1323–7.
6. Lau B, DiFronzo LA. An acute care surgery model improves timeliness of care and reduces hospital stay for patients with acute cholecystitis. Am Surg. 2011;77(10):1318–21.
7. Papi C, Catarci M, D'Ambrosio L, Gili L, Koch M, Grassi GB, et al. Timing of cholecystectomy for acute calculous cholecystitis: a meta-analysis. Am J Gastroenterol. 2004;99(1):147–55.
8. Siddiqui T, MacDonald A, Chong PS, Jenkins JT. Early versus delayed laparoscopic cholecystectomy for acute cholecystitis: a meta-analysis of randomized clinical trials. Am J Surg. 2008;195(1):40–7.
9. Brunt LM, Quasebarth MA, Dunnegan DL, Soper NJ. Outcomes analysis of laparoscopic cholecystectomy in the extremely elderly. Surg Endosc. 2001; 15(7):700–5.
10. Kapan M, Onder A, Tekbas G, Gul M, Aliosmanoglu I, Arikanoglu Z, et al. Percutaneous cholecystostomy in high-risk elderly patients with acute cholecystitis: a lifesaving option. Am J Hospice and Palliat Med. 2013;30(2):167–71.
11. Li M, Li N, Ji W, Quan Z, Wan X, Wu X, et al. Percutaneous cholecystostomy is a definitive treatment for acute cholecystitis in elderly high-risk patients. Am Surg. 2013;79(5):524–7.
12. McGillicuddy EA, Schuster KM, Barre K, Suarez L, Hall MR, Kaml GJ, et al. Non-operative management of acute cholecystitis in the elderly. Br J Surg. 2012;99(9):1254–61.
13. Morse BC, Smith JB, Lawdahl RB, Roettger RH. Management of acute cholecystitis in critically ill patients: contemporary role for cholecystostomy and subsequent cholecystectomy. Am Surg. 2010;76(7):708–12.
14. Nielsen LBJ, Harboe KM, Bardram L. Cholecystectomy for the elderly: no hesitation for otherwise healthy patients. Surg Endosc. 2014;28(1):171-177.
15. Qasaimeh GR, Banihani MN. Laparoscopic cholecystectomy in the elderly and young: A comparative study. Hepatogastroenterology. 2012;59(113):22–5.
16. Vracko J, Markovic S, Wiechel KL. Conservative treatment versus endoscopic sphincterotomy in the initial management of acute cholecystitis in elderly patients at high surgical risk. Endoscopy. 2006;38(8):773–8.
17. Ambe PC, Weber SA, Christ H, Wassenberg D. Primary cholecystectomy is feasible in elderly patients with acute cholecystitis. Aging Clin Exp Res. 2015; 27(6):921-6.
18. Borzellino G, Sauerland S, Minicozzi AM, Verlato G, Di Pietrantonj C, de Manzoni G, et al. Laparoscopic cholecystectomy for severe acute cholecystitis. A meta-analysis of results. Surg Endosc. 2008;22(1):8–15.
19. Simorov A, Ranade A, Parcells J, Shaligram A, Shostrom V, Boilesen E, et al. Emergent cholecystostomy is superior to open cholecystectomy in extremely ill patients with acalculous cholecystitis: A large multicenter outcome study. Am J Surg. 2013;206(6):935–41.
20. Tarragón AV, Soria JSA, Lens V, Manzoni D, Fabiano P, Goergen M. Two staged minimally invasive treatment for acute cholecystitis in high risk patients. Hepatogastroenterology. 2013;60(123):466–9.
21. Zerem E, Omerović S, Imširović B. Is surgical cholecystectomy better than percutaneous in treatment of acute cholecystitis in patients unfit for surgery? J Gastrointest Surg. 2013;17(8):1542–3.
22. Yokoe M, Takada T, Strasberg SM, Solomkin JS, Mayumi T, Gomi H, et al. TG13 diagnostic criteria and severity grading of acute cholecystitis (with videos). J Hepatobiliary Pancreat Sci. 2013;20(1):35–46.
23. Yokoe M, Takada T, Strasberg SM, Solomkin JS, Mayumi T, Gomi H, et al. New diagnostic criteria and severity assessment of acute cholecystitis in revised Tokyo guidelines. J Hepatobiliary Pancreat Sci. 2012;19(5):578–85.
24. Ambe PC, Christ H, Wassenberg D. Does the Tokyo guidelines predict the extent of gallbladder inflammation in patients with acute cholecystitis? A single center retrospective analysis. BMC Gastroenterol. 2015;15(1):142.
25. Kimura Y, Takada T, Kawarada Y, Nimura Y, Hirata K, Sekimoto M, et al. Definitions, pathophysiology, and epidemiology of acute cholangitis and cholecystitis: Tokyo Guidelines. J Hepatobiliary Pancreat Surg. 2007;14(1):15–26.
26. Wolters U, Wolf T, Stutzer H, Schroder T. ASA classification and perioperative variables as predictors of postoperative outcome. Br J Anaesth. 1996;77(2):217–22.
27. Dindo D, Demartines N, Clavien PA. Classification of surgical complications: a new proposal with evaluation in a cohort of 6336 patients and results of a survey. Ann Surg. 2004;240(2):205–13.
28. Lau H, Lo CY, Patil NG, Yuen WK. Early versus delayed-interval laparoscopic cholecystectomy for acute cholecystitis: a metaanalysis. Surg Endosc. 2006; 20(1):82–7.
29. Ambe P, Esfahani BJ, Tasci I, Christ H, Köhler L. Is laparoscopic cholecystectomy more challenging in male patients? Surg Endosc and Other Interventional Techniques. 2011;25(7):2236–40.
30. Botaitis S, Polychronidis A, Pitiakoudis M, Perente S, Simopoulos C. Does gender affect laparoscopic cholecystectomy? Surg Laparosc Endosc Percutan Tech. 2008;18(2):157–61.
31. Ibrahim S, Hean TK, Ho LS, Ravintharan T, Chye TN, Chee CH. Risk factors for conversion to open surgery in patients undergoing laparoscopic cholecystectomy. World J Surg. 2006;30(9):1698–704.
32. Kanakala V, Borowski DW, Pellen MG, Dronamraju SS, Woodcock SA, Seymour K, et al. Risk factors in laparoscopic cholecystectomy: a multivariate analysis. Int J Surg (London, England). 2011;9(4):318–23.
33. Lee HK, Han HS, Min SK, Lee JH. Sex-based analysis of the outcome of laparoscopic cholecystectomy for acute cholecystitis. Br J Surg. 2005;92(4):463–6.
34. Fagan SP, Awad SS, Rahwan K, Hira K, Aoki N, Itani KM, et al. Prognostic factors for the development of gangrenous cholecystitis. Am J Surg. 2003; 186(5):481–5.
35. Hunt DR, Chu FC. Gangrenous cholecystitis in the laparoscopic era. Aust N Z J Surg. 2000;70(6):428–30.
36. Merriam LT, Kanaan SA, Dawes LG, Angelos P, Prystowsky JB, Rege RV, et al. Gangrenous cholecystitis: analysis of risk factors and experience with laparoscopic cholecystectomy. Surgery. 1999;126(4):680–5. discussion 685–686.
37. Wilson AK, Kozol RA, Salwen WA, Manov LJ, Tennenberg SD. Gangrenous cholecystitis in an urban VA hospital. J Surg Res. 1994;56(5):402–4.
38. Zhu B, Zhang Z, Wang Y, Gong K, Lu Y, Zhang N. Comparison of laparoscopic cholecystectomy for acute cholecystitis within and beyond 72 h of symptom onset during emergency admissions. World J Surg. 2012;36(11):2654–8.
39. Kortram K, van Ramshorst B, Bollen TL, Besselink MGH, Gouma DJ, Karsten T, Kruyt PM, Nieuwenhuijzen GAP, Kelder JC, Tromp E et al.. Acute cholecystitis in high risk surgical patients: Percutaneous cholecystostomy versus laparoscopic cholecystectomy (CHOCOLATE trial): Study protocol for a randomized controlled trial. Trials. 2012, 13. doi:10.1186/1745-6215-13-7.
40. Yamashita Y, Takada T, Strasberg SM, Pitt HA, Gouma DJ, Garden OJ, et al. TG13 surgical management of acute cholecystitis. J Hepatobiliary Pancreat Sci. 2013;20(1):89–96.
41. Gurusamy KS, Davidson C, Gluud C, Davidson BR. Early versus delayed laparoscopic cholecystectomy for people with acute cholecystitis. Cochrane Database Syst Rev. 2013;6:CD005440.

9

The learning curve of single-port laparoscopic appendectomy performed by emergent operation

YongHun Kim[1] and WooSurng Lee[2*]

Abstract

Background: Single-port laparoscopic appendectomy (SPLA) has the advantage of minimizing abdominal incision scars with patient satisfaction. However, it has the following disadvantages: it provides a narrower surgical field than conventional laparoscopic appendectomy, which requires a considerably longer operative time to achieve surgical skills. This study was conducted to evaluate the learning curve for SPLA.

Methods: This study included a total of 120 patients with acute abdomen who visited our emergency department and were diagnosed with acute appendicitis between March 2013 and February 2015. They underwent SPLA by a single surgeon. Patients were divided into 4 groups of 30 patients each according to operation dates. Operative time, time to resume oral intake, length of hospital stay, and postoperative complications were analyzed.

Results: The mean operative time was 59.9 ± 19.9 min. It was shortened after completion of 30 operations and remained unchanged until it was further shortened after completion of 90 operations. There was no significant difference in time to resumption of oral intake or length of hospital stay between the 4 groups. Postoperative complications occurred in 18 patients, but the frequency of the complications was not significantly different between the 4 groups.

Conclusions: The results of this study suggest that surgeons can achieve surgical skills for SPLA after completion of 30 operations and more experienced surgical skills by SPLA successfully after completion of 90 operations.

Keywords: Learning curve, Laparoscopy, Appendectomy, Emergencies

Background

Laparoscopic appendectomy is minimally invasive compared to conventional open appendectomy and has the advantages of decreased postoperative pain, shortened hospital stay, fewer postoperative complications, and better cosmesis. It has replaced conventional open appendectomy in the treatment of acute appendicitis [1, 2]. Therefore, this laparoscopic appendectomy is currently the gold standard operation for acute appendicitis and provides similar surgical outcomes as conventional open appendectomy, even in cases of complicated appendicitis [3]. Recently, advances in laparoscopic instruments and optical systems enabled surgeons to perform intra-abdominal operation through a single incision around the umbilicus; in particular, single-port laparoscopic appendectomy (SPLA), which minimizes visible scars in the abdominal wall, satisfies patients [4, 5]. In addition, previous randomized controlled studies reported that SPLA has surgical outcomes similar to those of three-port laparoscopic appendectomy (TPLA) [6, 7]. However, since SPLA has the disadvantages of limited surgical field and difficult access to the operation site through a small incision compared to TPLA, it requires more experience with surgical cases and more skills than TPLA, especially in emergency cases. For this reason, to achieve surgical outcomes similar to those of TPLA, SPLA demands additional training programs. Recent preliminary studies have not yet completely elucidate the learning curve of SPLA [8, 9]. Thus, the aims of this study were

* Correspondence: timesgoby@naver.com
[2]Department of Thoracic and Cardiovascular Surgery, School of Medicine, Konkuk University, Konkuk University Chungju Hospital, 82, Gugwon-daero, Chungju-si, Chungbuk, Republic of Korea
Full list of author information is available at the end of the article

to analyze the learning curve of SPLA over a longer period and to assess its surgical safety and feasibility.

Methods

This study included a total of 122 patients with acute abdomen who visited our emergency department and were diagnosed with acute appendicitis between March 2013 and February 2015. They underwent SPLA. To make a definite diagnosis of acute appendicitis, all patients were evaluated using a comprehensive history taking, physical examination, laboratory findings, and abdominal computed tomography with contrast enhancement. Each patient gave informed consent to SPLA. Two patients had undergone right hemicolectomy for peritonitis with severe cecal inflammation and diverticular perforation, who were excluded from the study. All operations were performed by a single surgeon in the same surgical team who had experience with more than 500 TPLA cases and more than 500 conventional open appendectomy cases. Patients were consecutively assigned to 4 groups of 30 patients each: group A (the first 30 patients), group B (the second 30 patients), group C (the third 30 patients), and group D (the fourth 30 patients). Clinical data on age, gender, body mass index (BMI), severity of appendicitis, and previous history of abdominal surgery was collected and analyzed with regard to operative time, postoperative complications, length of hospital stay, time to resume oral intake, and conversion rate.

Surgical procedure

SPLA was performed under general anesthesia. The patent lay on the operating table in the supine position, with both arms lying outside. Both the surgeon and assistant stood on the patient's left side. After a 2-cm mid-line linear incision was made just above the umbilicus, the abdominal wall was opened using the Hassan technique. Once proper umbilical access has been obtained, a Glove Port (Nelis, Seoul, Korea) was positioned and secured within the incision, providing both 360° wound protection and circumferential atraumatic retraction. Pneumoperitoneum was maintained at 10–12 mm Hg using CO_2. SPLA was conducted using a 5-mm Flexible EndoEYE laparoscope (Olympus Surgical & Industrial America Inc, Center Valley, PA, USA) and a 5-mm HiQ™ Curved Instrument (Olympus Surgical & Industrial America Inc, Center Valley, PA, USA). The appendix was grasped and pulled with a 5-mm HiQ™ Curved Instrument immediately on its tip, if visible, or starting from its base or proximal third and gradually mobilizing the entire body of the appendix. When the appendix was stuck by surrounding dense and thick inflammatory adhesions, the use of a blunt suction device could be extremely safe and useful for creating a plane for dissection and mobilization from the surrounding inflamed viscera and tissues. Once the appendix was fully mobilized and its base on the cecum was identified, the mesentery was carefully dissected and coagulated using a Harmonic scalpel (Ethicon, Blue Ash, OH, USA). Once the base of the appendix on the cecum was reached and the mesenteric tissues were fully cleansed, the appendix base was ready to be knotted using a Surgitie™ loop (Covidien, Mansfield, MA, USA). Finally, after cutting the appendix, the specimen was retrieved under direct vision and extracted through the umbilical glove port. The operation was terminated with aspiration and eventual cautious lavage, especially in the right iliac fossa and Douglas pouch, checking hemostasis on the mesentery and good closure of the appendiceal stump (Fig. 1).

Statistical analysis

Data analysis was performed using MedCalc for Windows version 12.3.0 (MedCalc Software, Ostend, Belgium). In statistical testing, a two-sided P value of >0.05 was considered statistically significant. Continuous variables are expressed as mean ± standard deviation. Categorical variables are presented as frequency and percentage. In univariate analysis, Fisher's exact test and one-way analysis of variance were used as appropriate for group comparisons. Then, multivariate analysis was conducted by fitting multiple linear regression models to identify important predictors of operative time.

Results

The mean age of the patients was 45.1 ± 16.1 years (range, 19.0–87.0 years), and there were 67 males and 53 females. The mean BMI was 23.38 ± 3.20 (range, 17.0–34.8). Of the 120 patients, 16 had a history of abdominal surgery: 1 had cholecystectomy, 9 had cesarean section, 3 had myomectomy, and 3 had tubal ligation. There was no significant difference in age, gender, BMI, or history of abdominal surgery between the 4 groups (Table 1). The types of appendicitis classified according to severity were as follows: the suppurative ($n = 83$), gangrenous ($n = 24$), and perforated ($n = 13$) types. The appendices were categorized according to their location as follows: the retrocecal ($n = 18$), subcecal/pelvic ($n = 76$), and retroileal ($n = 26$) types. The mean operation time was 59.9 ± 19.9 min, and there was no intra-abdominal injury or massive bleeding during operation. Of the 120 patients, 4 required additional port insertion, all of whom belonged to group A. There were no patients who required conversion to open appendectomy. The mean time to resume oral intake was 1.5 ± 0.7 days, but it was not significantly different between the 4 groups ($P = 0.418$) Postoperative complications occurred in 18 patients, and most of them were wound complications ($n = 11$, 9.1 %). There were four patients (3.3 %) with intra-abdominal inflammation which was resolved by antibiotics therapy, without percutaneous drainage. Postoperative ileus occurred in three patients

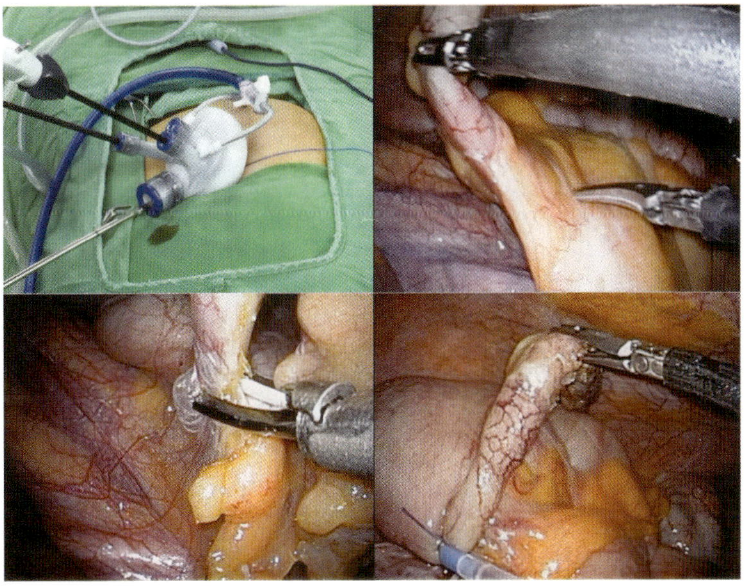

Fig. 1 Surgical procedure of single-port laparoscopic appendectomy

(2.5 %), which was improved by conservative treatment. There was no significant difference in postoperative complications between the 4 groups ($p = 0.853$) (Table 1). Mean operative times were 67.0 ± 23.9 min in group A, 61.7 ± 23.9 min in group B, 60.4 ± 17.5 min in group C, and 50.6 ± 16.8 min in group D. Mean operative times were longest in group A and shortest in group D. One-way analysis of variance (ANOVA) showed significant correlations between groups A and D, and between groups B and C ($P = 0.012$). The mean operative time was shortened after completion of 30 operations and remained unchanged until it was further shortened after completion of 90 operations (Fig. 2). In multiple linear regression analysis, the severity of appendicitis was significantly associated with operative time; however, history of abdominal surgery, location of the appendix, or BMI was not significantly associated with operative time (Table 2).

Discussion

Single puncture tubal ligation via a laparoscopic single-opening approach was first introduced by Wheeless in 1969 [10]. Thereafter, this approach has been employed in the treatment of complicated gynecological diseases and applied for appendectomy, placement of peritoneal dialysis catheters, and resection of intra-abdominal cysts [11, 12]. Despite such applications in various clinical conditions, single-port laparoscopic surgery (SPLS) has not yet been widely performed in real-world practice.

Table 1 Patients demographics and comparisons of learning curve-related variables

	Overall	Group A	Group B	Group C	Group D	*P value*
Age (years)	45.1 ± 16.1	43.8 ± 17.3	44.9 ± 10.8	44.6 ± 15.2	47.1 ± 17.8	0.297
Gender (M/F)	67/53	14/16	14/16	20/10	19/11	0.245
BMI (kg/m^2)	23.38 ± 3.2	23.58 ± 3.3	23.02 ± 3.4	23.63 ± 3.1	23.30 ± 2.9	0.874
Previous history of AS	16	5	4	3	4	0.901
Operation time (minutes)	59.9 ± 19.9	67.0 ± 23.9	61.7 ± 17.9	60.4 ± 17.5	50.6 ± 16.8	0.012
Additional port insertion	4	4	0	0	0	0.006
Time to ROI (days)	1.5 ± 0.7	1.5 ± 0.8	1.6 ± 0.8	1.5 ± 0.6	1.6 ± 0.8	0.966
Hospitalization (days)	5.1 ± 2.5	5.3 ± 2.7	5.2 ± 2.3	4.9 ± 1.9	4.8 ± 2.0	0.418
Complications	18	5	5	5	3	0.853
wound problem	11	3	3	4	1	0.230
intraabdominal infection	4	1	1	1	1	1.000
ileus	3	1	1	0	1	0.890

Abbreviations: *M/F* male/female, *BMI* body mass index, *AS* abdominal surgery, *ROI* resumption of oral intake

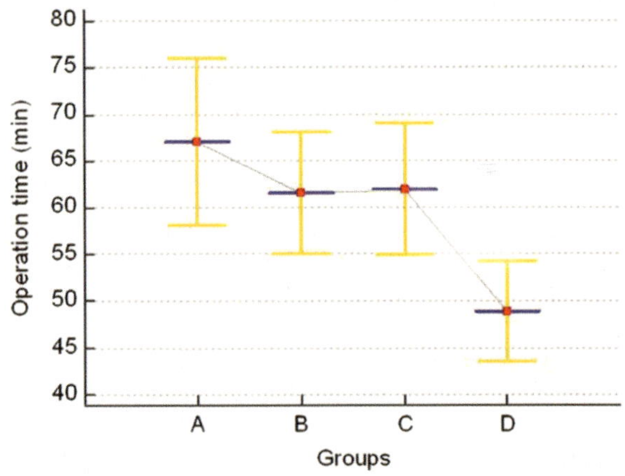

Fig. 2 Changes in operative time according to operation dates

The reasons for this may be the limitations of SPLS to clinical indications and the steep learning curve to overcome. A major problem is difficulty in manipulating the laparoscope and the instruments introduced through a single port because surgeons should avoid extra- and intracorporeal conflict between the laparoscope and the instruments. Such drawbacks frequently lead to the loss of triangulation and difficult instrumentation during SPLS, unlike conventional multiport laparoscopic surgery. SPLS requires the surgeon and the assistant to maintain a poor ergonomic position different from that in conventional laparoscopic surgery. SPLS may be more difficult to perform than conventional laparoscopic surgery, prolong operative time, require a steep learning curve, and have low feasibility and safety [11–13]. For addressing these issues, many improved devices have been used in real-world practice: longer laparoscopes (45 cm in length), laparoscopes with various angles, improved port systems, such as Home-made Glove port, SILS™ Port (Covidien Inc, Norwalk, CT, USA), Uni-X™, AirSeal (SurgiQuest, Orange, CT, USA), Glove port (Nelis, Seoul, South Korea), and laparoscopic instruments specifically designed for SPLS, such as Roticulator™ (Covidien Inc, Norwalk, CT, USA), HiQ LS™ Curved instrument (Olympus Surgical & Industrial America Inc, Center Valley, PA, USA) [11, 12]. Despite such advances in laparoscopes and instruments, surgeons should have a substantial learning curve to perform SPLS.

Recently, SPLA has been extensively performed because of the superior cosmesis with no visible scarring [14]. Most of the previous studies have reported that the clinical outcomes of SPLA are the same as those of TPLA [4–7]. Meanwhile, some studies have reported that SPLA requires a longer operative time and a substantial learning curve [15]. Liao et al. [8] analyzed 30 cases of non-complicated appendicitis undergoing SPLA and documented that the operative time for SPLA was shortened after experience with 10 cases of SPLA, which became the same as that for TPLA. Validad et al. [9] investigated 65 pediatric cases of acute appendicitis undergoing SPLA and showed that the operative time for SPLA was equal to that for TPLA, regardless of board certification. These studies may have some limitations to interpret their results in that they excluded cases of complicated appendicitis. However, our study analyzed 120 cases of acute appendicitis which included cases of complicated appendicitis, so that it has clinical implications in such aspects. Moreover, since our study included only SPLA cases during the study period, with exclusion of TPLA cases, we avoided selection bias and obtained more general data on the learning curve for SPLA. The learning curve for SPLA can be assessed by various parameters, such as blood loss, complication rates, conversion rates, operative time, and length of hospital stay, of which operative time and length of hospital stay are more important [16, 17]. In this study, the operative time for SPLA was shortened after completion of 30 SPLA cases, remained unchanged, and was further shortened significantly after completion of 90 SPLA cases. Since previous studies on the learning curve for SPLA had a relatively small sample size (n = 20–50), they may have some limitations to generalize their results [16–19]. Pan et al. [20] divided 180 consecutive single-incision laparoscopic cholecystectomies into 9 groups according to operation dates, and each group included 20 patients operated on consecutively in each time period. They also reported that the operative time was significantly longer in group 1 than in the other groups.

Table 2 Multivariate analysis of predictors of operative time

	Coefficient	Standard error	*T* value	*P* value
Group	-5.26	1.52	-3.45	0.0008
Severity of appendicitis	7.95	2.53	3.14	0.0021
BMI	1.14	1.78	0.63	0.524
Location of appendix	-0.89	2.75	-0.32	0.746
Past history of abdominal surgery	-2.99	5.01	-0.59	0.552

By the multiple linear regression model: $n = 120$, residual standard error = 18.6, $R^2 = 0.126$, overall F test statistic = 4.448, $P = 0.001$ ($df = 5, 114$)
Abbreviation: *BMI* body mass index

Lee et al. [21] divided 160 cases of myoma uteri requiring single-port laparoscopic myomectomy into 4 groups according to operation dates and reported that the operative time declined significantly in the last 3 groups compared to the first group. Our results on the progressive decrease in the operative time for SPLA can provide useful information on a general learning curve for SPLA. Further studies are needed to confirm our results.

In this study, the learning curve for SPLA showed no significant changes in the length of hospital stay between the 4 groups, which is similar to the results of previous studies [8, 22, 23] Additionally, there was no significant difference in the occurrence of postoperative complications between the 4 groups, which is similar to the results of previous studies [8, 23]. In TPLA, the complication rates have been shown to decreases to <10 % with the mastery of the TPLA technique [18, 24]. In this study, the complication rate of SPLA turned out to be 15 %, mainly including wound complications such as seroma ($n = 9$), which may have attributed to longer umbilical incisions and a larger proportion of cases of complicated appendicitis. The complication rates of SPLA was acceptable with the exclusion of seroma (9/120, 7.5 %).

There have been only a few studies on clinical predictors associated with the operative time for SPLA. Liao et al. [8] have documented that operative time for SPLA is related to the severity of appendicitis, BMI > 21 kg/m^2, and use of endoloops. Lee et al. [24] have shown that the operative time for SPLA is not associated with leukocyte count or duration of symptoms; however, it is associated with BMI and pathology of the appendix. In this study, the operative time for SPLA was associated with the severity of appendicitis, but not with BMI or the location of the appendix. However, BMI seems more likely to be a significant factor that can affect the operation time. In our study, it was found that there was a less reduction in the operative time in the obese and extremely obese patients compared to normal weight patients, but it was not so in underweight patients (Fig. 3), suggesting that BMI may not be significantly associated with operative time. Based on these results, it is conceivable that the severity of appendicitis may affect the operative time for SPLA. Another considerable limitation of SPLA is related to costs. The increased costs of SPLA compared to TPLA are still a considerable disadvantage that limits the use of SPLA [5, 25]. Di Saverio et al. [26] analyzed 45 cases of single-incision laparoscopic appendectomy using a self-made surgical-glove port and showed that the postoperative results from their surgical method were comparable to those from conventional single-incision laparoscopic appendectomy. They suggested that their surgical-glove port, single-incision laparoscopic appendectomy could be considered as a cost-effective alternative to conventional SPLA using commercially available devices.

This study has a limitation because all the SPLA cases were performed by a single surgeon in the same surgical team. Further studies are needed to achieve a general learning curve for SPLA.

Conclusions

The results of this study suggest that equipment conflict, difficulty in manipulating the laparoscope and the laparoscopic instruments through a small umbilical incision, and limited surgical field may hamper the clinical

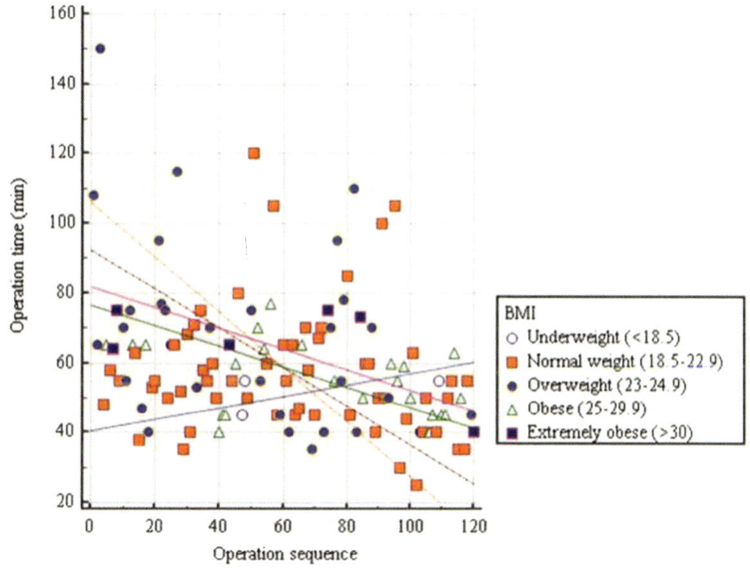

Fig. 3 Correlation of operation time and BMI

application of SPLA, but that the surgical outcome can be the same as that of TPLA. Even surgeons proficient in TPLA will need a substantial learning curve to safely perform the SPLA technique.

Abbreviations

BMI, body mass index; SPLA, single-port laparoscopic appendectomy; SPLS, single-port laparoscopic surgery; TPLA, three-port laparoscopic appendectomy.

Acknowledgments

This paper was supported by Konkuk University in 2016.

Funding

Not applicable

Authors' contributions

YHK and WSL drafted the manuscript, searched the literature, interpreted findings, and prepared for manuscript writing/editing and submission of the manuscript. WSL and YHK critically reviewed the manuscript. All authors have read and approved the final manuscript submission.

Competing interests

The authors declare that they have no competing interests.

Author details

[1]Department of Surgery, School of Medicine, Konkuk University, Konkuk University Chungju Hospital, 82, Gugwon-daero, Chungju-si, Chungbuk, Republic of Korea. [2]Department of Thoracic and Cardiovascular Surgery, School of Medicine, Konkuk University, Konkuk University Chungju Hospital, 82, Gugwon-daero, Chungju-si, Chungbuk, Republic of Korea.

References

1. Faiz O, Clark J, Brown T, Bottle A, Antoniou A, Farrands P, et al. Traditional and laparoscopic appendectomy in adults: outcomes in English NHS hospitals between 1996 and 2006. Ann Surg. 2008;248:800–6. doi:10.1097/SLA.0b013e31818b770c.
2. Wei HB, Huang JL, Zheng ZH, Wei B, Zheng F, Qiu WS, et al. Laparoscopic versus open appendectomy: a prospective randomized comparison. Surg Endosc. 2010;24:266–9. doi:10.1007/s00464-009-0563-7.
3. Tiwari MM, Reynoso JF, Tsang AW, Oleynikov D. Comparison of outcomes of laparoscopic and open appendectomy in management of uncomplicated and complicated appendicitis. Ann Surg. 2011;254:927–32. doi:10.1097/SLA.0b013e31822aa8ea.
4. Cai YL, Xiong XZ, Wu SJ, Cheng Y, Lu J, Zhang J, et al. Single-incision laparoscopic appendectomy vs conventional laparoscopic appendectomy: systematic review and meta-analysis. World J Gastroenterol. 2013;19:5165–73. doi:10.3748/wjg.v19.i31.5165.
5. St Peter SD, Adibe OO, Juang D, Sharp SW, Garey CL, Laituri CA, et al. Single incision versus standard 3-port laparoscopic appendectomy: a prospective randomized trial. Ann Surg. 2011;254:586–90. doi:10.1097/SLA.0b013e31823003b5.
6. Hua J, Gong J, Xu B, Yang T, Song Z. Single-incision versus conventional laparoscopic appendectomy: a meta-analysis of randomized controlled trials. J Gastrointest Surg. 2014;18:426–36. doi:10.1007/s11605-013-2328-9.
7. Markar SR, Karthikesalingam A, Di Franco F, Harris AM. Systematic review and meta-analysis of single-incision versus conventional multiport appendicectomy. Br J Surg. 2013;100:1709–18. doi:10.1002/bjs.9296.
8. Liao YT, Lin TH, Lee PC, Chou TH, Liang JT, Lin MT. Learning curve of single-port laparoscopic appendectomy for noncomplicated acute appendicitis: a preliminary analysis compared with conventional laparoscopic appendectomy. J Laparoendosc Adv Surg Tech A. 2013;23:441–6. doi:10.1089/lap.2012.0265.
9. Vahdad MR, Nissen M, Semaan A, Klein T, Palade E, Boemers T, et al. Experiences with LESS-appendectomy in Children. Arch Iran Med. 2016;19:57–63. doi: 0161901/AIM.0011.
10. Wheeless Jr CR. A rapid, inexpensive, and effective method of surgical sterilization by laparoscopy. J Reprod Med. 1969;3:65–9.
11. Tsai AY, Selzer DJ. Single-port laparoscopic surgery. Adv Surg. 2010;44:1–27. doi:10.1016/i.yasu.2010.05.017.
12. Lee WJ. Single port laparoscopic surgery. J Korean Med Assoc. 2010;53:793–806. doi:10.5124/jkma.2010.53.9.793.
13. Chouillard E, Dache A, Torcivia A, Helmy N, Ruseykin I, Gumbs A. Single-incision laparoscopic appendectomy for acute appendicitis: a preliminary experience. Surg Endosc. 2010;24:1861–5. doi:10.1007/s00464-009-0860-1.
14. Ahmed K, Wang TT, Patel VM, Nagpal K, Clark J, Ali M, et al. The role of single-incision laparoscopic surgery in abdominal and pelvic surgery: a systematic review. Surg Endosc. 2011;25:378–96. doi:10.1007/s00464-010-1208-6.
15. Kim HJ, Lee JI, Lee YS, Lee IK, Park JH, Lee SK, et al. Single-port transumbilical laparoscopic appendectomy: 43 consecutive cases. Surg Endosc. 2010;24:2765–9. doi:10.1007/s00464-010-1043-9.
16. Lin YY, Shabbir A, So JB. Laparoscopic appendectomy by residents: evaluating outcomes and learning curve. Surg Endosc. 2010;24:125–30. doi:10.1007/s00464-009-0691-0.
17. Meinke AK, Kossuth T. What is the learning curve for laparoscopic appendectomy? Surg Endosc. 1994;8:371–5. discussion 376.
18. Jaffer U, Cameron AE. Laparoscopic appendectomy: a junior trainee's learning curve. JSLS. 2008;12:288–91.
19. Kim SY, Hong SG, Roh HR, Park SB, Kim YH, Chae GB. Learning curve for a laparoscopic appendectomy by a surgical trainee. J Korean Soc Coloproctol. 2010;26:324–8. doi:10.3393/jksc.2010.26.5.324.
20. Pan MX, Liang ZW, Cheng Y, Jiang ZS, Xu XP, Wang KH, et al. Learning curve of transumbilical suture-suspension single-incision laparoscopic cholecystectomy. World J Gastroenterol. 2013;19:4786–90. doi:10.3748/wjg.v19.i29.4786.
21. Lee HJ, Kim JY, Kim SK, Lee JR, Suh CS, Kim SH. Learning Curve Analysis and Surgical Outcomes of Single-port Laparoscopic Myomectomy. J Minim Invasive Gynecol. 2015;22:607–11. doi:10.1016/j.jmig.2015.01.009.
22. Burjonrappa SC, Nerkar H. Teaching single-incision laparoscopic appendectomy in pediatric patients. JSLS. 2012;16:619–22. doi:10.4293/108680812X13462882737339.
23. Lee J, Lee SR, Kim HO, Son BH, Choi W. Outcomes of a single-port laparoscopic appendectomy using a glove port with a percutaneous organ-holding device and commercially-available multichannel single-port device. Ann Coloproctol. 2014;30:42–6. doi:10.3393/ac.2014.30.1.42.
24. Lee J, Baek J, Kim W. Laparoscopic transumbilical single-port appendectomy: initial experience and comparison with three-port appendectomy. Surg Laparosc Endosc Percutan Tech. 2010;20:100–3. doi:10.1097/SLE.0b013e3181d84922.
25. Chow A, Purkayastha S, Nehme J, Darzi LA, Paraskeva P. Single incision laparoscopic surgery for appendicectomy: a retrospective comparative analysis. Surg Endosc. 2010;24:2567–74. doi:10.1007/s00464-010-1004-3.
26. Di Saverio S, Mandrioli M, Birindelli A, Biscardi A, Di Donato L, Gomes CA, et al. Single-Incision Laparoscopic Appendectomy with a Low-Cost Technique and Surgical-Glove Port: "How To Do It" with Comparison of the Outcomes and Costs in a Consecutive Single-Operator Series of 45 Cases. J Am Coll Surg. 2016;222:e15–30. doi:10.1016/j.jamcollsurg.2015.11.019.

10

The importance of open emergency surgery in the treatment of acute mesenteric ischemia

Mansur Duran*, E. Pohl, K. Grabitz, H. Schelzig, T. A. Sagban and F. Simon

Abstract

Objective: Acute mesenteric ischemia (AMI) is a complex disease with a high mortality rate. A patient's chance of survival depends on early diagnosis and rapid revascularization to prevent progression of intestinal gangrene. We reviewed our experience with open surgery treatment in 54 cases of AMI.

Methods: A monocentric retrospective study was conducted between 01/01/2001 and 04/30/2014; 54 AMI patients with a mean age of 56.6 years underwent surgery (26 women and 28 men). Retrospectively, the risk factors, management until diagnosis, vascular therapy and follow-up were evaluated.

Results: The symptom upon admission was an acute abdominal pain event. The delay time from admission to surgery was, on average, 13.9 h ($n = 34$). The therapeutic procedures were open surgical operations. The complication rate was (53.7 %) ($n = 29$). The 30-day mortality was 29.6 % ($n = 16$). The late mortality rate was 24.1 % ($n = 13$), and the cumulative survival risk was 44.6 %. Survival was, on average, 60.54 months, however, in the over 70-year-old patient subgroup, the survival rate was 9.5 months ($p = 0.035$). The mortality rate was 27 % ($n = 22$) in the <12 h delay group, 20 % ($n = 5$) in the 12–24 h delay group, and 50 % ($n = 7$) in the > 24 h delay group.

Conclusions: The form of therapy depends on the intraoperative findings and the type of occlusion. Although the mortality rate has decreased in the last decade, in patients over 70 years of age, a significantly worse prognosis was seen.

Keywords: Mesenteric ischemia, Mesenteric infarction, Superior mesenteric artery, Vascular reconstruction, Endovascular treatment

Introduction

Cardiac arrhythmia with embolism is a frequent cause of acute mesenteric ischemia (AMI). An acute closure of the superior mesenteric artery (SMA) frequently leads to irreversible damage of the intestinal mucosa within 6 h [1]. The status of the celiac and SMA - celiac collaterals as well as the hemodynamic status of the patient can be important for AMI. Patients primarily present with an acute pain event, which is followed by an interval of reduced pain intensity due to the decline of intramural pain receptors arising from the hypoperfusion of the intestinal wall. As a result, this disease is often not initially recognized as a vascular emergency, which leads to the possibility of delays in making the appropriate diagnosis and initiating treatment. Further along the course of the disease, intestinal wall gangrene develops due to the destruction of the mucosal barrier, followed by bacterial translocation, which may lead to peritonitis, sepsis and multi-organ failure. Therefore, AMI comes with a high mortality rate (50–70 %) [2]. Prognostic factors include delays in diagnosis and in the revascularization of the intestine, age of the patient and comorbidities [1]. AMI increases up to 10 % in patients older than 70 years with an acute abdomen [1]. Predisposing risk factors include heart failure, coronary heart disease (CHD), hypertension, peripheral arterial disease (PAD) and location of the occlusion.

The mortality rate is directly correlated with the delay interval, and in the case of rapid therapy, it is approximately 0–10 %. The mortality rate increases to 50–60 %, with a delay of 6–12 h, and then to 80–100 % in cases where the delay interval is greater than 24 h [3]. Peripheral vessel occlusion is associated with lower mortality

* Correspondence: mansur.duran@uni-duesseldorf.de
Clinic for Vascular- and Endovascular Surgery, Heinrich-Heine-University, Moorenstr. 5, 40225 Düsseldorf, Germany

than is central vessel occlusion because of the better collateralization [3]. Non-occlusive mesenteric ischemia (NOMI) represents a special form of vessel occlusion that is caused by vasospasms of the mesenteric arterial vessels. This form is more difficult to diagnosis than the occlusive form and may therefore entail further delays.

The aim of this retrospective study is to describe AMI as a vascular emergency in an effort to sensitize primary clinicians in all disciplines. The study illustrates the evaluation of risk factors, management until diagnosis, vascular therapy and outcome.

Methods

In a retrospective study, 54 patients with AMI between 01/01/2001 and 04/30/2014 are presented. Patients who developed AMI as a complication of other operations or interventions were excluded from the study.

Mortality, morbidity, risk factors, management until diagnosis, vascular therapy and outcome were retrospectively evaluated. Institutional Review Board approval was waived because of the retrospective nature of the study. All patients gave their written and informed consent prior to surgery.

The patient characteristics (risk factors, cause of occlusion, operational procedure, complications) are summarized in Tables 1, 2 and 3.

Statistical analysis

Statistical analysis was performed in a logistic regression for risk factors. The relationships between bypass, delay interval and survival were assessed using the Fisher, Kruskal-Wallis- and χ^2-tests, as well as by cross tables. Survival curves and survival distributions were determined using the Kaplan-Meier method and the log-rank test. The level of significance was defined at p <0.05. The SPSS statistical package (IBM Corp. Released 2013. IBM SPSS Statistics for Windows, Version 22.0. Armonk, NY: IBM Corp.) was used for all statistical analyses.

Table 1 Risk factor- dependent analysis of survival was performed in a logistic regression

Variable	$n = 54$ (%)	*P* value
Age (mean ± SD)	56.61 ± 16.21	0.035
Gender	54 (100)	0.451
Arterial hypertension	31(57.4)	0.172
Coronary heart disease	15 (27.8)	0.959
Diabetes mellitus	11 (20.4)	0.567
Hyperlipidemia	10 (18.5)	0.564
Peripheral vascular disease	8 (14.8)	0.036
Smoking history	11 (20.4)	0.222
Arrhythmias	8 (14.8)	0.480
Second look	23 (42.6)	0.121

The level of significance was defined at p <0.05
SD Standard deviance

Table 2 Operational procedure and cause of occlusion of patients ($n = 54$) undergoing open surgical therapy

Parameter	*n* (%)
Operational procedure	
TEA	22 (40.7)
Thrombectomy/embolectomy	14 (25.9)
Bypass	13 (24.1)
Resection of the dissection membrane	11 (20.3)
SMA-transposition	7 (13.0)
Visceral surgery	8 (14.8)
Explorative laparotomy	3 (5.6)
Cause of occlusion	
Arterial embolism	16 (29.6)
Arteriosclerosis combined with local thrombosis	13 (24.0)
Arterial thrombosis	12 (22.2)
Arterial dissection	9 (16.7)
Local dissection	2 (3.7)
Unclear cause of occlusion	2 (3.7)

Results

Patients presented at the clinic with an acute pain event of the abdomen. The average age was 56.6 years (11–85 years, of which 12 patients (22.2 %) were over 70 years old). The youngest patient (11 years old) had cardiac arrhythmia with embolism and occlusion of the abdominal aorta and SMA.

Diagnosis was provided by CT angiography with contrast medium (83.3 %, $n = 45$), conventional angiography (53.7 %, $n = 29$), duplex sonography (27.8 %, $n = 15$) or magnetic resonance imaging (MRI) (1.9 %, $n = 1$). Altogether, a total of 45 out of 54 patients (83.3 %) had leukocytosis (>10 000 /μl), 48 out of 52 patients (92.3 %) had an increase of C-reactive protein (>0.5 mg/dl) and 18 out of 26 patients (69.2 %) had an increase of L-lactate

Table 3 Complications after surgery

Parameter	*n* (%)
Vascular occlusion	8 (14.8)
Ischemia of the gut	8 (14.8)
Acute kidney failure	6 (11.1)
Multi-organ failure	5 (9.2)
Wound healing disorder	5 (9.2)
Arrhythmias	3 (5.6)
Septic shock, respiratory failure, abdominal compartment syndrome, rebleeding; each $n = 2$	8 (14.8)
Peritonitis, ileus, Leriche syndrome, Non occlusive disease, liver failure, delirium, cholecystitis; each $n = 1$	7 (13.0)

(>1.6 mmol/l). The delay from admission to surgery was, on average, 13.9 h ($n = 34$, 63 %). In 20 patients, the delay could not be determined. Logistical regression revealed that PAD ($p = 0.036$) and age ($p = 0.035$) were the factors with the greatest influence on survival (Table 1). The 30-day mortality was 30.8 % ($n = 16$), the late mortality was 25 % ($n = 13$) and the overall mortality was 53.7 % ($n = 29$). For the <12 h delay group, the mortality was 27.2 % ($n = 22$), and the mortality in the group with 12–24 h delay was 20 % ($n = 5$) and was 57.1 % ($n = 7$) in the > 24 h after admission group. The delay interval was known in 34 cases. Statistical analysis of the delay interval using the crosstab test and the χ^2 test did not reveal statistical significance on survival ($p = 0.42$).

The cumulative survival risk was 44.6 %, with an average survival of 60.5 months (men: 70.2 months, women: 42.8 months) (Fig. 1). The log-rank test did not show a significant effect of gender on survival ($p = 0.529$).

The under-70-year-old patient group had a survival-time of 72.6 months, in contrast to the over 70 age group, which only had a survival-time of 9.5 months. Statistical analysis (log rank test) showed a significant difference between the age groups ($p = 0.035$) (Fig. 2).

The causes of death during the early phase (<30 days) included necrosis of the gut ($n = 6$), multi-organ failure ($n = 5$), and other causes ($n = 5$). In the late phase (>30 days), the causes of death included ischemia of the gut ($n = 2$), other causes ($n = 3$), and unclear cause of death ($n = 8$).

The primary patency rates were 80 % for transposition, 62 % for bypass, 53 % for TEA, and the secondary rates were 77 % for grafts and 79 % for TEA. Overall, there was no significant relationship (cross-tab, Fisher test, χ^2 test and Kruskal-Wallis test) between the choice of the bypass ("French bypass" or other bypass) and the choice of the material (vein or alloplastic material) used in terms of survival.

Twenty-five patients survived the AMI, whereas 7 patients could not be located for follow-up and 3 patients refused the investigation.

The long-term results are based on 15 patients in the follow-up (4 months - 9 years). During follow-up, one patient complained about diarrhea and another patient suffered from nausea and vomiting. A total of 13 patients (86.7 %) were asymptomatic and stated a positive quality of life.

Discussion

The mortality in patients with AMI remains high despite the diagnostic, surgical and endovascular developments in recent decades. There was a decline in mortality rate from 80–100 % in the 1970s to 50–70 % in the last decade. The decrease has been attributed to the better management of diagnosis and therapy [4]. The cause of visceral ischemia is an important factor. The mortality rate after surgical therapy for arterial embolism (54.1 %) and venous thrombosis (32.1 %) in a meta-analysis of Schoots et al. [5] was very high. This number rose after surgical treatment for arterial thrombosis (77.4 %) and NOMI (72.7 %). In our study, the 30-day mortality rate was 30.8 %. Decisive factors that contribute to the severity of the disease are a late diagnosis, the resulting delay in vascular therapy and the pre-existing co-morbidities of many patients. An early diagnosis, prior to the

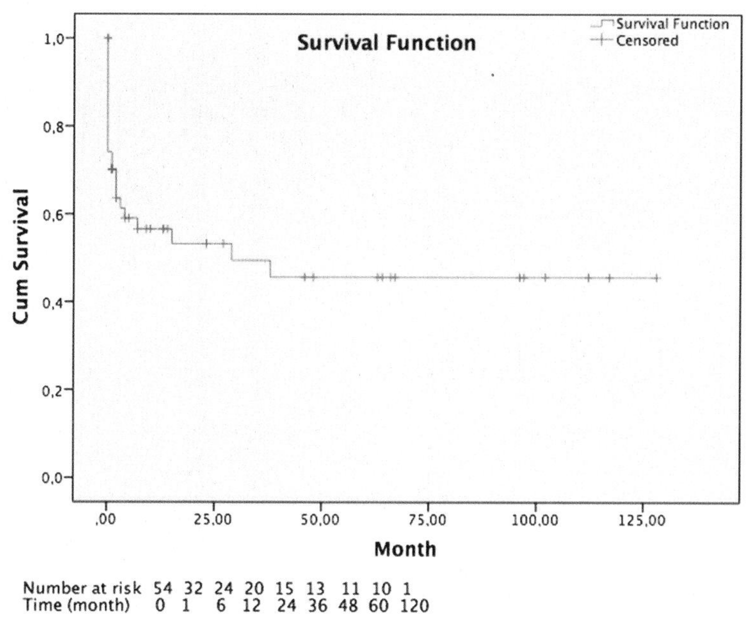

Fig. 1 Survival status of 54 patients with open surgical therapy

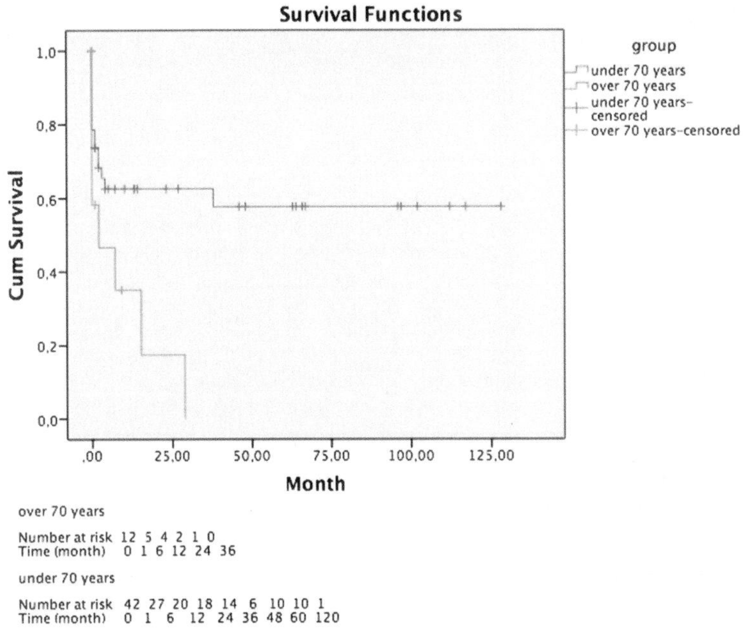

Fig. 2 Survival status oft he groups under and over 70 years of age

development of bowel necrosis with peritonitis, is one of the most important prognostic factors [6]. Statistical analysis of the delay interval did not reveal statistical significance on survival in our study because of the low number of cases ($n = 34$).

CT scanning with contrast agents is the current gold standard in instrument-based diagnostic testing, providing both high sensitivity and specificity. In contrast and despite its high sensitivity and specificity, MRI requires further development because of the longer duration of the investigation and its low availability. It therefore plays only a minor role in the diagnosis of peripheral embolisms of the SMA, NOD and of acute mesenteric ischemia [7, 8].

In cases of suspected AMI, the emergency diagnosis should include biphasic contrast computed tomography (CECT) with multi-planar reconstruction at 3 levels. The venous phase of the CT is necessary for the diagnosis of mesenteric vein thrombosis [9]. In our study, CT with contrast agents was the gold standard in instrument-based diagnostic testing, having replaced conventional angiography as our imaging modality of choice.

Non-specific serum lactate is often used as a diagnostic parameter. An elevated lactate level (>2.2 mmol/l) reflects the late phase of AMI with a transmural bowel infarction, where release of lactate into the bloodstream is caused by anaerobic metabolism with bacterial translocation. Serum lactate, however, cannot detect the early phase where there is only damage to the intestinal mucosa [10, 11]. Another serum parameter that can be used for diagnosis is the D-dimer, which, although sensitive to the early phase, has very low specificity [4].

As future biomarkers for the early phase of AMI, intestinal fatty acid-binding protein (I-FABP), α-glutathione S-transferase (GST) and D-lactate may play an important role. I-FABP and GST are localized in the small intestinal mucosa, whereas D-lactate is a natural degradation product of intestinal bacteria. These markers may appear early in the bloodstream if damage to the mucosa of the small intestine occurs, leading to a loss of enterocytes as the first sign of ischemia. However, the reliability of these serum markers has yet to be demonstrated in randomized controlled prospective studies [12]. In our daily clinical practice we used only L-lactate, leukocytosis and C-reactive protein as parameters for AMI. Biochemical markers, such as I-FABP, GST and D-lactate, must be further studied to determine their roles as valid biomarkers for AMI, and therefore, they cannot be used in daily clinical practice [11, 12]. L-lactate, currently the most commonly used marker, is not specific enough, however, and is only present during the late phase of AMI [13].

In a thrombectomy or embolectomy, the thrombus is recovered through a transaortic or transmesenteric arteriotomy. The arterial occlusion is closed by either direct suture or vein patch depending on the vessel diameter. As atherosclerotic plaques cause occlusion of the visceral arteries, these plaques can be removed either indirectly transaortally or directly via an open endarterectomy (TEA). Surgical access can be performed by a laparotomy or through a thoracoabdominal approach

[14]. An SMA transposition can be used for short segment stenosis and occlusions of the SMA. Here, the artery is discontinued and reinserted further distally into the infrarenal aorta [15].

On the other hand, in cases of stenoses extending to a large portion of the vessel wall, the bypass procedure is the method of choice. The great saphenous vein or an alloplastic material (PTFE, Dacron) are available as bypass materials that may be applied antegrade or retrograde. In the retrograde procedure, where the origin of the bypass is located distal to the SMA, the vessel substitutes should be guided behind the left renal vessels. The renal vessels serve as a fulcrum to prevent kinking of the bypass. Due to its complex correct anatomic description, this bypass is called the "French bypass". The "French bypass" combines the advantages of ante- and retrograde visceral bypasses. The procedure allows distal segments of the SMA to be reconstructed [16–18]. If the lumen of the SMA is occluded due to a dissection membrane that separates the true from the false lumen, the membrane can be resected transaortally following direct suturing of the aorta. In our center, we used all of these surgical procedures (Table 1) and saw the best results for transposition, with a primary patency rate of 80 %. Overall, there was no significant relationship between the choice of the bypass and the choice of the material used in terms of survival. The results from the first case series of 64 patients (1979–2000) were published in 2002 [19]. Compared to our 2002 study [19], no difference in terms of age, gender, risk profile or cause of occlusion could be found in the present work. However, the new study showed a reduction in the overall mortality rate, from 67 to 30 %, due to the improved management of the diagnostic and treatment options.

The modern treatment of AMI should primarily be performed by revascularization of the intestine.

A visceral surgical operation with bowel resection of necrotic parts can be performed afterwards. In modern vascular surgery, both endovascular and open surgical treatment options should be considered.

Preoperatively, both clinical and CT morphological aspects must be considered, whether the patient presents with peritonitis or an embolic or thrombotic occlusion of the SMA. The endovascular treatment option is recommended only in patients without peritonitis [1].

In the case of an AMI in combination with peritonitis, exploratory laparotomy with vascular therapy is the method of choice.

Five non-randomized studies have reported a comparison between open and endovascular surgery. In a retrospective study conducted within a single center, no difference in mortality between the two methods could be shown [4]. However, another study reported lower morbidity and mortality using the endovascular method [20]. Three other multicenter studies were national supra-regional studies: lower rates of bowel resection and lower mortality and morbidity were seen in these studies for the endovascular method [21, 22]. Therefore, if endovascular therapy appears to be possible, this method should be carried out whenever possible after the physician has excluded peritonitis.

Open surgery can also be used in patients with peritonitis in the late phase of AMI.

The poorer outcomes compared to endovascular procedures are due to the poorer conditions of a late phase AMI.

Our study is, however, limited by its retrospective nature and as a single center study in general validity.

Conclusions

AMI is an important differential diagnosis in acute abdomen. The diagnosis should be made by CT angiography without a delay interval. The type of therapy depends on the intraoperative findings and the type of occlusion. In patients over 70 years of age, a significantly worse prognosis was seen.

Competing interests

The authors declare that they have no competing interests.

Authors' contributions

MD, EP, KG, HS, TAS, FS: MD contributed substantially to the conception and design of the manuscript. He drafted the article, analyzed the data and revised them critically. TAS helped to concept the manuscript and contributed in data acquisition and interpretation. EP helped to write the article and contributed to its design. She participated in essential data interpretation. FS helped to improve the quality of the discussion as he revised this part critically. HS and KG helped to draft the manuscript. They participated in conceiving and designing the manuscript. All authors approved the final version of the manuscript.

Acknowledgements

No grant support.

A part of this study was presented in the plenary International Forum at the 2013 Vascular Annual Meeting of the German, Austrian and Swiss Society for Vascular Surgery "29. Jahrestagung der Deutschen Gesellschaft für Gefäßchirurgie und Gefäßmedizin - DGG 2013; Dreiländertagung ÖGG, DDG, SGG" Linz, September 04–07, 2013.

References

1. Klar E, Rahmanian PB, Bücker A, Hauenstein K, Jauch KW, Luther B. Acute mesenteric ischemia: a vascular emergency. Dtsch Arztebl Int. 2012;109(14):249–56.
2. Acosta S. Epidemiology of mesenteric vascular disease: clinical implications. Semin Vasc Surg. 2010;23:4–8.
3. Paes E, Vollmar JF, Hutschenreiter S, Schoenberg MH, Schölzel E. Diagnostik und Therapie des akuten Mesenterialinfarktes. Chir Gastroenterol. 1990;6:473–80.
4. Ryer EJ, Kalra M, Oderich GS, Duncan AA, Gloviczki P, Cha S, et al. Revascularization for acute mesenteric ischemia. J Vasc Surg. 2012;55:1682–9.
5. Schoots IG, Koffeman GI, Legemate DA, Levi M, van Gulik TM. Systematic review of survival after acute mesenteric ischaemia according to disease aetiology. Br J Surg. 2004;91:17–27.
6. Aliosmanoglu I, Gul M, Kapan M, Arikanoglu Z, Taskesen F, Basol O, et al. Risk Factors Effecting mortality in acute mesenteric ischemia and mortality rates: a single center experience. Int Surg. 2013;98:76–81.

7. Menke J. Diagnostic accuracy of multidetector CT in acute mesenteric ischemia: systemic review and meta-analysis. Radiology. 2010;256:93–101.
8. Oliva IB, Davarpanah AH, Rybicki FJ, Desjardins B, Flamm SD, Francois CJ, et al. ACR appropriateness criteria imaging of mesenteric ischemia. Abdom Imaging. 2013;38:714–9.
9. Kellow ZS, MacInnes M, Kurzencwyg D, Rawal S, Jaffer R, Kovacina B, et al. The role of abdominal radiography in the evaluation of the nontrauma emergency patient. Radiology. 2008;248:887–93.
10. Björnsson S, Resch T, Acosta S. Symptomatic mesenteric atherosclerotic disease – lessons learned from the diagnostic workup. J Gastrointest Surg. 2013;17:973–80.
11. van den Heijkant TC, Aerts BAC, Teijink JA. Challenges in diagnosing mesenteric ischemia. World J Gastroenterol. 2013;19(9):1338–41.
12. Acosta S, Nilsson T. Current status on plasma biomarkers for acute mesenteric ischemia. J Thromb Thrombolysis. 2012;33:355–61.
13. Demir IH, Ceyhan GO, Friess H. Beyond lactate: is there a role for serum lactate measurement in diagnosing acute mesenteric ischemia? Dig Surg. 2012;29:226–35.
14. Kazmers A. Operative management of chronic mesenteric ischemia. Ann Vasc Surg. 1998;12:299–308.
15. Kieny R, Batellier J, Kretz JG. Aortic reimplantation of the superior mesenteric artery for atherosclerotic lesions of the visceral arteries: sixty cases. Ann Vasc Surg. 1990;4:122–5.
16. Leschi JP, Coggia M, Goeau-Brissonniere O. Retrograde aortomesenteric bypass with tunneling behind the left renal pedicle. Ann Vasc Surg. 2001;15:503–6.
17. Pourhassan S, Grotemeyer D, Fürst G, Sandmann W. Das chronisch viszerale Ischämiesyndrom, Klinik, Diagnostik und Therapieoptionen. Gefässchirurgie. 2006;11:173–87.
18. Grotemeyer D, Iskandar F, Voshege M, Blondin D, Pourhassan S, Grabitz K, et al. Der retrograde aorto-mesenteriale Bypass mit links retrorenalem Verlauf ("französischer Bypass") bei der Behandlung der akuten und chronischen viszeralen Ischämie. Klinische Erfahrung und Langzeitverlauf bei 27 Patienten. (Retrograde Aortomesenteric Loop Bypass behind the Left Renal Pedicle ("French Bypass") in the Treatment of Acute and Chronic Mesenteric Ischemia. Clinical Experiences and Long-Term Follow-Up in 27 Patients). Zentralbl Chir. 2009;134:338–44.
19. Luther B, Moussazadeh K, Müller BT, Franke C, Harms JM, Ernst S, et al. Die akute mesenteriale Ischämie-unverstanden oder unheilbar? The Acute Mesenteric Ischemia - Not Understood or Incurable? Zentralbl Chir. 2002;127:674–84.
20. Arthurs ZM, Titus J, Bannazadeh M, Eagleton MJ, Srivastava S, Sarac TP, et al. A comparison of endovascular revascularization with traditional therapy for the treatment of acute mesenteric ischemia. J Vasc Surg. 2011;167:308–11.
21. Schmerhorn ML, Giles KA, Hamdan AD, Wyers MC, Pomposelli FB. Mesenteric revascularization: management and outcomes in the United States, 1988–2006. J Vasc Surg. 2009;50:341–8.
22. Block TA, Acosta S, Björck M. Endovascular and open surgery for acute occlusion of the superior mesenteric artery. J Vasc Surg. 2010;52:959–66.

Poor prognostic factors in patients who underwent surgery for acute non-occlusive ischemic colitis

Minsu Noh[1], Song Soo Yang[1*], Seok Won Jung[2], Jae Ho Park[2], Yeong Cheol Im[1] and Kyu Yeol Kim[1]

Abstract

Introduction: Ischemic colitis (IC) is a disease with high postoperative morbidity and mortality. Knowledge of the risk factors for postoperative mortality could be helpful in clinical decision making and in optimizing postoperative treatment.

Methods: From a prospective database, we conducted a retrospective medical record review of 50 patients who underwent surgery for IC between 2003 and 2011 at our institution. We analyzed the causes and potential risk factors for early mortality after surgery for IC.

Results: The early postoperative mortality and morbidity rates were 30.0% (15/50) and 54% (27/50), respectively. The two most common causes of death were multi-organ failure (66.7%, 10/15) and fulminant septic shock (20.0%, 3/15). Univariate analysis showed that postoperative mortality was significantly associated with preoperative nephropathy, coronary artery disease, a previous history of cardiovascular surgery, an ASA score ≥ 4, surgical delay ≥ 3 days, preoperative hemodynamic instability, and use of pre- and intraoperative adrenergic vasopressors. In the multivariate analysis, a previous history of cardiovascular surgery (odds ratio [OR], 8.2; 95% confidence interval [CI], 1.2–56.5) and surgical delay ≥ 3 days (OR, 5.7; 95% CI, 1.2–27.9) were identified as independent risk factors for postoperative mortality.

Conclusions: Because surgical delay is an avoidable determinant of early mortality, a high index of suspicion and early surgical intervention can increase survival. A routine postoperative evaluation for IC may be helpful in patients with a previous history of cardiovascular surgery.

Keywords: Ischemic colitis, Surgery, Postoperative mortality, Risk factors

Introduction

Despite improvements in perioperative care, the postoperative mortality rate after surgery for ischemic colitis (IC) remains high, and has been reported to be more than 30% [1-4]. This excess mortality rate is highest during the immediate postoperative period, however, patients who survive the initial acute IC event can achieve long-term survival. The median long-term survival after the initial acute IC event is more than 40 months [2,4]. Previous studies, which aimed to develop a predictive risk score for postoperative mortality of IC, suggest that the excess mortality is due to the difficulty in reaching a timely diagnosis and the effects of pre-existing medical conditions [1,5]. Recently, Reissfelder et al. reported on the predictive risk score by looking at various perioperative variables (acute renal failure, nonocclusive ischemic colitis, subtotal/total colectomy, serum lactate > 2.5 mmol, and pre- and intraoperative administration of catecholamines) that were predictive of postoperative mortality in patients undergoing surgery for ischemic colitis [2]. Additionally Anthony et al. demonstrated the effectiveness of this scoring system in predicting the postoperative mortality of IC [4].

However, the risk factors included in the scoring system and the other well-known risk factors such as age, gender, and pre-existing comorbidities that contribute to the postoperative mortality of IC are unavoidable. Because there is

* Correspondence: paul913@hanmail.net
[1]Department of Surgery, Ulsan University Hospital, 290-3 Jeonha-dong, Dong-gu, Ulsan 682-714, Korea
Full list of author information is available at the end of the article

lack of information on the avoidable risk factors, identifying them will allow researches and physicians to develop focused strategies aimed at reducing the risk and improving outcomes.

The aim of this study was to assess the incidence of morbidity and mortality in patients undergoing surgical treatment for IC at our institution. We also aimed to assess the causes and predictive factors of early mortality, and to determine whether a delay in surgery was associated with higher postoperative mortality of patient who undergo an operation for IC.

Materials and methods

We retrospectively reviewed our prospectively collected database of patients with IC, and identified 50 consecutive patients who underwent abdominal surgery for histologically established IC between January 2003 and May 2011 at the Ulsan University Hospital. The Ulsan University Hospital Institutional Review Board approved this study. Patients who underwent surgery for occlusive colitis secondary to volvulus, herniation, trauma, or cancer were excluded. Patients who underwent reoperations for early postoperative complications and concomitant small bowel ischemia were also excluded.

The following patient characteristics were recorded: age, gender, smoking history, alcohol consumption, body mass index (BMI), the presence of significant comorbidities (i.e., diabetes mellitus, hypertension, coronary heart disease, respiratory disease, nephropathy, and liver cirrhosis), American Society of Anesthesiologists (ASA) classification, history of previous abdominal surgery and cardiovascular surgery, initial presenting symptoms, delay in surgical intervention, preoperative laboratory data (white blood count, c-reactive protein, serum urea, serum creatinine, and serum lactate), preoperative SIRS/sepsis, preoperative hypotension, preoperative use of adrenergic vasopressors, localization of colonic ischemia (i.e., right, transverse, left, entire colon), indications for surgical intervention (i.e., stenosis, gangrene, or failure to respond to medical treatment), emergency surgery, type of operation (i.e., segmental colonic resection, subtotal/total colectomy, or colostomy), presence of peritonitis at the time of surgery, intra-operative blood loss (measured by collecting blood in the suction minus the rinsing fluid), intraoperative blood transfusion, covering stoma, operative time, and intraoperative use of adrenergic vasopressors.

Surgical delay was defined as surgical intervention performed ≥ 3 days after the first clinical symptoms appeared (abdominal pain, hematochezia, diarrhea, peritoneal signs, radiographic findings of ileus or free air, unexplained leukocytosis, or lactic acidosis). Intra-operative blood loss was assessed using the anesthetic protocol. Intraoperative blood transfusion was defined as an allogeneic blood transfusion during the surgical procedure. Transfusion was performed at the discretion of the operating surgeon and anesthesiologist. Hemodynamically significant intraoperative blood loss or a hemoglobin level of 8 to 10 g/dL was used as a threshold for transfusion, depending on the patient's comorbidities. In the present study, we defined hemodynamic instability as low blood pressure (<90 mmHg) requiring infusion without the use of vasopressors [6,7]. Sepsis was assessed in every patient who presented and was diagnosed if two or more of the following conditions were present: (1) temperature > 38°C or < 36°C; (2) heart rate > 90 beats per minute; (3) respiratory rate > 20 breaths per minute or $PaCO2 < 32$ mmHg; and (4) white blood cell count > 12,000/cu mm, or < 4,000/cu mm, or > 10% immature bands [8]. The use of vasopressors corresponded to the use of catecholamines (dopamine, dobutamine, dopexamine, noradrenaline, or adrenaline), and was administrated when patients had low blood pressure/heart rate due to decreased blood volume.

Surgical outcomes were determined on the basis of the postoperative follow-up. Postoperative mortality was defined as in-hospital death. Complications occurring within 30 days were classified as septic or non-septic. Septic complications included wound infections, persistent bowel ischemia, anastomotic leak, leakage of rectal stump, pneumonia, and septic shock. Anastomotic leak and leakage of rectal stump were confirmed by re-laparotomy or percutaneous drainage. Non-septic complications included intestinal obstruction, pulmonary edema and effusion, acute myocardial infarction, and acute renal failure.

The main analyses were based on comparing patients who experienced in-hospital postoperative mortality after surgery with those who did not. The chi-square test and Student's *t*-test were used for univariate analyses of categorical and continuous variables. Multivariate logistic regression models were used to identify independent predictors of postoperative mortality. A receiver operating characteristic (ROC) analysis was performed for assessing discriminative accuracy in predicting in-hospital mortality. Factors with a p value < 0.05 in the univariate analysis were included in the multivariate analysis. Statistical significance was defined as a p value < 0.05. Statistical analysis was performed using SPSS 18.0 software (SPSS, Chicago, IL, USA).

Results

Patients and characteristics

A total of 50 patients underwent surgery at our institution during the study period. The study population included 26 males (52%) and 24 females (48%). The mean age of all patients was 68 ± 14 years, and the mean postoperative hospital stay was 30 ± 3 days. Indications for the operation were bowel infarction (42.0%), free perforation (39.0%), failure of medical treatment (20.0%) and hemorrhage (2.0%).

Demographic characteristics and comorbid conditions of patients at the time of the surgery are summarized in Table 1. Thirty-nine patients (78%) had comorbidities including comorbid cancer, liver cirrhosis, coronary artery disease, history of previous abdominal and vascular surgery, diabetes mellitus, nephropathy, respiratory disease, and hypertension. Hypertension was the most common pre-existing condition (46%), followed by diabetes mellitus, nephropathy, and coronary artery disease. History of previous surgery was present in 24 (48%) patients; 12 patients underwent abdominal surgery including gastrointestinal surgery and abdominal aortic aneurysm surgery, and 9 patients (18%) underwent major cardiovascular surgery including coronary artery bypass surgery, aortoiliac surgery, and peripheral vascular surgery.

The main symptoms prompting patients to seek medical advice were abdominal pain (92%), followed by hematochezia (30%) and diarrhea (22%). During physical examination, the peritoneal sign was positive in 33 patients (66%), and 21 (42%) were hospitalized when the symptoms appeared. We also analyzed the surgical delay which was defined as mentioned above. The mean duration of surgical delay was 5 ± 9 days.

Seven (14%) patients were preoperatively classified with an ASA score of II, 8 (16%) had an ASA score III, 23 (46%) had an ASA score IV, and 12 (24%) had an ASA score V. Twenty-five (50%) patients showed signs of systemic inflammatory response syndrome (SIRS). Of the 27 (54%) patients with hemodynamic instability, 18 (66.7%) suffered from severe septic shock and required vasopressors.

Table 1 Demographic characteristics and comorbid conditions in the study population

	No. of patients (n = 50)	Proportion (%)
Age (years) ± SD	68.68 ± 14.14	-
Gender (male)	26	52.0
Smoking	20	40.0
Alcohol habit	16	32.0
Mean BMI (kg/m^2) ± SD	22.62 ± 3.48	-
Comorbidities	39	78.0
History of cancer	9	18.0
Diabetes mellitus	14	28.0
Hypertension	23	46.0
Liver cirrhosis	5	10.0
Coronary artery disease	13	26.0
Atrial fibrillation	11	22.0
Nephropathy	14	28.0
Respiratory disease[a]	2	4.0
Previous history of surgery	24	48.0
Cardiovascular surgery	9	18.0
Abdominal surgery	12	24.0
Others	8	16.0

[a]Respiratory disease included chronic obstructive pulmonary disease, bronchial asthma.
SD, standard deviation; BMI, body mass index.

Forty-four patients (88%) underwent emergency surgery, which was defined as surgery within the first 24 h after hospital admission or in the first 24 h after presentation to our emergency department. Eighteen patients (36%) were found to have a perforated colon, and the median operative time was 192 min (range, 110-465 min) with a median blood loss of 650 ml (range, 100-8000 ml). Twenty-six patients (52%) were given blood transfusions due to the indications as defined above. Ischemia involving the left colon was observed in 33 patients (66%), ischemia of the transverse colon was seen in 3 (6%), and ischemia of the right colon was seen 11 patients (22%). Three patients (6%) had ischemia involving the entire colon. A right hemicolectomy was performed in 8 patients (16%), a transverse colon segmentectomy was performed in 3 patients (6%), a left hemicolectomy was performed in 8 patients (16%), a sigmoid resection was performed in 18 patients (36%), and a subtotal/total colectomy was performed in 11 patients (22%). In 2 patients, a transverse colostomy was performed. A total of 34 patients (68%) received a stoma. Continuity of the bowel was not restored in any of the patients, so a Hartmann's pouch was created. A total of 16 patients (32.0%) was performed an anastomosis, of which 13 patients (81.2%) were hemodynamically stable during surgery. We considered a second look surgery in patient who was suffered from septic shock and required vasopressors. In our study, six patients were planned a second look surgery. In these patients, four received planned surgery and two did not due to hemodynamic instability.

We also analyzed the pre- and intra-operative use of adrenergic vasopressors. A total of 19 patients (38%) received adrenergic vasopressor infusion due to septic shock intra-operatively. Nine (18%) of them had previously received adrenergic vasopressors at our institution the day before surgery.

Within 30 days of the procedure, 27 patients (54%) experienced postoperative complications (Table 2). Of the 27 patients who experienced postoperative complications, 22 patients (44%) experienced septic complications and 5 (10%) experienced non-septic complications. The three most common major life-threatening complications were septic shock (20%), persistent bowel ischemia (8%), and wound infection (8%).

Eleven patients (22.0%) who had septic complications required reoperation, and 6 (54.5%) of them died. Reoperation itself did not influence the in-hospital mortality rate ($p = 0.143$). Two out of ten patients with septic shock received surgical intervention due to clinical deterioration that required re-exploration. Four patients developed persistent bowel ischemia, and all of them required additional

Table 2 Outcomes of surgery for ischemic colitis

	No. of patients (%)		
Type of complications	**Number N = 27 (54.0)**	**Re-operation N = 11 (22.0)**	**Mortality N = 15 (30.0)**
Septic complications	22 (44.0)	11 (22.0)	14 (28.0)
Wound infection	4 (8.0)	2 (4.0)	0
Persistent ischemia	4 (8.0)	4 (8.0)	3 (6.0)
Anastomotic leakage	2 (4.0)	2 (4.0)	0
Leakage of rectal stump	1 (2.0)	1 (2.0)	1 (2.0)
Pneumonia	1 (2.0)	0 (0)	0 (0)
Septic shock	10 (20.0)	2 (4.0)	10 (20.0)
Non-septic complications	5 (10.0)	0 (0)	1 (2.0)
Intestinal obstruction	2 (4.0)	0	0
Acute myocardial infarction	2 (4.0)	0	1 (2.0)
Acute renal failure	1 (2.0)	0 (0)	0 (0)

ischemic bowel resection. Two patients with anastomotic leakage and 1 patient with rectal stump leakage needed reoperation due to generalized peritonitis. Two patients required reoperation due to wound infection.

Postoperative mortality rate was high, with 15 patients (30.0%) dying during the postoperative period. The median survival until death in these patients was 16 days (range: 2-62 days).

The most common causes of early postoperative mortality were MOF in ten patients (66.7% and fulminant septic shock in three patients (20%). Fourteen of the 15 patients who died (93.3%) experienced septic complications. Of the ten patients (20.0%) who experienced septic shock, eight of them eventually died due to multiple organ failure and two died of fulminant septic shock, even though 2 underwent reoperation. Three patients (6%) with persistent bowel ischemia died due to MOF (n = 2) and fulminant septic shock (n = 1), and 1 patient with rectal stump leakage died due to pneumonia. Another reason for postoperative mortality was cardiac arrest due to acute myocardial infarction.

Thirty-five (70%) patients were discharged alive from the hospital, and the median time from surgery to discharge was 24 days (range: 9-127 days). Among these patients, those with postoperative complications had a significantly longer mean hospital stay (42 days vs. 28 days, $p < 0.045$).

Univariate analysis showed that postoperative mortality was significantly associated with preoperative nephropathy ($p = 0.029$), coronary artery disease ($p = 0.023$), a previous history of cardiovascular surgery ($p = 0.006$), an ASA score ≥ 4 ($p = 0.039$), surgical delay ≥ 3 days ($p = 0.021$), preoperative hemodynamic instability ($p = 0.021$), and severe hemodynamic instability requiring adrenergic vasopressors ($p = 0.043$). No other preoperative factors were associated with an increased risk of postoperative mortality, including patient age, gender, smoking history, hypertension, atrial fibrillation, respiratory disease, previous abdominal surgery, and localization of ischemia. The two groups did not differ in terms of clinical presentation, including abdominal pain, hematochezia, diarrhea, peritoneal sign, and preoperative SIRS. Moreover, intraoperative factors such as emergency surgery, type of surgery, bowel perforation, stoma formation, operative time, intraoperative blood loss, and blood transfusion were not associated with postoperative mortality (Table 3). In the multivariate analysis, a previous history of cardiovascular surgery (odds ratio [OR], 8.2; 95% confidence interval [CI], 1.2–56.5) and a surgical delay ≥ 3 days (OR, 5.7; 95% CI, 1.2–27.9) were identified as independent risk factors for postoperative mortality (Table 4). The rate of early postoperative mortality was 80.0% in patients who had both significant risk factors compared with the rate of early postoperative mortality of 8.7% in patients who had none of these risk factors ($p = 0.003$). These independent risk factors led to discriminative accuracy in predicting in-hospital mortality based on the area under the receiver operating characteristic curve of 0.825 (Figure 1).

Discussion

In our retrospective study of 50 consecutive patients who underwent surgery for IC, 15 patients (30.0%) died within 30 days of surgery. Multi-organ failure and fulminant septic shock were the most common causes of early death, followed by cardiac arrest.

High rates of postoperative morbidity and mortality have been reported in patients with ischemic colitis who require surgery [1,2,9-12]. The mortality rates have been reported to range from 28% to 54%, and high morbidity rates ranging from 21% to 85% have been reported in patients with ischemic colitis requiring surgery [1-3,9,12,13].

In our study, a relatively lower postoperative mortality rate of 30% was demonstrated, which is in line with the published data. The overall postoperative complication rate of

Table 3 Comparison of patient-related factors associated with postoperative mortality

	No. of patients (%)		
	Died (n = 15)	**Survived (n = 35)**	***P*-value[a]**
Mean age (years) ± SD	67.33 ± 12.87	69.26 ± 14.79	0.664
Gender			0.545
Male	9 (60.0)	17 (48.6)	
Female	6 (40.0)	18 (51.4)	
Smoking	7 (46.7)	13 (37.1)	0.547
Alcohol habit	3 (20.0)	13 (37.1)	0.328
Mean BMI (Kg/m^2) ± SD	23.18 ± 2.86	22.39 ± 3.74	0.468
Liver cirrhosis	2 (13.3)	3 (8.6)	0.629
Nephropathy	8 (53.3)	6 (17.1)	**0.016**
Diabetes	4 (26.7)	10 (28.6)	1.000
Hypertension	7 (46.7)	16 (45.7)	1.000
Respiratory disease[b]	0 (0)	2 (5.7)	1.000
Coronary artery disease	7 (46.7)	6 (17.1)	**0.040**
Atrial fibrillation	4 (26.7)	7 (20.0)	0.713
Previous abdominal surgery[c]	6 (40.0)	6 (17.1)	0.146
Previous cardiovascular surgery[d]	6 (40.0)	3 (8.6)	**0.015**
ASA score (≥4)[e]	14 (93.3)	20 (57.1)	**0.019**
Localization of ischemia			0.445
Right colon	2 (13.3)	9 (25.7)	
Transverse colon	0 (0)	3 (8.6)	
Left colon	10 (66.7)	23 (60.0)	
Entire colon	1 (6.7)	2 (5.7)	
Preoperative initial symptoms			
Abdominal pain	14 (93.3)	32 (91.4)	1.000
Hematochezia	4 (26.7)	11 (31.4)	1.000
Diarrhea	3 (20.0)	8 (22.9)	1.000
Surgical delay (≥3 days)	11 (73.3)	12 (34.3)	**0.015**
Peritoneal irritation	11 (73.3)	22 (62.9)	0.533
Preoperative SIRS	10 (66.7)	15 (42.9)	0.217
Hemodynamic instability	12 (80.0)	15 (42.9)	**0.029**
Preoperative use of vasopressors	9 (60.0)	9 (25.7)	**0.028**
Preoperative laboratory data			
WBC (k/uL)	1315 ± 6.59	1421 ± 9.16	0.687
CRP (mg/dL)	13.56 ± 7.92	10.47 ± 11.62	0.353
Urea (mg/dL)	41.98 ± 25.01	26.08 ± 20.77	**0.024**
Creatinine (mg/dL)	4.64 ± 9.74	1.54 ± 1.30	0.068
Lactate (mmol/L)	2.84 ± 2.69	3.08 ± 2.88	0.791
Type of surgery			0.492
Rt. Hemicolectomy	1 (6.7)	7 (20.0)	
T-colon segmental resection	0 (0)	3 (8.6)	
Lt. hemicolectomy	3 (20.0)	5 (14.3)	
Sigmoid resection	7 (46.7)	11 (31.4)	
Subtotal/Total colectomy	4 (26.7)	7 (20.0)	

Table 3 Comparison of patient-related factors associated with postoperative mortality *(Continued)*

Colostomy	0 (0)	2 (5.7)	
Emergency surgery	14 (93.3)	29 (82.9)	0.659
Bowel perforation	6 (40.0)	12 (34.3)	0.754
Stoma formation	12 (80.0)	22 (62.9)	0.328
Operative time (min)	236.1 ± 86.0	213.0 ± 81.4	0.370
Estimated blood loss (>1000 mL)	7 (46.7)	10 (28.6)	0.329
Intraoperative blood transfusion	9 (60.0)	17 (48.6)	0.545
Intraoperative use of vasopressors	9 (60.0)	10 (28.6)	0.056

[a]Cross-table analysis using Fisher's exact test.
[b]Respiratory disease included chronic obstructive pulmonary disease, bronchial asthma.
[c]Previous abdominal surgery included gastrointestinal surgery, abdominal aortic aneurysm surgery.
[d]Previous cardiovascular surgery included coronary artery bypass surgery, aortoiliac surgery, peripheral vascular surgery.
[e]ASA score according to the American Society of Anesthesiologists
BMI, body mass index; SIRS, systemic inflammatory response syndrome; SD, standard deviation
Bold print, P < 0.05.

54% in our study was also favorable when compared to the ranges reported in recent studies.

This study shows that sepsis and organ failure are common complications after surgery for IC. In almost all of the patients who died, the development of MOF and septic shock were significantly associated with postoperative mortality. These findings are in agreement with those in recent studies involving more than 100 patients who underwent surgery for IC, MOF and sepsis were found to be the principle causes of death [2,3]. Sepsis is a common postoperative complication in IC patients, and has been shown to be associated with postoperative mortality [4,14]. Our findings concur with those of previous studies, and we found that the development of postoperative sepsis is associated with up to a fifty-fold increase in mortality following surgery for IC.

In our study, septic complications, including wound infection, persistent bowel ischemia, anastomotic leakage, and septic shock were the most common postoperative complications. Septic shock was the most serious complication closely related to postoperative mortality, and occurred concurrently with or before MOF in most cases.

These findings highlight the observation that the development of MOF is strongly associated with sepsis. It has been postulated that progression to MOF exists in continuum with SIRS. Given that most of the patients with complications meet the criteria for SIRS, it is not surprising that MOF is common in IC patients.

Although the development of MOF does not predict mortality, a recent study found a greater than 50% prevalence of MOF among non-survivors of IC [2]. Two-thirds of postoperative mortality occurrences in our study were due to MOF.

The progression from the SIRS to MOF is not well explained, although some of the mechanisms responsible for it have been recognized. A surgery performed too late will favor MOF occurrence because of the inflammatory factors released by the necrotic intestine [15]. To prevent MOF, early surgical intervention and an aggressive approach may decrease the inflammation associated with IC.

Despite constant advances, IC patients' postoperative mortality and morbidity rates remains high [16,17]. To achieve better outcomes, many studies have demonstrated which predictive factors are associated with postoperative mortality. We aimed to determine the predictors of early postoperative mortality of IC and found that two variables were independent predictors of 30-day mortality; surgical

Table 4 Multivariate analysis of the risk factors associated with mortality

	Odds ratio	95% confidence interval	*P*-value[a]
Gender, male	1.433	0.363-5.649	0.607
Age, ≥65 years	1.712	0.410-7.139	0.461
Nephropathy	3.002	0.559-16.118	0.200
Previous history of cardiovascular surgery	8.182	1.184-56.538	**0.033**
Surgical delay, ≥3 days	5.692	1.159-27.967	**0.032**
Preoperative hemodynamic instability	1.438	0.148-13.948	1.438
Preoperative use of vasopressors	1.071	0.126-9.067	0.950

[a]Cross-table analysis using binary logistic regression.
Bold print, P < 0.05.

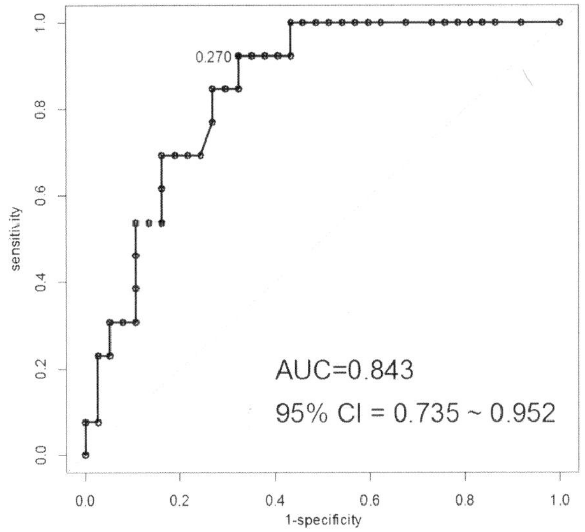

Figure 1 Receiver operating characteristic curve for prediction of early postoperative mortality.

delay of 3 days or more and a previous history of cardiovascular surgery.

Several patient- and surgery-related characteristics have been previously found to be associated with in-hospital mortality in patients undergoing surgery for IC; preoperative lactate level, ASA classification, emergency surgery, acute renal failure, elevated intraoperative blood loss, allogeneic blood and fresh plasma transfusions, occlusion of the mesenteric artery, low output heart failure, catecholamine administration, and a previous history of cardiovascular surgery [1-4].

Recently, researchers have also attempted to validate a scoring system to predict postoperative mortality after surgery for IC [2]. In doing so, they identified that acute renal failure, serum lactate, intraoperative catecholamine, non-occlusive etiology, and total/subtotal colectomy are the components of the score. Although our findings are similar in some respects, that study only looked at a selective group of comorbidities and did not include surgical delay as a variable. We showed that a surgical delay of 3 days or more is a significant predictor of postoperative mortality. Our findings are supported by studies suggesting that early surgery is associated with lower mortality rates in patients requiring surgery for IC [2,17].

However, one of the main problems of ischemic colitis is the difficulty in reaching an adequate, early diagnosis. The clinical need for sensitive and specific non-invasive tests for detecting IC was highlighted in a recent review of the condition because its diagnosis still represents a challenge for physicians [18,19]. Absence of typical clinical findings because of old age, underlying disease, altered mental state, or medications has long been recognized as a reasons for the delay in surgical evaluation and intervention [20]. In such patients, the important issue is how to identify the more critically ill patients and make the most appropriate diagnostic and therapeutic decisions. In our study, more than two-thirds of deaths due to surgical delay occurred in patients who were bedridden, had an altered mental status, had no peritoneal signs, antecedent opioid analgesia, needed mechanical ventilation, and were in the postoperative state. Our study confirms the diagnostic difficulties and extremely poor prognosis in patients with underlying IC. High clinical suspicion, repeated abdominal exams, radiologic investigation, and most importantly, early surgical intervention, are recommended to reduce the significantly high mortality rates associated with surgical delay [21,22].

Additionally, we analyzed surgical delay in patients who experienced in-hospital mortality. When we compared the surgical delay between hospitalized and non-hospitalized patients, although there was no statistically significant difference, we found that the mean surgical delay was longer in the hospitalized group than in the non-hospitalized group (12 vs. 3 days, $p = 0.397$). These findings show that the physician's suspicion of acute IC should not be restricted only to patients who are newly admitted to the emergency unit, but should also include patients currently in the hospital.

According to the previously published data, the incidence of IC varies from 1.2-4.6% after cardiovascular surgery [6,7,23-26]. Although the incidence is relatively low, IC has been recognized as a common determinant of mortality after cardiovascular surgery. This was also observed in our study, in which 6 of 9 patients (67%) who underwent cardiovascular surgery died due to IC. A previous retrospective study in a cohort of more than 600 patients who underwent aortic aneurysm repair showed that postoperative IC occurred in 4.1% patients within 2 days of surgery, with a subsequent mortality rate of 58.8%.

Postoperative diagnosis of IC should be systematically suspected after every cardiovascular surgery whenever digestive symptoms, unexplained sepsis, or hemodynamic instability occur [6]. As demonstrated in the Bjorck series, early passage of stools or hemodynamic instability are suggestive of postoperative IC [6]. These signs should be followed up by an endoscopic examination [27]. On the other hand, in one large study including almost 5000 patients, the mean time to diagnosis was 5.5 days following aortic surgery, regardless of the presentation [28]. Therefore, recommendations have been made for the routine performance of a postoperative colonoscopy, despite the absence of symptoms, as an in-hospital preventive strategy to reduce IC-related mortality [29,30].

This study had several limitations. First, because of small number of patients in our study, the mortality rate might not be representative of all patients who underwent surgery for IC and it could have relatively favorable outcomes in comparison. The limitation of small number of patients also affects out results in regards to the prognostic factors of patients who underwent surgery for IC, but we included almost all variables and identified parameters that had emerged in other studies [5,17]. Second, owing to its retrospective design, we could not be sure whether other factors may have influenced the postoperative outcomes, including intraoperative fecal spillage and tension on the anastomosis. Moreover, the surgeon's assessment of the state of ischemic tissue at the time of surgery is important when deciding how much of the intestine should be resected and whether to perform an anastomosis. This assessment is subjective and difficult to quantify. However, all patients in this study were followed-up in the same unit by the same group of physicians, who used similar guidelines and made decisions collectively.

Conclusion

Our study shows that the mortality and morbidity rates remain high after surgery for IC. The predominant causes of postoperative mortality after surgery for IC were MOF and fulminant septic shock. Patients at greatest risk of early postoperative mortality are those who have a previous history of cardiovascular surgery and a delay of 3 or more days from symptom onset to surgery. Because surgical delay is an avoidable determinant of early mortality, especially in hospitalized patients, a high index of suspicion and early surgical intervention can increase survival. Moreover, the correlation observed between a previous history of cardiovascular surgery and death from IC in the early postoperative period may provide the rationale for routine evaluation of IC in selected high-risk patients. A prospective study is needed to predict the risk of postoperative mortality in patients with ischemic colitis.

Consent

Written informed consent was obtained from the patient for the publication of this report and any accompanying images.

Abbreviations

IC: Ischemic colitis; BMI: Body mass index; ASA: American Society of Anesthesiologists; SIRS: Systemic inflammatory response syndrome; MOF: Multiple organ failure; CI: Confidence interval; OR: Odds ratio; SD: Standard deviation.

Competing interests

The authors declare that they have no competing interests.

Authors' contributions

MN carried out conception and design, acquisition of data, analysis, interpretation, and writing manuscript; SSY carried out conception and design, data analysis, interpretation, and writing manuscript; SWJ carried out data extraction, interpretation and drafting manuscript, JHP carried out data extraction, interpretation and drafting manuscript; YCI carried out data extraction, interpretation and drafting manuscript; KYK carried out data extraction, interpretation and drafting manuscript. All authors read and approved the final manuscript.

Author details

[1]Department of Surgery, Ulsan University Hospital, 290-3 Jeonha-dong, Dong-gu, Ulsan 682-714, Korea. [2]Department of Digestive medicine, Ulsan University Hospital, Ulsan, Korea.

References

1. Antolovic D, Koch M, Hinz U, Schottler D, Schmidt T, Heger U, et al. Ischemic colitis: analysis of risk factors for postoperative mortality. Langenbecks Arch Surg. 2008;393:507–12.
2. Reissfelder C, Sweiti H, Antolovic D, Rahbari NN, Hofer S, Buchler MW, et al. Ischemic colitis: who will survive? Surgery. 2011;149:585–92.
3. Genstorfer J, Schafer J, Kettelhack C, Oertli D, Rosenthal R. Surgery for ischemic colitis: outcome and risk factors for in-hospital mortality. Int J Colorectal Dis. 2014;29:493–503.
4. Castleberry AW, Turley RS, Hanna JM, Hopkins TJ, Barbas AS, Worni M, et al. A 10-year longitudinal analysis of surgical management for acute ischemic colitis. J Gastrointest Surg. 2013;17:784–92.
5. Acosta-Merida MA, Marchena-Gomez J, Hemmersbach-Miller M, Roque-Castellano C, Hernandez-Romero JM. Identification of risk factors for perioperative mortality in acute mesenteric ischemia. World J Surg. 2006;30:1579–85.
6. Bjorck M, Bergqvist D, Troeng T. Incidence and clinical presentation of bowel ischaemia after aortoiliac surgery–2930 operations from a population-based registry in Sweden. Eur J Vasc Endovasc Surg. 1996;12:139–44.
7. Van Damme H, Creemers E, Limet R. Ischaemic colitis following aortoiliac surgery. Acta Chir Belg. 2000;100:21–7.
8. Bone RC, Balk RA, Cerra FB, Dellinger RP, Fein AM, Knaus WA, et al. Definitions for sepsis and organ failure and guidelines for the use of innovative therapies in sepsis. The ACCP/SCCM Consensus Conference Committee. Am Coll Chest Phys Soc Crit Care Med Chest. 1992;101:1644–55.
9. Scharff JR, Longo WE, Vartanian SM, Jacobs DL, Bahadursingh AN, Kaminski DL. Ischemic colitis: spectrum of disease and outcome. Surgery. 2003;134:624–9. discussion 629-630.
10. Guttormson NL, Bubrick MP. Mortality from ischemic colitis. Dis Colon Rectum. 1989;32:469–72.
11. Abel ME, Russell TR. Ischemic colitis. Comparison of surgical and nonoperative management. Dis Colon Rectum. 1983;26:113–5.
12. Guivarc'h M, Roullet-Audy JC, Mosnier H, Boche O. Ischemic colitis. A surgical series of 88 cases. J Chir (Paris). 1997;134:103–8.
13. Longo WE, Ward D, Vernava 3rd AM, Kaminski DL. Outcome of patients with total colonic ischemia. Dis Colon Rectum. 1997;40:1448–54.
14. Medina C, Vilaseca J, Videla S, Fabra R, Armengol-Miro JR, Malagelada JR. Outcome of patients with ischemic colitis: review of fifty-three cases. Dis Colon Rectum. 2004;47:180–4.
15. Cabie A, Farkas JC, Fitting C, Laurian C, Cormier JM, Carlet J, et al. High levels of portal TNF-alpha during abdominal aortic surgery in man. Cytokine. 1993;5:448–53.
16. Endean ED, Barnes SL, Kwolek CJ, Minion DJ, Schwarcz TH, Mentzer Jr RM. Surgical management of thrombotic acute intestinal ischemia. Ann Surg. 2001;233:801–8.
17. Ritz JP, Germer CT, Buhr HJ. Prognostic factors for mesenteric infarction: multivariate analysis of 187 patients with regard to patient age. Ann Vasc Surg. 2005;19:328–34.
18. Theodoropoulou A, Koutroubakis IE. Ischemic colitis: clinical practice in diagnosis and treatment. World J Gastroenterol. 2008;14:7302–8.
19. Chaudhary BN, Sharma H, Nadeem M, Niayesh MH. Ischemic colitis or melanosis coli: a case report. World J Emerg Surg. 2007;2:25.
20. Gregor P, Prodger JD. Mead Johnson Critical Care Symposium for the Practising Surgeon. 4. Abdominal crisis in the intensive care unit. Can J Surg. 1988;31:331–2.
21. Kollef MH, Allen BT. Determinants of outcome for patients in the medical intensive care unit requiring abdominal surgery: a prospective, single-center study. Chest. 1994;106:1822–8.

22. Liolios A, Oropello JM, Benjamin E. Gastrointestinal complications in the intensive care unit. Clin Chest Med. 1999;20:329–45.
23. Sandison AJ, Panayiotopoulos Y, Edmondson RC, Tyrrell MR, Taylor PR. A 4-year prospective audit of the cause of death after infrarenal aortic aneurysm surgery. Br J Surg. 1996;83:1386–9.
24. Dadian N, Ohki T, Veith FJ, Edelman M, Mehta M, Lipsitz EC, et al. Overt colon ischemia after endovascular aneurysm repair: the importance of microembolization as an etiology. J Vasc Surg. 2001;34:986–96.
25. Jarvinen O, Laurikka J, Sisto T, Tarkka MR. Intestinal ischemia following surgery for aorto-iliac disease. A review of 502 consecutive aortic reconstructions. Vasa. 1996;25:148–55.
26. Jarvinen O, Laurikka J, Salenius JP, Lepantalo M. Mesenteric infarction after aortoiliac surgery on the basis of 1752 operations from the National Vascular Registry. World J Surg. 1999;23:243–7.
27. Bjorck M, Troeng T, Bergqvist D. Risk factors for intestinal ischaemia after aortoiliac surgery: a combined cohort and case-control study of 2824 operations. Eur J Vasc Endovasc Surg. 1997;13:531–9.
28. Longo WE, Lee TC, Barnett MG, Vernava AM, Wade TP, Peterson GJ, et al. Ischemic colitis complicating abdominal aortic aneurysm surgery in the U.S. veteran. J Surg Res. 1996;60:351–4.
29. Forde KA, Lebwohl O, Wolff M, Voorhees AB. The endoscopy corner: reversible ischemic colitis–correlation of colonoscopic and pathologic changes. Am J Gastroenterol. 1979;72:182–5.
30. Houe T, Thorboll JE, Sigild U, Liisberg-Larsen O, Schroeder TV. Can colonoscopy diagnose transmural ischaemic colitis after abdominal aortic surgery? An evidence-based approach. Eur J Vasc Endovasc Surg. 2000;19:304–7.

12

Retrospective one-million-subject fixed-cohort survey of utilization of emergency departments due to traumatic causes in Taiwan, 2001–2010

Nan-Ping Yang[1,2,3†], Dinh-Van Phan[4,5†], Yi-Hui Lee[6], Jin-Chyr Hsu[7], Ren-Hao Pan[4,5], Chien-Lung Chan[4,5], Nien-Tzu Chang[6,8†] and Dachen Chu[2,3,9,10*]

Abstract

Background: Epidemiological study was needed to evaluate trends in emergency department (ED) utilization that could be taken into account when making policy decisions regarding the delivery and distribution of medical resources.

Methods: A retrospective fixed-cohort study of emergency medical utilization from 2001 to 2010 was performed based on one-million people sampled in 2010 in Taiwan. Focusing on traumatic cases, the annual incidences in various groups split according to sex and age were calculated, and further information regarding location of trauma and type of trauma was obtained.

Results: In 2010, significantly greater proportions of male and younger subjects were visitors to EDs with a traumatic injury. During 2001–2010, the number of both traumatic cases and non-traumatic cases presenting at EDs significantly increased (average annual percentage change, AAPC 4.7 and 3.6, respectively) and a significantly greater direct medical cost associated with traumatic cases than non-traumatic cases was noted. Focusing on traumatic cases, most of these cases were directed to highest-level hospitals, accounting for 73.5–78.8 % of all traumatic cases, with a significant AAPC of 5.6. The traumatic ED visit annual incidence in males was 58.63 in 2001, which significantly increased to 69.35 per 1000 persons in 2010 (AAPC 1.5); and in females was 38.96 in 2001, which significantly increased to 50.73 per 1000 persons in 2010 (AAPC 2.5). Most of the traumatic cases treated in EDs were minor injuries, such as contusion with the skin intact, open wound of the upper limbs, open wound of the head, neck, or trunk, and other superficial injury (accounting for about 60 % of all cases). The traumatic categories of sprains/strains of joints and adjacent muscles, fractures of upper limbs, fractures of lower limbs, and fractures of the spine/trunk required greater medical resources and significantly positive AAPC values (4.3, 4.0, 4.5 and 6.8, respectively).

Conclusions: Increased ED utilization due to traumatic causes, as assessed by the annual number of cases and incidence, average direct medical cost and highest-level hospital utilization, was observed from 2001 to 2010. Orthopedic-related injuries, including soft tissue trauma of extremities and various fractures, were the categories with the greatest increase in incidence.

Keywords: Emergency department, Trauma, Utilization

* Correspondence: dad57@tpech.gov.tw
†Equal contributors
[2]Faculty of Medicine, School of Medicine, National Yang-Ming University, Taipei, Taiwan
[3]Institute of Public Health and Community Medicine Research Center, National Yang-Ming University, Taipei, Taiwan
Full list of author information is available at the end of the article

Background

Globally, injury is a major cause of death and disability. The burden of injury is greatest in developing countries, and trauma registries are known to be integral in the monitoring and improvement of trauma care [1]. There remains great international variability in terms of patient mix, process of care, and performance of different pre-hospital trauma care systems [2]. To date, the classification, measurement and improvement of data quality in trauma registries have been inconsistent [3]. There is no doubt that injury is a large issue for the health care system, and in particular for emergency management units.

Usually, patients suffering a traumatic injury and other acute diseases constitute the majority of ambulance transports, and adult patients aged 15–60 years are the principal users of Emergency Medical Services (EMSs) [4]. Furthermore, triage, inter-hospital transfer processes and protocols for inter-hospital transfer are also central to trauma systems [5, 6]. From the viewpoints of public health and health policy, epidemiological study is needed in order to evaluate trends in health care utilization, which could inform policy decision-making for the re-distribution of medical resources, especially in developing countries.

Methods

Data source, security, and quality control

Taiwan launched a single-payer National Health Insurance (NHI) program on March 1, 1995. As of 2014, 99.9 % of Taiwan's population was enrolled [7]. Foreigners in Taiwan are also eligible for this program. The database of this program contains registration files and original claim data for reimbursement. Large computerized databases derived from this system by the National Health Insurance Administration (the former Bureau of National Health Insurance, BNHI), Ministry of Health and Welfare (the former Department of Health, DOH), Taiwan and maintained by the National Health Research Institutes (NHRI), Taiwan, are provided to scientists in Taiwan for research purposes. Only citizens of the Republic of China who fulfill the requirements of conducting research projects are eligible to apply for the National Health Insurance Research Database (NHIRD). The NHIRD includes nationwide population-based data with good quality control and representation and is provided to scientists in Taiwan for research purposes [8–12].

Ethics approval, and consent for participation or publication

The study design was a retrospective health data analytic study. The protocol was evaluated and approved by the Institutional Review Board (IRB) of Taipei Hospital, Ministry of Health & Welfare, Taiwan, which has been certificated by the Ministry of Health and Welfare, Taiwan (IRB Approval Number: TH-IRB-0015-0003).

The information related to all subjects is encrypted using a double scrambling protocol for research purposes to protect the privacy of patients. Theoretically, it is impossible to query the data alone to identify individuals at any level using this database. No any individual informed consent of all the insured is requested. All researchers who wish to use the NHIRD are required to sign a written agreement declaring that they have no intention of attempting to obtain information that could potentially violate the privacy of patients or care providers. The use of NHIRD is limited to research purposes only. Applicants must follow the Computer-Processed Personal Data Protection Law and related regulations of National Health Insurance Administration and NHRI, and an agreement must be signed by the applicant and his/her supervisor upon application submission.

The application of the present study was reviewed by the NHI Administration, who gave their agreement to the planned analysis of the NHIRD and released the data. (Data approval Number: NHIRD-104-183).

Source and definition of study population

In this retrospective fixed-cohort study, the records of 1 million people in the NHIRD sampled in 2010 were used to perform an epidemiological and descriptive study of emergency medical utilization in Taiwan from 2001 to 2010. This specific longitudinal health insurance dataset (LHID) is the latest cohort data in Taiwan that was named LHID2010 (see Fig. 1) [13]. LHID2010, used as the study population in the present study, contains the entire original claim data of 1,000,000 beneficiaries enrolled in year 2010 randomly sampled from the year 2010 Registry for Beneficiaries (ID) of the NHIRD, where registration data of everyone who was a beneficiary of the National Health Insurance program during the period of Jan. 1st 2010 to Dec. 31 2010 were drawn for random sampling. There are approximately 27.38 million individuals in this registry. All the registration and claim data of these 1,000,000 individuals collected by the National Health Insurance program constitute the LHID2010. There was no significant difference in the gender distribution (p-value = 0.796) between the patients in the LHID2010 and the original NHIRD [13].

The entire medical claim data of the patients enrolled in LHID2010 was collected in the year 2010 and during the period of 2001–2009 retrospectively. All incident ED visits of the 1,000,000 studied subjects in each calendar year were evaluated. The causes of ED visits were divided into 2 groups: traumatic (ICD-9-CM diagnostic codes ranging from 800.X to 959.X) and non-traumatic. Traumatic cases were defined as subjects who visited an ED due to a trauma event once or more in 1 year, while

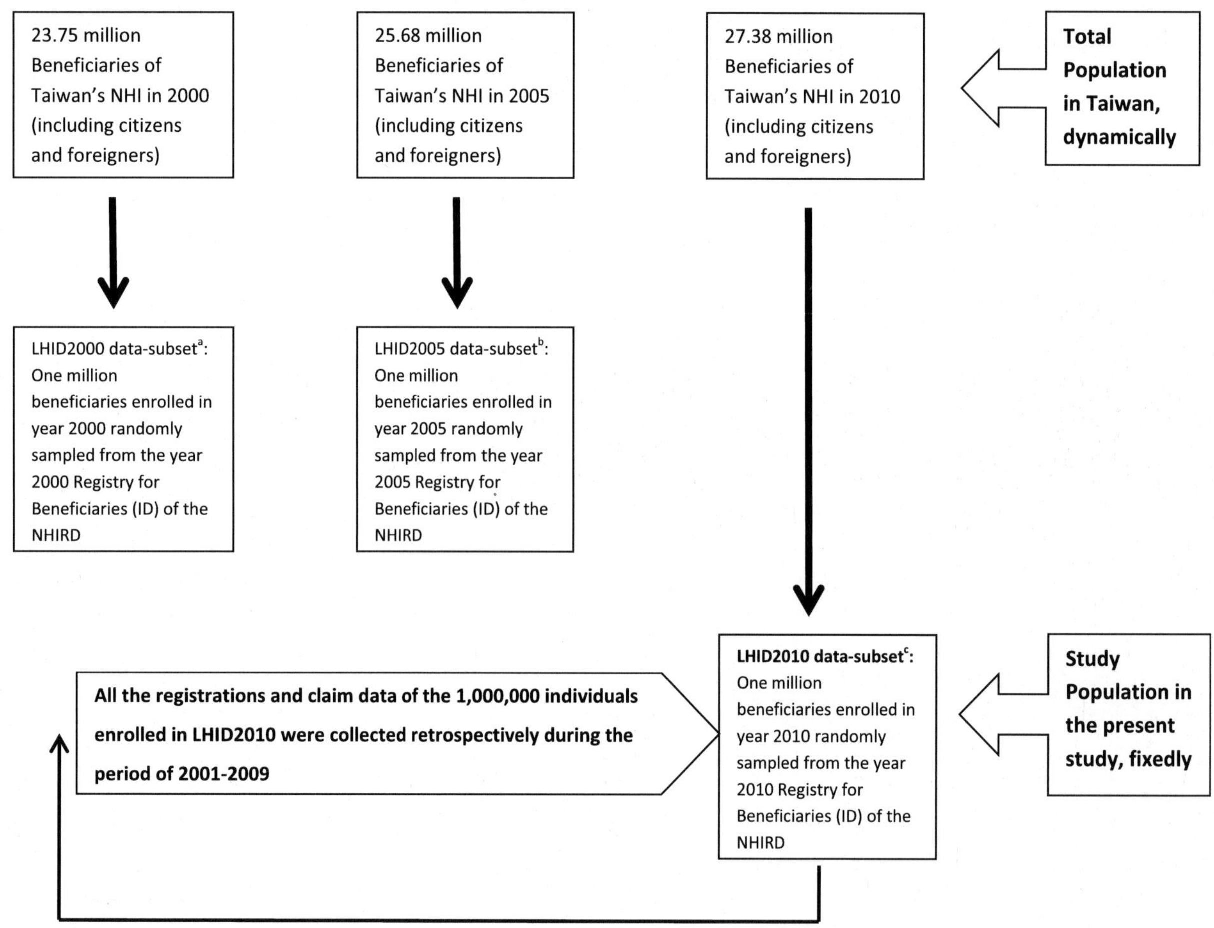

Note:

[a] There was no significant difference in the gender distribution (p=0.187) between the patients in the LHID2000 and the original NHIRD.

[b] There was no significant difference in the gender distribution (p=0.931) between the patients in the LHID2005 and the original NHIRD.

[c] There was no significant difference in the gender distribution (p=0.796) between the patients in the LHID2010 and the original NHIRD.

These three datasets (LHID2000, LHID2005 and LHID2010) are isolated and not traced back to their original NHIRD.

Fig. 1 The relationship of study population and total population in the present study

the non-traumatic cases were defined as subjects who visited an ED for reasons entirely due to a non-traumatic event. Furthermore, each ED visit of the subjects was analyzed to assess the number of annual ED visits and the direct medical cost per ED case. Focusing on traumatic ED cases, the distribution of hospital level, annual incidence by gender, annual incidence by age strata, and detailed information regarding traumatic location/type (classified into 20 categories) [11] were studied.

Statistical analysis

Descriptive statistics are represented by numbers of cases, percentages, and means with standard deviation (SD). The chi-square test or independent *t*-test was used to analyze significant differences between groups for categorical or continuous variables, respectively. The average annual percentage change (AAPC) and its 95 % confidence interval (CI) was calculated using the Join-point Regression Program Ver.4.2.0.2 in order to test for time trends. 95 % CI of cumulative incidence (ci) cab be calculated as the followed formula: $ci \pm 1.96\sqrt{ci(1-ci)/N}$. All analyses of data were conducted using the Hadoop big data distributed computing environment and the Impala massive parallel processing (MPP) SQL query engine (Cloudera Corporation), and statistical calculations were performed using the Statistical Package for Social Sciences for Windows (SPSS Ver.22.0).

Results

Of the enrolled 1 million people sampled in 2010, 176,126 subjects visited an ED, who were classified into 59,900 traumatic subjects (34 %) and 116,226 non-traumatic subjects (66 %). Significantly greater proportions of male subjects (57 %) and younger patients (64 %) presented as traumatic ED cases (see Table 1).

All ED visits of the subjects were analyzed as individual cases, and the annual number of ED visits, average direct ED medical cost per case, and time trends were evaluated, as shown in Table 2. During 2001–2010 in Taiwan, the numbers of both traumatic cases and non-traumatic cases sent to EDs significantly increased (average annual increase ratio 4.7 % (95 % CI: 3.2–6.2 %) and 3.6 % (95 % CI: 1.0–6.4 %), respectively). Although fewer traumatic cases were seen in EDs than non-traumatic cases, the direct medical cost of traumatic cases was significantly greater than that of non-traumatic cases, and a significant increasing trend of the direct medical cost was observed for both types of case. Focusing on traumatic cases, most (i.e., 73.5–78.8 % of all traumatic cases) were taken to highest-level hospitals, this incidence exhibiting a significant increasing annual trend of 5.6 % during 2001–2010 in Taiwan.

Furthermore, still focusing on traumatic cases, the annual ED visit incidence and the annual trend were analyzed by gender and age. The point estimation of incidence was calculated by the number of subjects visiting ED due to traumatic causes divided by the numbers of various gender and age stratums among the one million study population in each calendar year. Because the study population of 1,000,000 subjects was randomly sampled in 2010 whose information could not be traced back to their original NHIRD, point estimates of cumulative incidences were calculated and their 95 % CIs could be predicted only in 2010. Even though the same fixed one-million subjects were studied during 2001–2009, all the 95 % CIs of point estimates of incidence were not projected accounting for actually dynamic total population rather than an assumedly fixed total population in Taiwan for the past 10 years. As shown in Table 3, the annual incidence of traumatic ED visitors in male subjects was 58.63 per 1000 persons, significantly increasing to 69.35 (95 % CI: 68.85–69.85) per 1000 persons from 2001 to 2010, with an average annual change of 1.5 % (95 % CI: 0.1–2.8 %); that in the female subjects was 38.96 per 1000 persons, significantly increasing to 50.73 (95 % CI: 50.30–51.16) per 1000 persons from 2001 to 2010, with an average annual change of 2.5 % (95 % CI: 1.3–3.7 %). Analyzing the subjects by age, significant increasing trends in the annual incidence of traumatic ED visitors were noted in subjects aged 29 years or under and ones aged 60 years or order. However, as illustrated in Fig. 2, a dramatically increasing linear trend of 43.61/1000 to 70.16/1000 during 2001–2010 was noted in the subject population aged 60 years or older, with an AAPC of 5.7 (95 % CI: 4.7–6.8), which was greater than that in other age strata groups.

Based on the ICD-9-CM diagnostic codes, the trauma locations of the traumatic cases in the present study were classified into 20 categories. Table 4 shows that most of the traumatic patients in EDs were treated for minor injuries, such as contusion with the skin intact, open wound of upper limb, open wound of the head, neck, or trunk, and other superficial injury (accounting for about 60 % of all cases, ranging from 58.5 to 63.3 %). Besides the above-listed and some unspecified injuries, the traumatic categories of sprains/strains of joints and adjacent muscles, fractures of upper limbs, fractures of lower limbs, and fractures of the spine/trunk required greater medical resources and significantly positive AAPC values (4.3, 4.0, 4.5 and 6.8, respectively).

Table 1 Retrospective one-million-subject fixed-cohort survey of utilization of emergency departments (EDs) due to traumatic or non-traumatic causes in Taiwan, 2010

Age (years)/Gender	Traumatic subjects		Non-traumatic subjects			ED-utilized subjects in 2010		One million study subjects based on LHID2010[a]	
	N	(%)	N	(%)	*p* value of χ^2 test	N	(%)	N (%)	
Total subjects who visited the ED	59,900	34.01	116,226	65.99		176,126	100.00	1,000,000	100
Age (years)									
0–29	25,801	43.07	46,062	39.63	.000	71,863	40.80	372,341	37.23
30–44	12,286	20.51	22,493	19.35		34,779	19.75	251,103	25.11
45–59	11,047	18.44	21,024	18.09		32,071	18.21	223,100	22.31
60+	10,766	17.97	26,647	22.93		37,413	21.24	153,456	15.35
Gender									
Female	25,750	42.99	60,968	52.46	.000	86,718	49.24	507,577	50.76
Male	34,150	57.01	55,258	47.54		89,408	50.76	492,423	49.24

[a]LHID2010: longitudinal health insurance dataset randomly selected in 2010

Table 2 Trends and comparisons of medical utilization in traumatic and non-traumatic ED cases in Taiwan, 2001–2010

	2001–2002	2003–2004	2005–2006	2007–2008	2009–2010	AAPC[a]	95 % CI[b] of AAPC
Annual ED visits, case numbers							
Traumatic cases	63,477	71,221	76,904	80,703	94,176	4.7	3.2, 6.2
Non-traumatic cases	127,988	133,837	141,391	145,217	175,571	3.6	1.0, 6.4
Direct medical cost (US$), per visit							
Traumatic cases, mean (SD)	53.51 (97.20)	60.98 (72.12)	67.86 (86.65)	72.08 (84.97)	78.61 (100.81)	4.8	3.6, 6.0
Non-traumatic cases, mean (SD)	40.53 (94.04)	46.37 (113.32)	56.11 (104.56)	65.24 (110.76)	75.49 (116.98)	8.2	7.5, 9.0
p value for *t* test	0.000	0.000	0.000	0.000	0.000		
Level of hospital visited by traumatic cases, per year							
Medical center, No. (%)	46,647 (73.49)	52,296 (73.43)	57,909 (73.91)	61,737 (76.50)	74,179 (78.77)	5.6	4.0, 7.3
Regional hospital, No. (%)	15,770 (24.84)	17,557 (24.65)	18,590 (23.73)	17,385 (21.54)	18,513 (19.66)	1.6	−1.0, 4.2
Local hospital or other, No. (%)	1061 (01.67)	1369 (01.92)	1852 (02.36)	1581 (01.96)	1484 (01.58)	4.2	−5.1, 14.3

Currency: USD: NTD = 1: 32
[a]*AAPC* average annual percentage change; the AAPC was significantly different from zero at alpha = 0.05
[b]*95 % CI* 95 % confidence interval

Discussion

In the US, publicly-available ED visit data from the National Hospital Ambulatory Medical Care Survey (NHAMCS) from 1997 through 2007 were assessed using codes from the International Classification of Diseases, Ninth Revision (ICD-9). ED visit rates increased from 352.8 to 390.5 per 1000 persons during that time ($P = .001$ for trend), and adults with Medicaid cover accounted for most of the increase in ED visits; in addition, the visit rate increased from 693.9 to 947.2 visits per 1000 enrollees ($p = 0.001$ for trend) between 1999 and 2007 [14]. According to NHAMCS data from 1997 to 2009, the overall adjusted probability of an ED visit being treatable in a primary care setting increased by 0.19 % (95 % CI = 0.10 to 0.28) per year. This probability increased at a rate of 0.52 % per year for Medicare patient visits (95 % CI = 0.38 % to 0.65 %), more than double that for Medicaid patient visits (0.25 % per year, 95 % CI = 0.13 % to 0.37 %). In contrast, there was no significant change from 1997 to 2009 in the average probability of an ED visit being treatable in a primary care setting in privately-insured patients (0.05 % per year, 95 % CI = −0.07 to 0.16) or uninsured individuals (0.00 % per year, 95 % CI = −0.12 to 0.13) [15]. In Taiwan, the ED visit rate, including traumatic and non-traumatic cases, was approximately 190 visits per 1000 persons in 2001, which increased significantly to 270 visits per 1000 persons in 2010 based on one-million sampled patients who were insured under the official Taiwan health insurance system. Therefore, a greater increase in the ED visit rate as measured by the AAPC, and in particular in the ED visit rate for cases due to traumatic causes, was observed in Taiwan, an Asian developing country.

In the US, older adults (aged 75 and over), non-Hispanic black persons, less wealthy people, and those with Medicaid coverage were more likely to have made at least one ED visit within a 12-month period than other subjects. Persons with Medicaid coverage were more likely to have made multiple visits to an ED within a 12-month period than those with private insurance

Table 3 Characteristics of traumatic ED visitors in terms of annual incidence* of the fixed one-million subjects in Taiwan, 2001–2010 retrospectively

	2001 Inc.	2002 Inc.	2003 Inc.	2004 Inc.	2005 Inc.	2006 Inc.	2007 Inc.	2008 Inc.	2009 Inc.	2010 Inc.	95 % CI of Inc. in 2010	AAPC	95 % CI of AAPC
Gender													
Male	58.63	57.09	61.80	68.42	68.59	64.68	64.63	62.44	66.52	69.35	68.85–69.85	1.5	0.1,2.8
Female	38.96	39.62	41.25	45.98	47.00	45.09	46.17	43.87	48.40	50.73	50.30–51.16	2.5	1.3,3.7
Age (years)													
0–29	55.99	56.45	60.65	67.59	67.25	63.54	63.58	61.61	66.20	69.29	68.80–69.79	2.8	0.3,5.3
30–44	42.52	41.65	43.99	48.75	49.84	46.32	45.96	43.29	46.88	48.93	48.51–49.35	2.0	−3.1,7.4
45–59	40.76	39.94	42.15	47.23	47.86	46.69	46.66	44.52	47.69	49.52	49.09–49.94	2.0	0.7,3.2
60 +	43.61	42.56	45.97	51.55	55.80	55.71	61.31	59.52	66.52	70.16	69.66–70.66	5.7	4.7, 6.8

*Incidence (Inc.): cumulative incidence, 1/1000

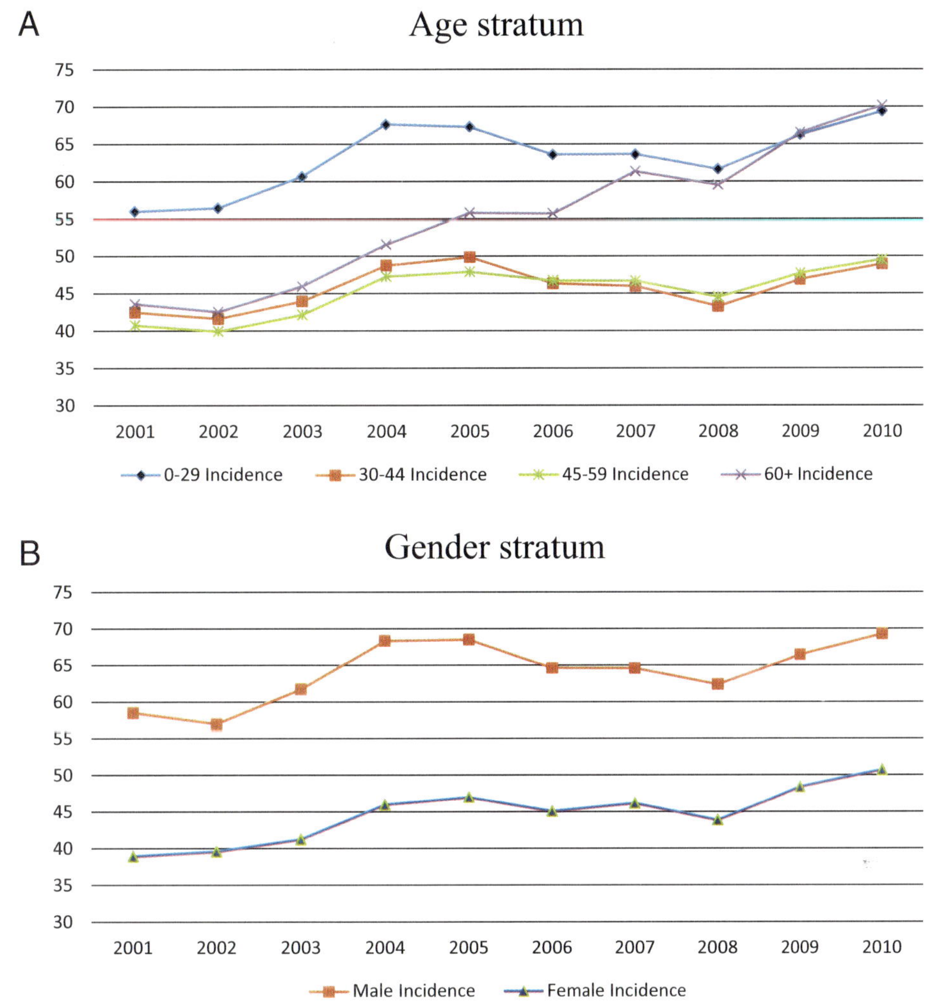

Fig. 2 a, b Linear trends of the annual incidence of traumatic ED visiting subjects in various subgroups

and the uninsured [16]. Based on data from the USA National Health Interview Survey in 2012, 18 % of children aged 0–17 years visited the ED, and children with Medicaid coverage were more likely than uninsured children and those with private coverage to have visited the ED at least once in the past year [17]. A recent systematic review concluded that in most healthcare systems, frequent ED users were more likely to be older, female, and have a mental health diagnosis, and previous hospitalizations and high primary care use were associated with future frequent ED use [18]. The main finding of the present study was that female subjects and the elderly (aged 65 years or more) exhibited a greater increase in the incidence of ED visits for traumatic reasons in Taiwan.

Overcrowding of EDs is an important issue, and in order to design strategies aimed at avoiding overcrowding, mathematical models used to predict ED patient volume are considered essential. Most of the models used to predict patient volume are linear regression models, including Poisson regression models or time series models that can include calendar- or climate-related variables. These models explain 31–75 % of the patient-volume variability [19–22]. A significantly increased rate of ED utilization was found in the present study, especially with regards to traumatic cases, of which cases of soft tissue trauma of extremities and various fractures were the categories that exhibited the greatest increasing tendencies. This information is useful to inform Taiwan's health authorities with regards to the delivery and distribution of medical resources.

In Singapore, a statistical report showed that 40.7 % of ambulance arrivals were attributable to trauma, versus 27.3 % of walk-in arrivals. The majority of trauma cases brought in by ambulance was because of road traffic accidents, followed by accidents in the home [23]. In India, traffic crashes and consequent injuries represent a growing public health concern. Open wounds and superficial

Table 4 Distributions of traumatic categories in traumatic ED cases in Taiwan, 2001–2010

Traumatic category*	ICD-9-CM code	2001–2002 No. (%)	2003–2004 No. (%)	2005–2006 No. (%)	2007–2008 No. (%)	2009–2010 No. (%)	AAPC	95 % CI of AAPC
1. Fracture of skull, intracranial injury	800–804 & 850–854	11,060 (11.66)	10,229 (9.77)	8650 (7.60)	7429 (6.47)	7688 (6.09)	−5.5	−8.0, −2.1
2. Fracture of spine and trunk	805–809	870 (0.92)	835 (0.80)	989 (0.87)	1133 (0.99)	1439 (1.14)	6.8	2.2, 11.6
3. Fracture of upper limb	810–819	3058 (3.22)	3305 (3.16)	3539 (3.11)	3819 (3.33)	4193 (3.32)	4.0	3.5, 4.4
4. Fracture of lower limb	820–829	2376 (2.51)	2511 (2.40)	2597 (2.28)	2875 (2.51)	3432 (2.72)	4.5	1.8, 7.2
5. Dislocation	830–839	963 (1.02)	821 (0.78)	846 (0.74)	938 (0.82)	1037 (0.82)	1.4	−3.5, 6.5
6. Sprains and strains of joints and adjacent muscles	840–848	3472 (3.66)	3998 (3.82)	4441 (3.90)	4482 (3.91)	4975 (3.94)	4.3	2.2, 6.3
7. Internal injury of chest	860–862	151 (0.16)	139 (0.13)	128 (0.11)	090 (0.08)	132 (0.10)	−3.5	−12.3, 6.2
8. Internal injury of abdomen and pelvis	863–869	158 (0.17)	144 (0.14)	137 (0.12)	133 (0.12)	153 (0.12)	−0.7	−4.6, 3.3
9. Open wound of head, neck and trunk	870–879	15,579 (16.43)	15,939 (15.22)	15,739 (13.83)	15,062 (13.12)	14,221 (11.26)	−1.2	−2.7, 0.3
10. Open wound of upper limb	880–887	14,278 (15.06)	15,498 (14.80)	16,147 (14.19)	15,072 (13.13)	15,768 (12.48)	0.9	−1.4, 3.2
11. Open wound of lower limb	890–897	7437 (7.84)	7506 (7.17)	7932 (6.97)	7853 (6.84)	8149 (6.45)	1.1	0.4, 1.9
12. Injury to blood vessels	900–904	660 (0.70)	944 (0.90)	671 (0.59)	232 (0.20)	194 (0.15)	−17.5	−33.1, 1.7
13. Late effects of injuries and other external causes	905–909	101 (0.11)	84 (0.08)	75 (0.07)	70 (0.06)	96 (0.08)	−1.4	−9.6, 7.6
14. Superficial injury	910–919	7429 (7.83)	8580 (8.19)	10,376 (9.12)	11,497 (10.02)	13,376 (10.59)	7.6	6.4, 8.8
15. Contusion with intact skin surface	920–924	18,229 (19.22)	23,468 (22.41)	28,704 (25.23)	30,963 (26.98)	36,358 (28.78)	8.6	5.6, 11.8
16. Crush injuries	925–929	1958 (2.06)	2190 (2.09)	2237 (1.97)	2070 (1.80)	2089 (1.65)	0.4	−2.6, 3.4
17. Effects of foreign body entering through orifice	930–939	2359 (2.49)	2661 (2.54)	2844 (2.50)	2794 (2.43)	3023 (2.39)	2.8	0.7, 4.9
18. Burns	940–949	3411 (3.60)	3369 (3.22)	3320 (2.92)	3226 (2.81)	3579 (2.83)	0.3	−1.9, 2.5
19. Injury to nerves and spinal cord	950–957	107 (0.11)	155 (0.15)	163 (0.14)	179 (0.16)	227 (0.18)	8.6	3.6, 13.8
20. Certain traumatic complications and unspecified injuries	958–959	1181 (1.25)	2343 (2.24)	4246 (3.73)	4850 (4.23)	6203 (4.91)	22.4	9.6, 36.7

*Accounting for the 1st main diagnostic code only

injuries to the head (69.3 %), upper extremities (27 %) and lower extremities (24 %) were found to be the most common injuries [24]. Based on data from the state-wide trauma registry in Queensland, Australia, from 2006 to 2010, moped/scooter riders sustained a greater percentage of head/neck (+8.6 %), facial (+3.0 %) and abdominal injuries (+2.3 %), whereas motorcycle riders sustained a greater percentage of upper extremity (+4.0 %), thoracic (+3.9 %), spinal (+3.6 %) and lower extremity injuries (+2.6 %) [25]. In Taiwan, the incidence of traffic accident-related hospitalization was between 9.17 and 11.54 %, and in all inpatients admitted due to road traffic accidents, the orthopedic fractures of (1) fracture of upper limb, (2) fracture of lower limb, and (3) fracture of spine/trunk were the most common injuries, accounting for 29.36 % of all injuries [26]. Road traffic accidents involving motorized two-wheeled vehicle (MTV) riders often result in severe morbidity and mortality. Many studies have focused on this specific issue [27, 28]. In the present study, which focused on traumatic injuries, most traumatic cases presenting at EDs had sustained superficial or open-wound injuries; however, the traumatic categories of sprains/strains of joints and adjacent muscles, fractures of upper limbs, fractures of lower limbs, and fractures of the spine/trunk exhibited significant annual increases in incidence. Most traumatic ED cases in the present study were sent to highest-level hospitals, which is contrary to another study performed in Taiwan showing the use of the ED service in the nearest community hospital to be more acceptable in an emergency situation than medical center treatment for dying cancer patients [29]. More detailed evaluation is needed in future studies to examine the causes of accidents and the subsequent morbidity or mortality.

Some limitations were still persisted in the present study. In Taiwan, no researchers can approach all the NHI beneficiaries' inpatient and ambulatory medical records. A longitudinal health dataset of one million fixed cohort populations, including their inpatient and ambulatory medical records, was the most popular research databank. However, more detailed personal information such as occupation, education level, living area, or healthy habitus were absent. Up to now, there were three isolated longitudinal datasets containing LHID2000, LHID2005 and LHID2010 that can provide only point estimates for epidemiological studies due to lack of available data of whole Taiwan's population in each calendar year. In another way, during the study period of 2001–2010, 10 separated cross-sectional surveys in each calendar year might be performed based on the truly dynamic total population but only 0.2 % of the ambulatory care records extracted by systematic sampling method have been allowed to be released to Taiwanese researchers [13]. Finally, the latest longitudinal health dataset (LHID2010) in Taiwan was chosen to perform a descriptive epidemiological analysis that was designed as a retrospective fixed-cohort study.

Conclusions

Focusing on traumatic visits of patients to EDs, increased ED utilization was observed between 2001 and 2010 in Taiwan, as evidenced by the increases in the annual number of cases, annual incidence assessed by gender and age, average direct medical cost, and highest-level hospital utilization. Of the 20 categories into which all traumatic causes were divided, orthopedic-related injuries, including soft tissue trauma of extremities and various fractures, were the categories in which the greatest increases in incidence were observed. Greater numbers of surgical and orthopedic physicians may be needed in EDs, especially in the highest-level hospitals in Taiwan,

Acknowledgments

This study was partially supported by MOST-102-2221-E-155-027-MY3 & MOST-104-2218-E-155-004. The authors would still like to thank Keelung Hospital and the Ministry of Health& Welfare for supporting the study.

Authors' contributions

The study was designed by NPY, CLC and DC; data were gathered and analyzed by NPY, DVP, NTC and RHP; the initial draft of the manuscript was written by NPY, DVP and NTC; the accuracy of the data and analyses was assured by YHL, JCH and DC. All authors participated in the preparation of the manuscript and approved the final version. All authors have read and approved the final manuscript. NPY, DVP and NTC contributed equally to this work.

Competing interests

The authors declare that they have no competing interests.

Author details

[1]Department of Surgery & Orthopedics, Keelung Hospital, Ministry of Health & Welfare, Keelung, Taiwan. [2]Faculty of Medicine, School of Medicine, National Yang-Ming University, Taipei, Taiwan. [3]Institute of Public Health and Community Medicine Research Center, National Yang-Ming University, Taipei, Taiwan. [4]Department of Information Management, Yuan Ze University, Taoyuan, Taiwan. [5]Innovation Center for Big Data and Digital Convergence, Yuan Ze University, Taoyuan, Taiwan. [6]Department of Nursing, School of Nursing, College of Medicine, Chang-Gang University, Taoyuan, Taiwan. [7]Department of Medicine, Taipei Hospital, Ministry of Health & Welfare, Taipei, Taiwan. [8]School of Nursing, College of Medicine, National Taiwan University, Taipei, Taiwan. [9]Department of Neurosurgery, Taipei City Hospital, Taipei, Taiwan. [10]Department of Health Care Management, National Taipei University of Nursing and Health Sciences, Taipei, Taiwan.

References

1. O'Reilly GM, Joshipura M, Cameron PA, Gruen R. Trauma registries in developing countries: a review of the published experience. Injury. 2013;44:713–21.
2. Roudsari BS, Nathens AB, Arreola-Risa C, Cameron P, Civil I, Grigoriou G, et al. Emergency Medical Service (EMS) systems in developed and developing countries. Injury. 2007;38:1001–13.
3. O'Reilly GM, Gabbe B, Moore L, Cameron PA. Classifying, measuring and improving the quality of data in trauma registries: a review of the literature. Injury. 2016;47:559–67.
4. Man Lo S, Min Yu Y, Larry Lee LY, Eliza Wong ML, Ying Chair S, J Kalinowski E, et al. Overview of the shenzhen emergency medical service call pattern. World J Emerg Med. 2012;3:251–6.
5. Kristiansen T, Lossius HM, Søreide K, Steen PA, Gaarder C, Næss PA. Patients Referred to a Norwegian Trauma Centre: effect of transfer distance on injury patterns, use of resources and outcomes. J Trauma Manag Outcomes. 2011;5:9.
6. Kristiansen T, Ringdal KG, Skotheimsvik T, Salthammer HK, Gaarder C, Naess PA, et al. Implementation of recommended trauma system criteria in south-eastern Norway: a cross-sectional hospital survey. Scand J Trauma Resusc Emerg Med. 2012;20:5.
7. National Health Insurance Administration, Ministry of Health and Welfare, Taiwan, R.O.C. Background of National Health Insurance Research Database. [http://nhird.nhri.org.tw/en/index.html]. Accessed 1 Aug 2016.
8. Yang NP, Deng CY, Chou YJ, Chen PQ, Lin CH, Chou P, et al. Estimated prevalence of osteoporosis from a Nationwide Health Insurance database in Taiwan. Health Policy. 2006;75:329–37.
9. Yang NP, Chan CL, Yu IL, Lee CY, Chou P. Estimated prevalence of orthopaedic fractures in Taiwan—a cross-sectional study based on nationwide insurance data. Injury. 2010;41:1266–72.
10. Chan CL, Lin W, Yang NP, Huang HT. The association between the availability of ambulatory care and non-emergency treatment in emergency medicine departments: a comprehensive and nationwide validation. Health Policy. 2013;110:271–9.
11. Yang NP, Chan CL, Chu D, Lin JS, Lin KB, Yu CS, et al. Epidemiology of hospitalized traumatic pelvic fractures and their combined injuries in Taiwan: 2000–2011 nationwide surveillance. BioMed Res Int. 2014. Article ID 878601. doi: 10.1155/2014/878601.
12. Lin KB, Lai KR, Yang NP, Chan CL, Liu YH, Pan RH, et al. Epidemiology and socioeconomic features of appendicitis in Taiwan: a 12-year population-based study. World J Emerg Surg. 2015;10:42.
13. National Health Insurance Administration, Ministry of Health and Welfare, Taiwan, R.O.C. Data subset of National Health Insurance Research Database. [http://nhird.nhri.org.tw/en/Data_Subsets.html]. Accessed 1 Aug 2016.
14. Tang N, Stein J, Hsia RY, Maselli JH, Gonzales R. Trends and characteristics of US emergency department visits, 1997–2007. JAMA. 2010;304:664–70.
15. Pukurdpol P, Wiler JL, Hsia RY, Ginde AA. Association of Medicare and Medicaid insurance with increasing primary care-treatable emergency department visits in the United States. Acad Emerg Med. 2014;21:1135–42.
16. Garcia TC, Bernstein AB, Bush MA. Emergency department visitors and visits: who used the emergency room in 2007? NCHS Data Brief. 2010;38:1–8.
17. Gindi RM, Jones LI. Reasons for emergency room use among U.S. children: National Health Interview Survey, 2012. NCHS Data Brief. 2014;160:1–8.

18. Soril LJ, Leggett LE, Lorenzetti DL, Noseworthy TW, Clement FM. Characteristics of frequent users of the emergency department in the general adult population: a systematic review of international healthcare systems. Health Policy. 2016;120:452–61.
19. Wargon M, Guidet B, Hoang TD, Hejblum G. A systematic review of models for forecasting the number of emergency department visits. Emerg Med J. 2009;26:395–9.
20. Au-Yeung SW, Harder U, McCoy EJ, Knottenbelt WJ. Predicting patient arrivals to an accident and emergency department. Emerg Med J. 2009;26: 241–4.
21. Schweigler LM, Desmond JS, McCarthy ML, Bukowski KJ, Ionides EL, Younger JG. Forecasting models of emergency department crowding. Acad Emerg Med. 2009;16:301–8.
22. McCarthy ML, Zeger SL, Ding R, Aronsky D, Hoot NR, Kelen GD. The challenge of predicting demand for emergency department services. Acad Emerg Med. 2008;15:337–46.
23. Seow E, Wong HP, Phe A. The pattern of ambulance arrivals in the emergency department of an acute care hospital in Singapore. Emerg Med J. 2001;18:297–9.
24. Fitzharris M, Dandona R, Kumar GA, Dandona L. Crash characteristics and patterns of injury among hospitalized motorised two-wheeled vehicle users in urban India. BMC Public Health. 2009;9:11.
25. White D, Lang J, Russell G, Tetsworth K, Harvey K, Bellamy N. A comparison of injuries to moped/scooter and motorcycle riders in Queensland, Australia. Injury. 2013;44:855–62.
26. Pan RH, Chang NT, Chu D, Hsu KF, Hsu YN, Hsu JC, et al. Epidemiology of orthopedic fractures and other injuries among inpatients admitted due to traffic accidents: a 10-year nationwide survey in Taiwan. ScientificWorldJournal. 2014;2014:637872.
27. Leijdesdorff HA, Siegerink B, Sier CF, Reurings MC, Schipper IB. Injury pattern, injury severity, and mortality in 33,495 hospital-admitted victims of motorized two-wheeled vehicle crashes in The Netherlands. J Trauma Acute Care Surg. 2012;72:1363–8.
28. Miggins M, Lottenberg L, Liu H, Moldawer L, Efron P, Ang D. Mopeds and scooters: crash outcomes in a high traffic state. J Trauma. 2011;71:217–22.
29. Lee YH, Chu D, Yang NP, Chan CL, Cheng SP, Pai JT, et al. Emergency visits among end-of-life cancer patients in Taiwan: a nationwide population-based study. BMC Palliat Care. 2015;14:25.

13

Etiology, treatment outcome and prognostic factors among patients with secondary peritonitis at Bugando Medical Centre, Mwanza, Tanzania

Amri Mabewa[1,2], Jeremiah Seni[3*], Phillipo L. Chalya[1,2], Stephen E. Mshana[3] and Japhet M. Gilyoma[1,2]

Abstract

Introduction: Secondary peritonitis due to perforation of the gastrointestinal tract is one of the most common surgical emergencies all over the world and is associated with significantly morbidity and mortality. Previous studies conducted at Bugando Medical Centre (BMC) were retrospective and each was focused on single etiology; therefore there was an obvious need to evaluate the etiologies, treatment outcome and their prognostic factors altogether.

Methods: This was a descriptive cross-sectional study involving patients with secondary peritonitis admitted at BMC from May 2014 to April 2015. Sociodemographic and clinical characteristics among consented patients were collected using questionnaires. Peritoneal aspirate, biopsy and blood were collected perioperatively and processed using standard operating procedures. Analysis was done using STATA version 11 software.

Results: The study enrolled 97 patients with the female to male ratio of 1:1.8 and approximately 41.2 % (40/97) were in their third and fourth decades of life. Only 3 (3.09 %) patients arrived to the hospital within 24 hours of onset of illness, 26 (26.80 %) patients presented with shock and HIV seropositivity among all patients was 13.40 % (13/97). The common etiologies of secondary peritonitis were perforated appendicitis 23 (23.71 %), peptic ulcer disease 18 (18.56 %), ischemia 18 (18.56 %) and typhoidal perforation 15 (15.46 %). Of the 97 patients, 35 (36.08 %) had complications and 15 (15.46 %) died. Presence of premorbid illness and post-operative complication were found to be associated with death (p values = 0.004 and <0.001 respectively).

Conclusions: The most common etiologies of secondary peritonitis at BMC are perforated appendicitis, peptic ulcer disease, ischemia and typhoidal perforation. Premorbid illness and postoperative complications in this setting are associated with death and as the matter of fact proper screening on admission should be done to identify patients with premorbid illness and confer prompt management.

Keywords: Etiology, Treatment outcome, Prognostic factors, Secondary peritonitis, Tanzania

Introduction

Peritonitis has a long historical background and is conventionally divided into three broad groups namely; primary, secondary and tertiary basing on the source and nature of the microbial contamination [1]. Secondary peritonitis which is due to perforation of the gastrointestinal tract is one of the most common surgical emergencies all over the world and it is associated with significantly morbidity and mortality [1–4]. Due to the loss of epithelial integrity, bacterial pathogens can traverse into the peritoneal cavity leading to a cascade of inflammatory response, sepsis, multisystem organ failure and death if not treated in a timely manner [1]. Aggressive resuscitation and early surgical intervention is therefore required in order to deliver optimal care for the patients and improve their treatment outcome [2–5].

The spectrum of gastrointestinal perforation have a wide geographical variations; with preponderance of lower gastrointestinal perforations western countries as

* Correspondence: senijj80@gmail.com
[3]Department of Microbiology and Immunology, Catholic University of Health and Allied Sciences, P.O. Box 1464, Mwanza, Tanzania
Full list of author information is available at the end of the article

opposed to upper gastrointestinal perforations in developing countries [3, 6–8].

At Bugando Medical Centre (BMC), primary bacterial peritonitis was recently reported to have a prevalence of 11.6 % among patients with portal hypertension and ascites [9]. Moreover, secondary peritonitis is the commonest indication for admission in the surgical wards resulting into increased workload, increased duration of hospital stays, and complications such as enterocutaneous fistula, surgical site infections and sepsis. Furthermore, the death rates attributable to secondary peritonitis in this settings has been shown to be 10.7 % and 23.1 % among patients with peptic ulcer and typhoid perforations respectively [10–12]. Despite advances in surgical techniques, antimicrobial therapy, and intensive care support; the management of peritonitis continues to be highly demanding, difficult, and complex [3, 13]. Early prognostic evaluation of peritonitis is desirable to provide objective classification of the severity of the disease and select high-risk patients for more aggressive therapeutic procedures [14, 15]; but this has been affected by late presentation to the health facilities by majority of patients, a situation which further complicates effective management [16].

Previous studies from BMC were retrospective and each focused on single etiology thus, lacking a holistic approach in addressing the implicated etiologies [10–12]; therefore the present study aimed at exploring the wide range of etiologies causing secondary peritonitis so as to identify factors responsible for the poor outcome and specifically address them in the context of reducing poor outcomes among patients with secondary peritonitis.

Methods

Study design, site and sampling procedures

A descriptive cross-sectional study involving patients with secondary peritonitis admitted at BMC from May 2014 to April 2015 inclusive was conducted. BMC is one of the four largest referral hospitals in the country, located in the northwestern part of Tanzania. It has a bed capacity of 1000 and serves a catchment population of approximately 13 million people. It is also a consultant and teaching hospital for the Catholic University of Health and Allied Sciences-Bugando (CUHAS). A minimum sample size of 93 was estimated basing on the Yamane Taro (1967) using previous local data which revealed 243 patients who were operated with secondary peritonitis in 2013 as well as accepted error of 8 %. Patients who met the inclusion criteria were offered explanations about the study and requested to provide a written informed consent before being enrolled into the study.

Preoperatively, all the patients recruited into the study were resuscitated with intravenous fluids to correct fluid and electrolyte deficits; nasogastric suction; urethral catheterization and broad-spectrum antibiotic coverage as per BMC protocol. Relevant preoperative investigations included hemoglobin estimation, blood grouping and cross-matching. In addition, provider initiated testing for HIV infection was offered to all patients according to National AIDS Control Program [17, 18]. For patients found to be HIV seropositive, CD4+ count using FACSCALIBUR (BD Biosciences, USA) was done. Radiological investigations included abdominal x-rays (erect and supine) as well as abdominal ultrasound were performed in all patients.

After resuscitation, all patients had to undergo preoperative anesthetic assessment using the American Society of Anesthetists (ASA) classification [19]. Patients who were clinically and hemodynamically stable for surgery were subjected to exploratory laparotomy under general anesthesia by the residents using the standard techniques.

The diagnosis of secondary peritonitis was established clinically based on guarding, rigidity, and tenderness on palpation of the abdomen, supported radiologically by detection of free air under the diaphragm and/or free intra peritoneal fluid on abdominal ultrasound and confirmed by intraoperative clinical and investigational findings.

Intraoperatively, purulent materials were aspirated from peritoneal cavity for Ziehl-Neelsen stain for Acid fast bacilli (AFB), tissue biopsy and regional lymph nodes were taken for histopathological analysis [20]. The primary outcome of the study was survival i.e. whether a patient died or was alive at the time of discharge.

Data management

A structured questionnaires were used to collect socio-demographic and clinical data preoperatively, intra-operatively and post-operatively. Data were entered into Microsoft excel and then exported to the STATA version 11.0 software for analysis according to the objectives of the study. The results are presented into percentages/ proportions for categorical variables whereas continuous variables are described as mean (± standard deviation) or median (interquantile range) depending on the distribution of data. The difference in distribution of a predictor variable was considered significant if p-value is less than 0.05.

Ethical considerations

Ethical clearance was obtained from the joint BMC/ CUHAS ethical committee. Written informed consent was obtained from every participant prior to be involved in the study. Anonymity of patients was ensured by use of codes. Laboratory results were timely reported to the attending doctors for specific management.

Results

A total of 112 patients were diagnosed to have secondary peritonitis and were admitted during the study period; of these 97 fulfilled the inclusion criteria and were enrolled whereas15 patients were excluded (samples were not taken in 10 and 5 did not fulfill inclusion criteria).

The female to male ratio of the study participants was 1:1.8. The median age (IQR) of the study was 32 (21–47) years, the youngest was 5 years old and the oldest was 86 years old. Moreover, approximately 41.2 % (40/97) were in their third and fourth decades of life, 51 (52.58 %) were from urban, and majority had primary school education (59.79 %) and were unemployed (62.89 %).

Clinical presentations

Majority of patients (96.91 %, 94/97) presented to hospital more than 24 hours since the illness started. Twenty seven (27.84 %) patients presented with co morbid illness, with HIV infection being the predominant co morbidity in about 46.43 % (13/28) of patients. Abdominal pain was found to be the most common presenting symptom in about 95 (97.6 %) patients and 93 (95.88 %) were diagnosed with generalized peritonitis. About 26 (26.80 %) patients presented with shock with systolic blood pressure bellow 90 mmHg and heart rate was above 100 beats per minute and 56 (57 .73 %) patients were febrile (Table 1).

Laboratory and radiological investigations

The median hemoglobin (IQR) of the 97 patients was 9.2 (7.3–11) gm/dl; ranging from 1.2 gm/dl to 17 gm/dl. Widal test was done in 71 patients and titers were high in 14 patients and were within normal range in 57 patients. Thirteen patients (13.40 %) were found to be HIV seropositive; with the median CD4 count of 250 (150–330) and lowest level was 95 and highest was 480.

Abdominal x ray supine and erect were normal in 51 (52.58 %) patients and abnormal in 46 (47.42 %). Pneumoperitoneum was found in 31 (31.96 %) and air fluid level in 35 (36.08 %) patients (Table 2).

Operative data

Majority of the patients were in ASA 2 and ASA 3 in about 58 (59.79 %) and 24 (24.74 %) respectively. The median waiting time (IQR) was 3 (2–6) hours. The common etiologies of secondary peritonitis were perforated appendicitis 23 (23.71 %), peptic ulcer disease 18 (18.56 %), ischemia 18 (18.56 %) and typhoidal perforation 15 (15.46 %). The median size of perforation (IQR) was 1 (0.8-1) cm. The minimum size perforation was 0.4 cm and maximum size was 3 cm.

The most common surgical interventions done were bowel resection and anastomosis in 27 (27.84 %),

Table 1 Clinical presentation of the patients with secondary peritonitis at BMC

Characteristic			Number (%)
Symptoms	Vomiting	Yes	30 (30.93)
		No	67 (69.07)
	Abdominal pain	Yes	95 (97.94)
		No	2 (2.06)
	Fever	Yes	65 (67.01)
		No	32 (32.99)
	Diarrhea	Yes	3 (3.09)
		No	94 (96.91)
	Constipation	Yes	17 (17.53)
		No	80 (82.47)
	Dehydration	Yes	2 (2.06)
		No	95 (97.94)
Type peritonitis	Generalized		93 (95.88)
	Localized		4 (4.12)
Signs	Systolic BP	≤90 mmHg	26 (26.80)
		>90 mmHg	71 (73.20)
	Heart rate	Below 100 bpm	30 (30.93)
		Above 100 bpm	67 (69.07)
	Respiratory rate	Below 30 brpm	87 (89.69)
		Above 30 brpm	10 (10.31)
	Temperature	Below 36 °C	2 (2.06)
		36-38 °C	39 (40.21)
		Above 38 °C	56 (57.73)
Comorbid illness[a]	Yes		27 (27.84)
	No		70 (72.16)

[a]HIV (12); Puerperal sepsis (4); Severe anemia (4); Hypertension (4); Tumor (1); Heart failure (1); Renal failure (1) and HIV & Hypertension (1)

Table 2 The investigation findings of patients with secondary peritonitis at BMC

Investigations		Number (%) or (IQR)
Hemoglobin		9.2 (7.3-11) g/dl
Widal test	Suggestive	14 (19.72)
	Not suggestive	57 (80.28)
HIV	Reactive	13 (13.40)
	Non reactive	84 (86.6)
CD_4[a]		250 (150–330)
X ray	Normal	51 (52.58)
	Abnormal	46 (47.42)
Ultrasound	Fluid seen	32 (32.99)
	No fluid	3 (3.09)
	Not done	62 (63.92)

[a]Only HIV positive patients were included

appendectomy in 21 (21.65 %), Grahams omental patch in 18 (18.56 %) patients and perforation were repaired in 16 (16.49 %). The median time for operation (IQR) was 2 (1.5-2) hours, with the shortest time being 45 minutes and longest time was 4 hours (Table 3).

The outcome of treatment

Of the 97 patients, 35 (36.08 %) had complications, of which 18 (51.43 %) had surgical site infections, 11 (31.43 %) wound dehiscence and 6 (17.14 %) developed septicemia. The median length of hospital stay (IQR) was 7 (5–11) days; the longest hospital stay was 60 days and shortest 1 day. Mortality rate was 15 (15.46 %) (Table 4).

The prognostic factors for mortality

There was no significant association between socio-demographic characteristics of patients with the outcome.

Table 3 The operative findings of patients with secondary peritonitis

Characteristic	Number (%) or median (IQR)	
Timing of operation	Less than 24	3 (3.09)
	More than 24	94 (96.96)
Waiting time	3(2–6) hours	
ASA	1	8 (8.25)
	2	58 (59.79)
	3	24 (24.74)
	4	6 (6.19)
	5	1 (1.03)
Site of perforation	Gastric	18 (18.56)
	Small intestine	28 (28.87)
	Appendix	23 (23.71)
	Large intestine	18 (18.56)
	Others[a]	10 (10.31)
Etiology of perforation	PUD	18 (18.56)
	Typhoid	15 (15.46)
	Appendicitis	23 (23.71)
	Trauma	11 (11.34)
	Neoplastic	2 (2.06)
	Ischemia	18 (18.56)
	Others[a]	10 (10.31)
Type of surgery	Repair of perforation	16 (16.49)
	Resection and anastomosis	27 (27.84)
	Grahams' omental patch	18 (18.54)
	Appendectomy	21 (21.65)
	Others[b]	15 (15.46 %)
Duration of operation	2(1.5-2) hours	

[a]Ruptured abscess (9) and Perforated gall bladder (1)
[b]Cholecystectomy (1); Diverting stoma (1) and Lavage (13)

Table 4 Outcome of treatment for the patients with secondary peritonitis at BMC

Parameter		Number (%) or median (IQR)
Complications	Yes	35 (36.08)
	No	62 (63.92)
Type of complication	Surgical site infection	18 (18.55)
	Wound dehiscence	11 (11.34)
	Septicemia	6 (6.19)
Survival	Yes	82 (84.54)
	No	15 (15.46)
Length of hospital stay (days)		7 (5–11)

Presence of premorbid illness and post-operative complications were found to be significantly associated with mortality (p value of 0.004 and <0.001 respectively) (Tables 5 and 6).

Discussion

The etiology of secondary peritonitis at BMC

The predominance of perforated appendicitis, peptic ulcer disease, ischemia and typhoidal perforation as the common etiologies of secondary peritonitis in this study are similar to the study done at St. Francis Hospital Nsambya Kampala-Uganda [21] and other two previous studies in the same hospital [10, 11]. Ruptured appendix and ischemia leading to gangrenous sigmoid volvulus may be due to poor health seeking behavior, as shown in this study whereby majority of patients (96 %) came to hospital more than 24 hours after the onset of illness or mismanagement in the lower health facilities. The reason for ruptured peptic ulcer and typhoidal perforations may be due to poor sanitary condition in developing countries, exposing the patients to Salmonella infection and *Helicobacter pylori* infection in the community, which in turn may result into perforations.

The treatment outcome of secondary peritonitis

Similar to another previous study [22], about 36.08 % of patients with secondary peritonitis in this study developed complications namely superficial surgical site infection, wound dehiscence and septicemia. Mortality rate was found to be 15.46 % and median length of hospital stay was 7 days. These findings are comparable to other studies [8, 22–24] but lower than what were reported in the same hospital four years ago by Chalya et al. [11] which showed complication rate to be 39.4 %, superficial surgical site infection 55.5 %, mortality 23.1 % and median length of hospital stay of 28 days in patients with typhoidal perforation [11]. The difference could be related to the recently renovated modern accident & emergency department and ICU which are well equipped

Table 5 Association of socio-demographic characteristics with outcome among patients with secondary peritonitis at BMC

Predictor variable		Outcome (N = 97)		Chi^2	p-value
		Survived (82)	Died (15)		
		n (%) or median (IQR)	n (%) or median (IQR)		
Median age (years)		32 (21–45)	34 (31–51)	-	0.4244
Sex	Female	28 (34.15)	7 (46.67)	0.8619	0.353
	Male	54 (65.85)	8 (53.33)		
Residence	Urban	45 (54.88)	6 (40.00)	1.1257	0.289
	Rural	37 (45.12)	9 (60.00)		
Education	Informal	12 (14.63)	2 (13.33)	-	0.444
	Primary	47 (57.32)	11 (73.33)		
	Secondary	23 (28.05)	2 (13.33)		
Occupation	Employed	19 (2317)	1 (6.67)	2.1153	0.347
	Unemployed	50 (60.98)	11 (73.33)		
	Under 18	13 (15.88)	3 (20.00)		

Table 6 Association of clinical characteristics with outcome among patients with secondary peritonitis at BMC

Predictor variable		Outcome (N = 97)		Chi^2	p value
		Survived (82)	Died (15)		
		n (%) or median (IQR)	n (%) or median (IQR)		
Duration of illness	≤24 hours	3 (3.66)	0 (0.00)	-	0.601
	>24 hours	79 (96.34)	15 (100.00)		
Temperature	≤36 °C	2 (2.44)	0 (0.00)	-	0.233
	36-38 °C	30 (36.59)	9 (60.00)		
	>38 °C	50 (60.98)	6 (40.00)		
Comorbid illness	Yes	19 (23.17)	9 (60.00)	8.3764	0.004
	No	63 (76.83)	6 (40.00)		
HIV	Reactive	9 (10.98)	4 (26.67)	2.6900	0.101
	Non reactive	73 (89.02)	11 (73.33)		
CD4[a]		315 (203–330)	172.5 (117.5-342.5)	-	0.4398
Hemoglobin ± SD[b]		9.6 ± 2.7 g/dl	8.6 ± 2.4 gm/dl	-	0.1866
X ray	Normal	44 (54.66)	7 (46.67)	0.2486	0.618
	Abnormal	38 (46.34)	8 (53.30)		
Etiology of perforation	PUD	15 (18.3)	3 (20.0)	-	0.491
	Typhoid	11 (13.4)	4 (26.7)		
	Appendicitis	20 (24.4)	3 (20.0)		
	Trauma	9 (11.0)	2 (13.3)		
	Neoplastic	1 (1.2)	1 (6.7)		
	Ischemia	17 (20.7)	1 (6.7)		
	Others	9 (11.0)	1 (6.7)		
Mean waiting time ± SD[b] (hours)		7.29 ± 1.09	3.667 ± 1.68	-	0.8043
Complication	Yes	23 (28.02)	12 (80.00)	-	<0.001
	No	59 (71.95)	3 (20.00)		

[a]CD4+ count was only done to patients with HIV infection
[b]Standard deviation

to provide emergence services. Moreover, in the previous studies initial assessments of patients were done by intern doctors as opposed to now where registrars who are experienced on accident & emergency services initially attend the patients. Surgical site infection found in this study (18.55 %) is similar to what is expected in contaminated wounds as reported previously (21 %); but lower than 26 % reported before in the same hospital by Mawala et al. [1, 25]. This could be due to the fact when the previous study was conducted, the department of surgery consisted of general surgery, urology, orthopedic & traumatology as well as otorhinolaryngology which are now separate departments, and thus more care can be offered timely as a result of this decentralization.

The prognostic factors for mortality among patients with secondary peritonitis

In this study, only premorbid illness and post-operative complications were statistically found to predict deaths. This is possible because less priority can be given to other premorbid illness in case of obvious surgical condition of the patient and thus, these premorbid illnesses may be overlooked resulting into poor outcome [19, 25–27]. As a result, the present study emphasizes on carefully screening of potential premorbid illnesses and also alert care providers to ensure that they make all efforts to prevent postoperative complications. The predominance of HIV among premorbid illnesses in this and previous study in the same hospital [28] worthy to be further explored using a long term prospective study with large sample size so as to specifically delineate the contribution of HIV in the outcome of patients with secondary peritonitis. But from this study, it is sufficing to reiterate that approximately 30.8 % of patients with HIV infections died and their median CD4+ count were relatively low (172.5 cells/mm^3) compared to HIV infected patients who survived (315 cells/mm^3). Development of complications postoperatively was strongly associated with death in the present study, similarly another study revealed that development of complication like sepsis can escalate mortality [22]. Sociodemographic factors such as age, gender, clinical symptoms such as vomiting and sign like fever in this study and another related study were not found to predict deaths [23].

The limitation of the study

The present study diagnosed peptic ulcer disease basing of clinical (site of perforation) and histology. Stool antigen test for *Helicobacter pylori* could have been of interest to ascertain the role of this point-of-care test and this is recommended in future studies.

Conclusions

The most common etiologies of secondary peritonitis at BMC are perforated appendicitis, peptic ulcer disease, ischemia and typhoid. Premorbid illnesses and postoperative complications in this setting are associated with death and as the matter of fact proper screening on admission should be done to identify patients with premorbid illness and confer prompt management to prevent postoperative complications and subsequent death. Moreover, a study to explore the long-term outcomes of patients with secondary peritonitis is recommended.

Competing interests

The authors declare that they have no competing interests.

Authors' contributions

AM, JS, PLC, SEM and JMG conceived, designed and executed the study; AM and JMG managed the patients; AM, JS and PLC analyzed the data; JS wrote the first draft of the manuscript which was critically reviewed by all authors. All authors have read and approved the final draft of the manuscript.

Acknowledgements

Authors are sincerely thankful to the members of staff in the Departments of Surgery, Pathology as well as Microbiology and Immunology of CUHAS and BMC for their support. Authors are also grateful for the technical assistance provided by Dr. Peter Rambau.

Author details

[1]Department of Surgery, Catholic University of Health and Allied Sciences, P.O. Box 1464, Mwanza, Tanzania. [2]Department of Surgery, Bugando Medical Centre, P.O. Box 1370, Mwanza, Tanzania. [3]Department of Microbiology and Immunology, Catholic University of Health and Allied Sciences, P.O. Box 1464, Mwanza, Tanzania.

References

1. Levison ME, Bush LM. Intra-abdominal Infection. In Mandell, Bennett, & Dolin's Principles and Practice of Infectious Diseases. In: Peritonitis and Intraperitoneal Abscesses. 6th ed. Churchill Livingstone: An Imprint of Elsevier; 2005.
2. Simmen H, Heinzelmann M, Largiader F. Peritonitis classification and causes. Dig Surg. 1996;13:381–3.
3. Malangoni MA, Inui T. Peritonitis - the Western experience. World J Emerg Surg. 2006;1:25.
4. Agarwall N, Saha N, Srivastava A, Chumber S, Dhar A, Garg S. Peritonitis 10 years experience in a simple surgical unit. Trop Gastroenterol. 2007;28(3):117–20.
5. Schein M. Surgical management of intra-abdominal infection: is there any evidence? Langenbecks Arch Surg. 2002;387(1):1–7.
6. Agarwal N, Saha S, Srivastava A, Chumber S, Dhar A, Garg S. Peritonitis: 10 years' experience in a single surgical unit. Trop Gastroenterol. 2007;28(3):117–20.
7. Afridi SP, Malik F, Ur-Rahman S, Shamim S, Samo KA. Spectrum of perforation peritonitis in Pakistan: 300 cases Eastern experience. World J Emerg Surg. 2008;3:31.
8. Jhobta RS, Attri AK, Kaushik R, Sharma R, Jhobta A. Spectrum of perforation peritonitis in India–review of 504 consecutive cases. World J Emerg Surg. 2006;1:26.
9. Mlwati A. Spontaneous bacterial peritonitis among patients with portal hypertension and ascitis attending Bugando Medical Centre. Tanzania. CUHAS MMed Dissertation: Mwanza; 2013.
10. Chalya PL, Mabula JB, Koy M, McHembe MD, Jaka HM, Kabangila R, et al. Clinical profile and outcome of surgical treatment of perforated peptic ulcers in Northwestern Tanzania: A tertiary hospital experience. World J Emerg Surg. 2011;6:31.

11. Chalya PL, Mabula JB, Koy M, Kataraihya JB, Jaka H, Mshana SE, et al. Typhoid intestinal perforations at a University teaching hospital in Northwestern Tanzania: A surgical experience of 104 cases in a resource-limited setting. World J Emerg Surg. 2012;7:4.
12. Mabula JB, Chalya PL, McHembe MD, Kihunrwa A, Massinde A, Chandika AB, et al. Bowel perforation secondary to illegally induced abortion: a tertiary hospital experience in Tanzania. World J Emerg Surg. 2012;7(1):29.
13. Marshall JC, Innes M. Intensive care unit management of intra-abdominal infection. Crit Care Med. 2003;31(8):2228–37.
14. Ranju S, Nishant K, Abhijit B, Homay V. Preoperative predictors of mortality in adult patients with perforation peritonitis. Indian Journal of Critical care Medicine. 2011;15(3):157–63.
15. Billing A, Frohlich D, Schildberg FW. Prediction of outcome using the Mannheim peritonitis index in 2003 patients. Peritonitis Study Group. Br J Surg. 1994;81(2):209–13.
16. Ersumo T, WM Y, Kotisso B. Perforated peptic ulcer in Tikur Anbessa Hospital: a review of 74 cases. Ethiop Med J. 2005;43(1):9–13.
17. NACP: National Guidelines for the Management of HIV and AIDS. Ministry of Health of and Social Welfare. The United Republic of Tanzania. In. Fourth edn. Dar-Es-Salaam; 2012
18. Lyamuya EF, Aboud S, Urassa WK, Sufi J, Mbwana J, Ndugulile F, et al. Evaluation of simple rapid HIV assays and development of national rapid HIV test algorithms in Dar es Salaam, Tanzania. BMC Infect Dis. 2009;9:19.
19. Wolters U, Wolf T, Stutzer H, Schroder T. ASA classification and perioperative variables as predictors of postoperative outcome. Br J Anaesth. 1996;77(2):217–22.
20. Koneman E, Allen S, Janda W, Schreckenberger PP, Lippincott PA. Color Atlas and Textbook of Diagnostic Microbiology. 5th ed. Williams & Wilkins Publishers: Lippincott; 1997.
21. Ojuka A, Ekwaro L, Kakande I. Causes and Patterns of Peritonitis at St. Francis Hospital Nsambya, Kampala-Uganda. East and Central African Journal of Surgery. 2015;19(3):99–106.
22. Fukuda N, Wada J, Niki M, Sugiyama Y, Mushiake H. Factors predicting mortality in emergency abdominal surgery in the elderly. World J Emerg Surg. 2012;7(1):12.
23. Samuel JC, Qureshi JS, Mulima G, Shores CG, Cairns BA, Charles AG. An Observational Study of the Etiology, clinical presentation and outcomes associated with peritonitis in Lilongwe, Malawi. World J Emerg Surg. 2011;6(1):37.
24. Singh R, Kumar N, Bhattacharya A, Vajifdar H. Preoperative predictors of mortality in adult patients with perforation peritonitis. Indian J Crit Care Med. 2011;15(3):157–63.
25. Mawalla B, Mshana SE, Chalya PL, Imirzalioglu C, Mahalu W. Predictors of surgical site infections among patients undergoing major surgery at Bugando Medical Centre in Northwestern Tanzania. BMC Surg. 2011;11:21.
26. Kujath P, Schwandner O, Bruch HP. Morbidity and mortality of perforated peptic gastroduodenal ulcer following emergency surgery. Langenbecks Arch Surg. 2002;387(7–8):298–302.
27. Mäkelä JT, Kiviniemi H, Ohtonen P, Laitinen SO. Factors that predict morbidity and mortality in patients with perforated peptic ulcers. European Journal of Surgery. 2002;168(8–9):446–51.
28. Giiti GC, Mazigo HD, Heukelbach J, Mahalu W. HIV, appendectomy and postoperative complications at a reference hospital in Northwest Tanzania: cross-sectional study. AIDS Res Ther. 2010;7:47.

14

Severe mutilating injuries with complex macroamputations of the upper extremity – is it worth the effort?

Katrin Stanger[1], Raymund E. Horch[2] and Adrian Dragu[3*]

Abstract

Introduction: An amputation of the upper extremity and the following replantation is still one of the most challenging operations in the field of reconstructive surgery, especially in extremely severe cases of combined mutilating macroamputations including avulsion and multilevel injuries. Specialists agree that macroamputations with sharp wound edges are an absolute indication for replantation. However, there is no agreement in disastrous cases including avulsion and multilevel injuries. The outcome of the operation is depending on several factors, including the type of accident, age and pre-existing disease of the patient, as well as time of ischemia and appropriate physical therapy.

Methods: Between January 1st 2003 and December 31st 2011 six patients underwent a macroreplantation with disastrous combined and complex injuries of the upper extremity in our department. We performed a follow up and evaluated the functional outcome of the upper extremity function using the DASH questionnaire (average follow up of 3.1 years).

Results: The mean time of ischemia was 04:50 h (02:46 h–06:17 h). The mean time for the operation was 05:30 h (01:55 h–08:20 h). The mean operations needed per patient were 7 (2–16). The average hospital stay was 29d (16–59d). According to the DASH-Score from five out of six patients the functional outcome of the replanted extremity has a mean score of 71 points. The versatility of the replanted extremity in the field of work had 95, and sport, music was assessed with a mean score of 96 points.

Conclusions: Severe and disastrous combined and complex macroamputations of the upper extremity may also have an absolute indication for replantation even though the functional outcome is poor. Not only the feeling of physical integrity can be restored, but the replantation of an amputated upper extremity enables complete or partial recovery of function and sensibility of the arm which is important for the individual. Although our results show a very high DASH-Score, those achievements justify time and person consuming operations. In most cases a replanted extremity is still superior to a secondary allotransplantation. Usually the use of prosthesis is not favored by the treated patients.

Keywords: Complex macroamputation, Avulsion, Replantation, Multiple injuries, Upper extremity, Functional outcome

Introduction

In 1914 the Austrian Ernst Jeger performed the first successful replantation of an amputated upper arm [1]. The two authors Malt and McKhann have operated successfully the first replantation of a hand with a 12 year old in 1962 [2].

Amputations of the upper extremity proximal to the radiocarpal joint or the ankle are referred to as macroamputations. Distal to these regions the amputations are specified as microamputation [3]. A macroamputation injury should be treated initially as a patient with a polytrauma [4]. An amputation of the upper extremity can be found in 0.2–3.0 % in a polytraumatized patient. In this context it is very important to differentiate between macroamputations with sharp wound edges and disastrous and severe complex cases including avulsion or

* Correspondence: adrian.dragu@sanktgeorg.de
[3]Department of Plastic and Hand Surgery, Klinikum St. Georg gGmbH, Leipzig, Germany
Full list of author information is available at the end of the article

multilevel injuries. The ischemic tolerance of the amputated part of the body depends on the content of muscle. An amputated finger tolerates a time of ischemia of up to 24 h, while a macroamputat containing a mass of muscles should not exceed a time of ischemia of more than eight hours [5].

The successful treatment of macroamputations of the upper extremity requires an expert knowledge and operating experience in the field of microsurgery [6–12]. Overall, the incidence of amputation injuries is declining due to modern safety precautions. Most accidents are industrial accidents, of which mainly work on machines with cutting surfaces and rollings can be classified as dangerous. An amputation of the upper limb results for the affected person in a significant functional, aesthetic and psychological impairment [7, 13]. Despite the impressive technical refinements of the artificial limbs the removable denture can only partially compensate for the functional limitations [13, 14]. Furthermore still the mental trauma remains due to the missing body integrity [13]. The ideal goal of revascularization or replantation of the upper extremity with the help of modern microsurgery is regaining a sensitive limb containing a protective sensibility with motorized gripping, holding and supporting function [7, 8, 13]. Due to a significantly better quality of life of these patients the indication for replantation is absolute, even with regard to higher costs, additional effort through serveral operations as well as longer postoperative care and non-productive time after reconstruction [13]. According to the current literature in up to 82 % of the affected patients a functional limb can be recuperated in macroamputations without avulsion and additional disastrous combined injuries.

The indication in favour or against the preservation of the affected upper extremity must take into account the individual circumstances of the patient and the case itself [15, 16]. As an additional support for making the decision the use of the mangled extremity scoring system "Ganga Hospital Score" first described by Shanmuganathan et al. and Rajasekaran et al. may be helpful [17, 18]. In addition the new OTA (Orthopaedic Trauma Association) open fracture classification may be of additional help [19]. On the other hand other scoring systems such as MESS ("mangled extremity scoring system") do not include any prediction regarding the functional outcome of replantation and therefore are not a validated scoring system for guidance of ampuations versus limb salvage in critical extremity injuries. "Life before limb" of course always remains a matter of principle [14, 20–22].

In case of life-threatening associated injuries of patients the replantation should be avoided or in appropriate cases (amputation of the hand or lower extremity) an interim solution can be discussed such as vascular connection to the axilla or the groin. As soon as the patient is stable enough a secondary replantation to the extremity is possible [21].

The success rate after replantation or revascularization depends on the extent of damage to the amputat, as well as the level of amputation, the soft tissue damage of the amputat and of the stump, the type and duration of ischemia, as well of the patient's age [6–8, 13, 23]. The level of amputation and the kind of trauma, as well as the patient's age seem to have the most important influences on the quality of the outcome (Table 1) [13]. All off our presented cases are mutilating severe and complex macroamputations with additional avulsion or multilevel injuries.

In the literature, the overall success rate of macroreplantationen is indicated with 76–100 % for total amputation, and indicated with 89.7 % for subtotal amputations [3, 4, 11]. Depending on the type of amputation injury the success rate for an even cutting damange injury averages 81.9 %, for localized crush injury it is 79.3 %, for amputation injuries with diffuse bruising it adds up to 87 % and for avulsion injuries it averages 68.0 % [11, 13]. With nowadays advanced strategies for replantations and microsurgical techniques for macroreplantation the exclusive claim for a viable and revascularized extremity may no longer prevail. Aspects such as functionality, aesthetics, painlessness and integration of the replanted limb into the overall picture of the patient and his profession need to be determining factors for the surgeon in deciding for the operation [9, 10, 24].

While in amputations of fingers the surgeon distinguishes between relative and absolute indications for replantation, in cases of macroamputations there is common

Table 1 Influencing factors for the functional outcomes of macroreplantations

Dependent relations of the functional outcome after macroreplantation of the upper extremity	
Therapy	-First aid at accident location
	-Transport to the hospital
	-Time of ischemia
	-Experience of the replanting team
Patient	-Diseases
	-Age
	-Compliance
	-Motivation
Amputat	-Level of amputation
	-Damage of the amputat (avulsion and/or multillevel injury)
	-Mechanism of trauma

agreement for an absolute indication for revascularization/replantation, as long as no relevant contraindications exist [21]. A relevant contraindication for example would be an unstable patient who would not survive a prolonged operation such is previewed for a replantation. Among others a warm ischemia over 12 h and a cold ischemia over 24 h, as well as a complex multilevel injury with massive destruction of amputated limb counts as a contraindications for replantation [10, 21, 22]. Some authors propagate, that only the amputated limb, which has the prospect of a successful revascularization, and obtaining a partial function of the limb should be chosen to operate on [12]. These authors say that a loose-hanging, functionless replanted limb is of no use to the patient and may lead to secondary request for amputation [7]. On the other side a subjective evaluation of results after replantation shows a high degree of bonding between the patient and his reconstructed limb no matter how the functional outcome is [25].

For the upper limb, in contrast to the lower limb the secondary amputation is an absolute exception [13]. The review of the literature reports an incidence of 2.5–8 % of affected patients. Obviously the artificial replacement of the upper limb with a prosthesis is only tolerated in only 20 to maximum 50 % of the cases. A situation of chronic pain is reported to occur in 5–10 % of the patients [13].

Technical aspects

Intraoperative management

One of the most important operational steps is the primary debridement of necrotic tissue [14, 8, 23]. This includes in the "zone of injury" not only the radical removal of foreign bodies and contaminations, but also involves the debridement of non-vital muscle, as well as the shortening of the fractured bone in the area of injury [7]. This is eminent to avoid postoperative infections caused by non-vital and necrotic structures. After debridement the decision for vascular, nervous or tendon grafts for a tension-free reconstruction can be determined. A stable and definitive bone fixation is desirable in primary care [21]. Macroamputations should primarily be fixed with plates and screws. An external fixation is advisable in complicated interjoint bony fractures with extensive debris zone [7]. After the treatment of the bone the tendon suture, the arterial and venous vascular suture and at last the nerve suture stands in line.

Due to the massive swelling of the almost always expected reperfusion injury and possible expansion of the demarcation zone, a complex soft tissue reconstruction as primary treatment is not indicated in most cases. Therefore a temporary coverage of the soft tissue with a negative pressure system is highly recommended. It enables further debridements in case of progressing necrosis as well as the final secondary soft tissue coverage under detumescent conditions later on [21, 23]. An initial adequate bony debridement with appropriate shortening of the bone may avoid the use of vascular, nervous or tendon grafts. In any case, the primary treatment is crucial for a good functional result. If tension-free sutures are not possible, the indication for a graft should always be made generously. The target is to reconstruct two veins for each reconstructed artery [7]. The compartments of the upper limb, the carpal tunnel as well as the Loge de Guyon should be split in order to avoid a postoperative compartment syndrome [26]. The two most common reasons for the failure of a replantation are the muscle necrosis and subsequent an infection, both can lead to a postoperative increasing swelling and thrombosis of the reconstructed vessels. It is therefore advisable to schedule the patient for a second look 48–72 h postoperatively in order to evaluate the viability of the soft tissues. An amputation of the upper extremity can lead to massive blood loss. The necessity for blood transfusion should be recognized timely [9].

Postoperative management

Ensuring a successful replantation depends on a stringent postoperative management [7]. After surgery, the hand has to be checked every hour for 72 h. The color of the skin of replanted extremity, the turgor, the vascular refill and temperature are crucial criteria. A closure of the arteries or veins, caused by a thrombus or due to severe swelling (compartment syndrome) should be diagnosed in time for early revision. A compartment syndrome, including swelling of the soft tissues or a hematoma may induce an increase of pressure, which can lead to hypoperfusion of the replanted extremity. Already the suspicion for a compartment syndrome should alert the surgeon to indicate an emergency revision.

An axillary plexus is ideally provided for the patient right from the beginning. The early sympatholysis is recommended for postoperative pain therapy and as well as a prophylaxe for developing an algodystrophy. The limb should be put up on a soft surface to reduce the swelling. Immobilization is achieved by a splint, which should be very loose at the beginning to avoid any pressure sores.

The level of hemoglobin should be monitored daily during the first postoperative days. A pre- and intraoperative blood loss can make a blood transfusion indispensable. A rapid drop of the hemoglobin may indicate the formation of a hematoma. Likewise the parameters myoglobin and creatine kinase should be monitored daily. Through the trauma and surgery large parts of the muscle are often bruised and injured, so the level of myoglobin may be increased. The clinical image of a crush kidney is likely to occur, which can lead to acute renal failure [7, 21]. Therefore the patient should be sufficiently provided with water in order to flush the kidneys. A urinary catheter is recommended to monitor the urine concentration and the excretion. Right from the beginning as well as in the medium and long-term postoperative follow-up an interdisciplinary psychosomatic should be initiated. The loss of a large body limbs is not only a significant turning point in the perception of the body, but also in the mental status. For the long term success of a replantation a well trained and experienced team is essential. Trained nursing staff, physiotherapists and occupational therapists, pain specialists and psychiatrists, as well as an experienced orthopaedic technicians should be part of this team. The rehabilitation is long, time consuming, costly and stressful [10, 27]. The patients should be attached to the clinic for many years. A regular follow-up by all members of the team, usually over years, is extremely important for the rehabilitation of the extremity into the overall picture of the patient and into the everyday life and work. Follow-up operations like arthrodesis, resection of a pseudarthrosis, a tenolysis or a nerve or tendon reconstruction may be necessary. Often the removal of metal, an improvement of a scar, a resection of a neuroma or a motoric reconstruction is required [7].

The affected patients should be informed that the replanted limb rarely achieves fully pretraumatic function. However, the possible achievable results are superior to any stump with subsequent prosthetic fitting or even secondary orthotropic transplantation with long life immunosuppressive therapy.

The functional outcome of a replantation depends on the level of amputation, the type of injury, the duration of ischemia, the sex and age of the patient, concomitant diseases, as well as on the existing noxious substances such as nicotine and alcohol consumption and the motivation of the patient. In particular the age of the patient appears to be of great importance for the possible functional outcome [6, 8, 28].

The ideal purpose of a limb replantation of the upper extremity is to achieve a sensitive extremity with motor function which contains gripping, holding and supporting function. If these achievements seem to be unrealistic, the indication for a replantation should be made very critically in each individual case [13]. However, even in disastrous cases with additional avulsion and multilevel injuries the patient may benefit from a replantation even though it is from the very beginning evident that the functional outcome may be poor. Such an assessment can only be made in a center of replantation. Still, if a replantation is possible, it should be the primary approach. The patient and the family should be informed that in case of a loss of the replanted limb the challenge of an orthotropic cadaver transplantation is possible. Therefore a lifelong immunosuppression is mandatory with possible severe systemic consequences. Only few long-term results are available regarding the immunosuppressive effect in replanted limbs [29, 30]. The initial higher costs, caused by the complex and interdisciplinary treatment have to be confronted with the benefits of a possible reintegration into the work and social life. An unemployed and socially isolated patient can cause significantly higher long-term costs for society. Therefore, we also believe from an economic point of view, that the replantation even in disastrous cases seems to be favorable [13].

Functional outcome

Upper arm

In patients with an amputation at the level of the upper arm securing the thoracohumeral pliers function, as well as active elbow flexion should be one of the principal achievements of therapy. Only the active elbow flexion allows the patient bimanual function of the hand.

Lower arm and wrist

At the forearm level the functional outcome depends mainly on the condition of the muscles in the proximal third and the quality of the reconstructed nerve [11]. The preservation of the wrist and adequate finger movement as well as the protective sensibility of the hand should be the principal achievements. According to the literature a functional limb can be restored in up to 41 % of the cases [11, 13]. In case of recovery of the grip function of the hand a power loss of up to 20–55 % compared to the contralateral non-injured side needs to be expected [27]. Often there is no regeneration of the intrinsic hand muscles, which may result in difficulties with fine mechanical work [27]. At this level of amputation about 20 % of the patients achieve a static two-point discrimination of <8 mm [27]. Regarding the functional results, a significant decline with increasing trauma, such as contusions or avulsions, multilevel injuries and age of the patient, must be expected. In addition to functional limitation such as ankylosis, capsulodesis, tenodesis, formation of a neuroma and lack of nerve regeneration may occur in over 20 %. In order to assess the function of the replanted limb German DASH questionnaire (Disability of Arm, Shoulder, Hand) can be used. The questionnaire measures the current subjective perception of the patient [31]. The patient himself assesses whether he meets the expected requirements according to rehabilitation and social reintegration. The assessment of functional impairment is calculated by the total score of the questions and the bandwidth of the questionnaire. A score of 0 represents a complete function without disability and a score of 100 an upper extremity without any function at all [31].

Role of the age in macroreplantation

The functional outcome of a replantation of the upper limb is closely related to the age of the patient [14, 32].

The results of this study, using the DASH questionnaire, show that replantation of the upper limb were technically possible for the patients in the group >50 years, but the functional result turned out to be worse in the group >50 years than in the group of patients <50 years.

Patients and methods

In the period from January 1st 2003 and December 31st 2011 six patients were replanted in our department after total or subtotal disastrous and complex macroamputation including additional injuries such as avulsion or multilevel injuries of the upper extremity. All patients have been treated by 4 senior plastic surgeons working in the same department with a standardized microsurgical treatment protocol. The only major changes within this period have been the implementation of new techniqual devices, e.g. new microscope or new microsurgical instruments. This retrospective clinical evaluation was approved by the local ethics committee of the University Hospital of Erlangen. The amputation was once at the level of the upper arm, once at the level of the elbow, three times the forearm was affected and once the wrist. All six patients were male. The average age was 49 years (25–73 years). Four patients had an accident at work, two of the patients were already pensioners who had an accident while performing private domestic work (Table 2). The accidents happened as followed: one patient had a smooth cut injury, one a convulsion injury, in three patients an avulsion injury was present with severe bruising and additional complex injuries of the amputated limb, one patient suffered a multilevel injury, a convulsion and avulsion injury of the forearm in addition to the amputation of three fingers (Fig. 1a–f).

Results

Five of the six disastrous and complex macroamputations were replanted successfully. In one of the patients the replanted limb needed to be amputated at the level of the middle third of the forearm. The operation was followed by an implantation of a vascular AV-loop, which allowed covering the defect with a free rectus flap and splitting skin graft to obtain as much length of the stump as possible. None of the patients wanted a secondary amputation of the replanted limb. The time of cold ischemia was < 7 h in all patients. A stable plate fixation was applied with adequate soft tissue coverage in 2 of 6 cases. In 4 of 6 cases the fracture was treated with an external fixator. The patient who received a re-amputation later on, was initially scheduled for an arthrodesis of the elbow by external fixator. Two patients received a wrist arthrodesis primarily; one of them got in addition an arthrodesis of a metacarpo-trapezium joint. In 5 of these patients a debridement and shortening of the bone between 2–4 cm was necessary. In 3 of 6 patients vascular grafts were used. Three times the artery was reconstructed and four times the vein. In all patients, a residual soft tissue defect was initially covered temporarily with a negative pressure dressing. After the swelling significantly reduced the residual soft tissue defect could be covered with a split skin graft.

The mean average time of cold ischemia of the amputated limb, calculated from the time of the accident until the restoration of the arterial circulation, was 4:50 h (2:46 h–06:17 h). The operation lasted an average of 5:30 h (1:55–08:20 h). While the patients were hospitalized each of them received 7 operations (2–16) till the day of discharge. One patient required three days postoperatively a re-amputation of the replanted limb as well as a debridement of necrotic tissue due to vascular congestion. The operation was followed by several

Table 2 Overview of the 6 presented patients from 2003–2011

Patient	Sex	Age (years)	Level of Amputation	Industrial accident	Time of ischemia	Operating time (h)	Number of operations	Time of hospitalization (days)	Job before → after replantation
1	m	70	Elbow	n	03:29	01:55 h	16	59	Retired
2	m	25	Distal third of the upper arm	y	05:51	05:05 h	10	30	Truck driver → wholesaler
3	m	73	Wrist	n	05:46	04:58 h	4	31	Retired
4	m	26	Distal lower arm	y	06:17	08:20 h	5	17	Occupational retraining mechanic → Computer technician
5	m	40	Proximal lower arm	y	02:46	05:33 h	2	16	Metalworker, up-to-date: rehabilitation
6	m	62	Middle lower arm	y	04:13	04:52 h	3	23	Locksmith, retired earlier

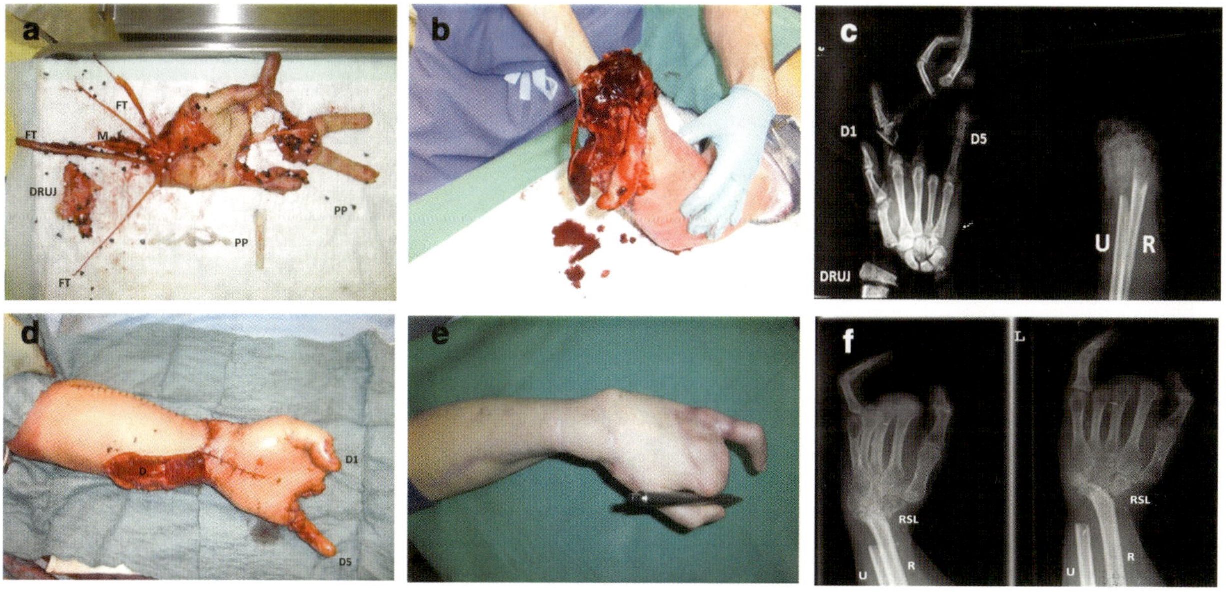

Fig. 1 **a**: Amputated left hand of a 26 year old male at the level of the wrist preoperatively with a multilevel and avulsion injury through a plastic pellet machine. It shows additional subtotal amputation of the index finger and complete amputation of the middle- and ringfinger. The thumb was not injured; the little finger had a radial soft tissue defect. (PP) = black/white plastic pallets. (DRUJ) = distal radioular joint. (FT) = Flexor tendons. (M) = N. medianus. **b**: Preoperative situation of the stump of the distal forearm of the same 26 year old male. **c**: X-Rays of the left lower upper extremity and the left amputated amputated hand. (D1) = digit 1. (D5) = digit 5. The left picture shows a complete fracture of the distal radius and the distal ulna, with the distal radio ulnar joint lying transverse (DRUJ). The right picture shows the lower upper extremity with a fracture of the radius (R) and the ulna (U). **d**: Replanted hand postoperatively: thumb (D1) and little finger (D5) could be preserved, the index, middle and ringfinger were not re-plantable, the remaining defect (D) was temporarily covered by a negative pressure wound dressing and in a second operation 5 days later covered with split-skin-grafts. **e**: Replanted hand 9 months postoperatively: the patient is able to perform minimal flexion and adduction of the thumb in order to grip objects. **f**: X-Ray of the replanted hand 9 months postoperatively. (U) = ulna. (R) = radius. (RSL) = atypical RSL-arthrodesis of the left wrist

interventions including a vascular loop and later on a free rectus flap with split skin graft in order to cover the defect and keep the length of the limb. One patient received three days after the initial treatment a free latissimus dorsi flap to cover the soft tissue defect of the forearm. An opening of the compartment had to be conducted twice. During follow-up procedures eight re-osteosynthesis were necessary, 13 times a changing of the negative pressure dressing was required, seven split-thickness skin grafts were transplanted, one arteriolysis, one neurolysis, one arthrolysis, seven removals of osthesyntheses materials and one resection of a pseudarthrosis was conducted. In another patient a scar contracture of the elbow was resolved which required subsequently free anterolateral thigh flap 14 months after the trauma. The average time of hospitalization right after the trauma was 29 days (16–59 days).

All six patients received rehabilitation after dismissal. Two patients received inpatient rehabilitation for six weeks and received subsequently outpatient physical therapy and occupational therapy for 18 weeks. Another patient was four weeks in outpatient rehabilitation, followed by seven months of outpatient physical therapy and occupational therapy. Due to severe pain this patient needed to be treated four weeks in a hospital. One patient received outpatient physiotherapy exercising for nine months after discharge from the clinic. Two patients performed inpatient rehabilitation for 9 months.

The average follow-up time was 3.1 years (max 8 years min. 9 months). Two patients were already pensioners before the accident. Two patients had trained for a new job and are back to 100 % operational work. One patient was in the retraining for his former profession. One patient retired earlier.

Five of the six presented patients had completed the DASH questionnaire. For Part 1, in which the patient assesses the functioning of the replanted limb, the average of points was 71 (SD ± 13). For Part 2, in which the patient assesses the applicability of his replanted hand for work, sports and music the mean was 95 points (SD ± 10) and 96 points (SD ± 5).

All five patients were complaining about chronic pain in the area of replanted limb at time of the follow-up. Two of them mentioned moderate pain and three of them severe pain (Visual Analog Scale, VAS). Two stated that they regularly need pain medication; three said they take pain medication as needed.

All 6 treated patients mentioned that even looking back they had not preferred a primary stump, especially not the older patients with significantly higher functional limitations.

Discussion

An amputation of the upper extremity and the following replantation is still one of the most challenging operations in the field of reconstructive surgery, especially in extremely severe cases of combined mutilating macroamputations including avulsion and multilevel injuries [8, 12]. Specialists agree that macroamputations with sharp wound edges are an absolute indication for replantation. However, there is no agreement in disastrous cases including avulsion and multilevel injuries. In these cases the chances for a good functional outcome are usually low as the outcome depends on several factors such as the type of accident and injury, the age and preexisting disease of the patient, as well as time of ischemia and compliance. In all cases however, the reconstruction or the replantation of a limb is secondary in severely injured patients "at risk" e.g. for traumatic-hemorrhagic shock, severe brain injuries, chest trauma or other acute life threatening injuries. In these cases, "life before limb" is the most important aspect of the interdisciplinary treatment plan and a contraindication for lengthy replant or even reconstructive procedures [33].

The presented cases show, that even in severe and disastrous combined and complex macroamputations of the upper extremity, there may be an absolute indication for replantation. Even though the functional outcome may be poor due to the severe and complex injuries, most patients may benefit due to other e.g. psychological effects. Not only the feeling of physical integrity can be restored, but the replantation of an amputated upper extremity enables complete or partial recovery of function and sensibiliy of the arm which is important for the individual. Although our results show a very high DASH-Score, those achievements justify in several cases time and person consuming operations. Due to the retrospective study design and the treatment of 4 senior plastic surgeons on 6 patients, the presented data has a poor evidence level. However, we believe that every clinical data for this very small and severely injured patient group may help to reevaluate our interdisciplinary treatment strategies.

A replanted extremity is still superior to a secondary allotransplantation. Cases of an allogeneic transplantation of the upper extremity of a brain-dead donor have been published and discussed on a global basis. Worldwide 41 hands and two fingers in 32 patients were transplanted allogeneic between 1998 and 2008 [29, 30]. The time between amputation and transplantation varied from six months up to 35 years. Allogeneic limb transplantation needs to be regard as an organ transplant and therefore has immunogenicity [29, 30]. Therefore, several different acting immunosuppressive drugs must be taken a lifetime to prevent rejection. The immunosuppressive therapy in combination with antiviral and antibacterial drugs can lead to infection, arterial hypertension, diabetes mellitus, to liver and kidney failure, and an increased risk of developing certain types of cancer [30]. In two cases of the above mentioned 41 transplanted hands a secondary amputation was necessary. Therefore the indication for an allogeneic transplantation should be made very cautiously. The patient and his family must be informed in detail about the long intense time of recovery, as well as the risks and side effects of lifelong immunosuppressive therapy [30].

Even the use of prosthesis is in most cases not favored by the treated patients [13]. The technique of myoelectric prostheses is nowadays very advanced, so in case of a stump a prosthesis could be an alternative. With the help of electrodes, which detect the muscle activity in the stump, electric motors are driven, which can control the hand grip and rotation movements of the hand and the elbow. The disadvantages of prostheses are the heavy weight, and the higher price compared to the cosmetic prosthesis. An intense training can convert the prosthesis to a very useful tool in everyday life. In addition, the prosthesis is often superior to the replanted upper extremity from an aesthetic point of view. According to the literature the artificial replacement of the upper limb with a prosthesis is tolerated in only 20 to maximum 50 % of the cases [13].

Finally, despite the scientific achievements in the field of tissue engineering and experimental ex vivo perfusion of tissue at the present time there is no clinical applicability for replantation surgery [34–36]. Therefore, such severe injuries are best treated in the hands of experienced trauma and emergency surgeons with knowledge on the field of microsurgery [37].

Conclusion

The presented cases show, that even in severe and disastrous combined and complex macroamputations of the upper extremity, there may be an absolute indication for replantation. The results of the DASH-Score in our patients are rather poor due to the severe and complex macroamputations including avulsion and multilevel injuries. Nevertheless all patients assure the usefulness of the replanted limb in their daily life. Although they cannot use the arm for very highly motoric movements, like playing an instrument with the hand and although they are highly limited with fine motoric movements in daily life, the limb seems be very helpful for them when it comes to gripping, holding and supporting function. The replanted limb gives them support in various daily requirements such as opening of doors. One patient mentioned that the limb is necessary for him to keep his body balance while he is walking or swimming.

The feeling of a still preserved sufficient physical integrity of a patient as well as the sensitive and significant functional advantages of replanted limb in comparison to dentures, justify the indication for a limb replantation with an enormous equipment and personal effort [10, 24]. After a realistic explanation of the functional prognosis of a formerly severely and complex injured replanted limb, the indication for replantation should not be limited by the age of the patient or the disastrous damage of tissue including avulsion and multilevel injuries, but by the patient's individual needs and wishes and the individual motivation to restore the physical integrity.

Statement

All three authors have read and complied with the instructions to authors and in particular the policy of our journal on ethical consent and standards of animal care.

Competing interests

The authors declare that they have no competing interests.

Authors' contribution

All authors declare that they performed essential work for this manuscript. KS performed the drafting and the acquisition of data. REH carried out the design and the revision of the manuscript and performed some of the operations. AD performed the drafting, the conception and design of the manuscript. In addition he performed some of the operations. All authors read and approved the final manuscript.

Author details

[1]Department of Plastic and Hand Surgery, OKM Orthopädische Klinik Markgröningen gGmbH, Markgröningen, Germany. [2]Department of Plastic and Hand Surgery, University Hospital of Erlangen, Friedrich-Alexander-University Erlangen-Nürnberg, Erlangen, Germany. [3]Department of Plastic and Hand Surgery, Klinikum St. Georg gGmbH, Leipzig, Germany.

References

1. Jeger E. Die Chirurgie der Blutgefäße und des Herzens. Berlin: Springer; 1913.
2. Rich RH, Knight PJ, Erickson EL, Broadhurst K, Leonard AS. Replantation of the upper extremity in children. J Pediatr Surg. 1977;12(6):1027–32.
3. O'Brien BM. Replantation and reconstructive microvascular surgery. Part I. Ann R Coll Surg Engl. 1976;58(2):87–103.
4. Upton J, Littler JW, Eaton RG. Primary care of the injured hand, part 2. Postgrad Med. 1979;66(2):127–31.
5. Delhey P, Huber S, Hanschen M, Haberle S, Trentzsch H, Deiler S et al. Significance of Traumatic Macroamputation in Severely Injured Patients—An Analysis of the TraumaRegister DGU (R). Shock. 2014. doi:10.1097/SHK.0000000000000292.
6. Baumgartner RF. The surgery of arm and forearm amputations. Orthop Clin North Am. 1981;12(4):805–17.
7. Beris AE, Lykissas MG, Korompilias AV, Mitsionis GI, Vekris MD, Kostas-Agnantis IP. Digit and hand replantation. Arch Orthop Trauma Surg. 2010;130(9):1141–7. doi:10.1007/s00402-009-1021-7.
8. Leclere FM, Mathys L, Juon B, Franz T, Unglaub F, Vogelin E. Macroreplantations of the upper extremity: a series of 11 patients. Arch Orthop Trauma Surg. 2012;132(12):1797–805. doi:10.1007/s00402-012-1590-8.
9. Prichayudh S, Verananvattna A, Sriussadaporn S, Sriussadaporn S, Kritayakirana K, Pak-art R, et al. Management of upper extremity vascular injury: outcome related to the Mangled Extremity Severity Score. World J Surg. 2009;33(4):857–63. doi:10.1007/s00268-008-9902-4.
10. Syrko M, Jablecki J. Quality of life-oriented evaluation of late functional results of hand replantation. Ortop Traumatol Rehabil. 2010;12(1):19–27.
11. Tamai S. Twenty years' experience of limb replantation–review of 293 upper extremity replants. J Hand Surg [Am]. 1982;7(6):549–56.
12. Wilhelmi BJ, Lee WP, Pagenstert GI, May Jr JW. Replantation in the mutilated hand. Hand Clin. 2003;19(1):89–120.
13. Hierner R, Berger A, Brenner P. Considerations on the management of subtotal and total macro-amputation of the upper extremity. Unfallchirurg. 1998;101(3):184–92.
14. Gabl M, Kropfl A. Subjective impairment after macroamputation of the upper extremity. Handchir Mikrochir Plast Chir. 2008;40(1):31–4. doi:10.1055/s-2007-989428.
15. Liang K, Zhong G, Yin J, Xiang Z, Cen S, Huang F. Cross-arm replantation for traumatic bilateral upper extremity amputations: a case report. Arch Orthop Trauma Surg. 2011;131(2):157–61. doi:10.1007/s00402-010-1112-5.
16. Ozcelik IB, Mersa B, Kabakas F, Sacak B, Kuvat SV. Crossover replantation as a salvage procedure following bilateral transhumeral upper limb amputation: a case report. Arch Orthop Trauma Surg. 2011;131(4):567–72. doi:10.1007/s00402-010-1217-x.
17. Rajasekaran S, Naresh Babu J, Dheenadhayalan J, Shetty AP, Sundararajan SR, Kumar M, et al. A score for predicting salvage and outcome in Gustilo type-IIIA and type-IIIB open tibial fractures. J Bone Joint Surg (Br). 2006;88(10):1351–60. doi:10.1302/0301-620X.88B10.17631.
18. Shanmuganathan R. The utility of scores in the decision to salvage or amputation in severely injured limbs. Indian J Orthop. 2008;42(4):368–76. doi:10.4103/0019-5413.43371.
19. Orthopaedic Trauma Association. Open Fracture Study G. A new classification scheme for open fractures. J Orthop Trauma. 2010;24(8):457–64. doi:10.1097/BOT.0b013e3181c7cb6b.
20. Drueckе D, Homann HH, Kutscha Lissberg F, Schinkel C, Steinau HU. Crossover extremity transfers. Limb salvage in amputations with segmental defects. Chirurg. 2007;78(10):954–8. doi:10.1007/s00104-006-1302-4.
21. Schadel-Hopfner M, Siebert H. Operative strategies for hand injuries in multiple trauma. A systematic review of the literature. Unfallchirurg. 2005;108(10):850–7. doi:10.1007/s00113-005-0996-y.
22. Schaller P, Geldmacher J. Hand injury in polytrauma. A retrospective study of 782 cases. Handchir Mikrochir Plast Chir. 1994;26(6):307–12.
23. Vanstraelen P, Papini RP, Sykes PJ, Milling MA. The functional results of hand replantation. The Chepstow experience. J Hand Surg (Br). 1993;18(5):556–64.
24. Unglaub F, Demir E, Von Reim R, Van Schoonhoven J, Hahn P. Long-term functional and subjective results of thumb replantation. Microsurgery. 2006;26(8):552–6. doi:10.1002/micr.20287.
25. Durham RM, Mistry BM, Mazuski JE, Shapiro M, Jacobs D. Outcome and utility of scoring systems in the management of the mangled extremity. Am J Surg. 1996;172(5):569–73. doi:10.1016/S0002-9610(96)00245-0. discussion 73–4.
26. Dragu A, Schnurer S, Surmann-Schmitt C, Unglaub F, Kneser U, Horch RE. Expression of HIF-1alpha in ischemia and reperfusion in human microsurgical free muscle tissue transfer. Plast Reconstr Surg. 2011;127(6):2293–300. doi:10.1097/PRS.0b013e318213a01f.
27. Russell RC, O'Brien BM, Morrison WA, Pamamull G, MacLeod A. The late functional results of upper limb revascularization and replantation. J Hand Surg [Am]. 1984;9(5):623–33.
28. Deubel U, Germann G. Micro – and macroreplantation of the upper and lower extremity. Aktuelle Traumatol. 1994;24(7):247–54.
29. Machens HG. [The First Bilateral Arm Transplantation in the Klinikum rechts der Isar, Technische Universitat Munchen.]. Handchir Mikrochir Plast Chir. 2008. doi:10.1055/s-2008-1038946.
30. Piza-Katzer H, Wechselberger G, Estermann D, Gabl M, Arora R, Hussl H. Ten years of hand transplantation experiment or routine? Handchir Mikrochir Plast Chir. 2009;41(4):210–6. doi:10.1055/s-0029-1225628.
31. Germann G, Wind G, Harth A. The DASH (Disability of Arm-Shoulder-Hand) Questionnaire—a new instrument for evaluating upper extremity

treatment outcome. Handchir Mikrochir Plast Chir. 1999;31(3):149–52. doi:10.1055/s-1999-13902.
32. Biemer E. Reimplantation of fingers and limb parts. Technics and results. Chirurg. 1977;48(6):353–9.
33. Stahel PF, Smith WR, Moore EE. Current trends in resuscitation strategy for the multiply injured patient. Injury. 2009;40 Suppl 4:S27–35. doi:10.1016/j.injury.2009.10.034.
34. Constantinescu MA, Knall E, Xu X, Kiermeir DM, Jenni H, Gygax E, et al. Preservation of amputated extremities by extracorporeal blood perfusion; a feasibility study in a porcine model. J Surg Res. 2011;171(1):291–9. doi:10.1016/j.jss.2010.01.040.
35. Merz K, Schweizer R, Schlosser S, Giovanoli P, Erni D, Plock JA. Distinct microhemodynamic efficacy of arteriogenesis and angiogenesis in critically ischemic skin flaps. Microvasc Res. 2012;83(2):249–56. doi:10.1016/j.mvr.2011.10.005.
36. Polykandriotis E, Popescu LM, Horch RE. Regenerative medicine: then and now—an update of recent history into future possibilities. J Cell Mol Med. 2010;14(10):2350–8. doi:10.1111/j.1582-4934.2010.01169.x.
37. Kruger A, Florido C, Braunisch A, Walther E, Yilmaz TH, Doll D. Penetrating arterial trauma to the limbs: outcome of a modified protocol. World J Emerg Surg. 2013;8(1):51. doi:10.1186/1749-7922-8-51.

15

Wells criteria for DVT is a reliable clinical tool to assess the risk of deep venous thrombosis in trauma patients

Shrey Modi[2], Ryan Deisler[2], Karen Gozel[1], Patty Reicks[1], Eric Irwin[1], Melissa Brunsvold[2], Kaysie Banton[1,2] and Greg J. Beilman[1,2*]

Abstract

Background: Deep Vein Thrombosis (DVT) is a common complication in trauma patients. Venous duplex surveillance is used widely for the diagnosis of DVT, however, there is controversy concerning its appropriate use. The Wells criterion is a clinically validated scoring system in an outpatient setting, but its use in trauma patients has not been studied. This study evaluated the application of the Wells scoring system in trauma population.

Methods: Wells scores were calculated retrospectively for all patients who were admitted to the trauma service and underwent Venous Duplex Scanning (VDS) at the author's institution between 2012 and 2013. Correlation of Wells score with DVT and its efficacy in risk stratifying the patients after trauma was analyzed using linear correlation and receiver operating characteristic (ROC) curve. Sensitivity and specificity of Wells score in ruling out or ruling in DVT were calculated in various risk groups.

Results: Of 298 patients evaluated, 18 (6 %) patients were positive for DVT. A linear correlation was present between Wells score and DVT with $R^2 = 0.88$ ($p = 0.0016$). Median Wells score of patients without DVT was 1 (1–3) compared to a median score of 2 (1–5) in those with DVT ($p < 0.0001$). In low risk patients (scores <1), Wells scoring was able to rule out the possibility of DVT with a sensitivity of 100 % and NPV of 100 %, while in moderate-high risk patients (scores ≥2), it was able to predict DVT with a specificity of 90 %. Area under ROC curve was 0.859 ($p < 0.0001$) demonstrating the accuracy of Wells scoring system for DVT risk stratification in post trauma patients.

Conclusions: A Wells score of <1 can reliably rule out the possibility of DVT in the trauma patients. Risk of developing DVT correlates linearly with Wells score, establishing it as a valid pretest tool for risk stratification.

Keywords: DVT risk assessment, Wells score, Trauma patients

Background

Venous thromboembolism (VTE), comprising of deep vein thrombosis (DVT) and pulmonary embolism (PE), is the third leading cause of death in hospitalized trauma patients, with an estimated incidence of 5–20 % with prophylaxis [1–3]. This wide range in incidence of VTE is attributed to variability in patients' risk factors, choice of prophylaxis and modalities of screening and detection of VTE [1, 4]. Thromboprophylaxis in trauma patients is complex for many reasons, one of them being the presence of an early coagulopathy present in 25 % of trauma patients at the time of admission [5], which is further complicated by hypo-perfusion, acidosis and resuscitative measures [4, 6]. This coagulopathy shifts to a pro-thrombotic state early after traumatic injury necessitating thromboembolism prophylaxis. Additionally, these patients have a high bleeding risk associated with the use of anticoagulants and limitation of use of compression devices due to extremity injuries [7]. DVT has been chosen as an important indicator of quality of care and pay for performance criteria, with an underlying assumption that all DVTs are preventable with appropriate detection and prophylaxis [8]. This has led to an

* Correspondence: beilman@umn.edu
[1]North Memorial Medical Center, Robbinsdale, MN, USA
[2]Department of Surgery, University of Minnesota Medical Center, Minneapolis, MN, USA

increased use of duplex ultrasound scanning for DVT in asymptomatic trauma patients, which may not be cost efficient or at times effective in preventing clinically relevant VTEs in a subset of these patients [7, 9]. Furthermore, there is immense variability in the utilization of duplex ultrasound screening among various trauma centers in the National Trauma Data Base (NTDB) [8]. Currently, screening is suggested for patients who are at high risk of developing DVT and have received suboptimal or no thromboprophylaxis. There are, however multiple opinions on what factors define a high risk trauma patient [1, 8] or what constitutes an optimal regimen for use in screening or prophylaxis against DVTs. Given this clinical dilemma, a means of increasing the pretest probability of screening algorithms is needed to optimize DVT detection and cost-effectiveness. Multiple tools are available to identify high-risk patients in the outpatient setting such as Wells Score, Geneva Score, Minaiti Score and Charlotte rule, of which the Wells score with its modification is the most widely used and accepted scoring system [10–12].

The aim of the current study was to evaluate if the Wells criteria for DVT (Table 1) [13] could be applied to the trauma population and aid clinicians in detection of DVTs.

Methods

This study was conducted at a Level I trauma center following review and approval by the North Memorial Institutional Review Board. All patients admitted to the trauma service at the authors' institution from January 2012 to July 2013 who underwent venous duplex scanning (VDS) were retrospectively identified. A standardized venous thromboembolism prophylaxis protocol using sequential compression devices, and early mobilization was followed for all patients admitted to the trauma service. Additionally, routine enoxaparin (or alternative anticoagulation) was started on post admission day 1 in patients determined to be at high risk for VTE, except when contraindicated. High risk patients are defined in our protocol as having one or more of these risk factors: spinal cord injury, traumatic brain injury, complex pelvic fractures, patients requiring multiple surgeries, solid organ injury, major venous injury, immobility >72 h, previous history of VTE and cancer.

Table 1 Wells criteria for the prediction of deep vein thrombosis (DVT)[a]

Clinical Characteristic	Score
Active cancer (patient either receiving treatment for cancer within the previous 6 months or currently receiving palliative treatment)	1
Paralysis, paresis, or recent cast immobilization of the lower extremities	1
Recently bedridden for ≥ 3 days, or major surgery within the previous 12 weeks requiring general or regional anesthesia	1
Localized tenderness along the distribution of the deep venous system	1
Entire leg swelling	1
Calf swelling at least 3 cm larger than that on the asymptomatic side (measured 10 cm below tibial tuberosity)	1
Pitting edema confined to the symptomatic leg	1
Collateral superficial veins (non-varicose)	1
Previously documented deep vein thrombosis	1
Alternative diagnosis at least as likely as deep vein thrombosis	-2

[a] Wells scoring system for DVT: -2 to 0: low probability, 1 to 2 points: Moderate probability, 3 to 8 points: high probability

VDS was performed on iU22 xMATRIX Ultrasound System (Philips Healthcare, Andover, MA), by trained ultrasound technologists. The diagnosis of DVT was based on final VDS reporting and classified as positive or negative.

The Wells score for each patient was calculated on the day of duplex ultrasound by a blinded reviewer (critical care fellow) based on a retrospective chart review of clinical symptoms and patient history factors from physicians', nurses' and other medical personnel notes. Wells score was calculated using Mdcalc.com's online calculator. Descriptive statistics and associations of the Wells score with incidence of DVT were calculated for the cohort. To calculate the sensitivity, specificity, positive predictive value (PPV) and negative predictive value (NPV) of the Wells scoring criteria, cut-off scores of 1 for low probability and cut-off scores of 2 for moderate and higher probability were used. The receiver operating characteristic (ROC) curve was analyzed and area under ROC curve (AUROCC) was used as a performance marker of the Wells scoring system in risk stratifying the trauma population.

Statistical analysis was performed using GraphPad Prism 6 (GraphPad Software Inc. La Jolla, CA). The statistical significance between proportions was determined by Chi-Square test, Mann-Whitney *U* test was used for ISS and Wells scores, correlation was calculated using Pearson *r* and coefficient of determination R^2, and an unpaired *t*-test was used for the rest.

Results

A total of 2712 patients were admitted to the trauma service at the authors' institution during the specified time period. Of these patients, the cohort consisted of 298 trauma patients, who underwent VDS for DVT evaluation. The median injury severity score of the cohort was 17 (1–66) and the median age was 58 (18–96) years. There were 197 (66 %) males and 101 (34 %) females in the cohort with a mean length of stay (LOS) of

13.5 days in the hospital and 6 days in the Intensive Care Unit (ICU) respectively. Of the 298 patients studied, a total of 18 patients (6 %) were positive for DVT. Wells score was used to define each patient's probability of developing DVT, patients were assigned a score and then categorized: -2 to 0 points: low probability, 1 to 2 points as moderate probability, and 3 to 8 points as high probability. When stratified into the above-mentioned categories, the incidence of DVT was found to be 0 % in low probability, 7.3 % in moderate probability and 66.6 % in high probability patients (Fig. 1a). There were no significant differences in the injury severity scores (ISS), age or sex between the patients developing DVT vs. those with no DVT. Median Wells score of patients without DVT was 1(1–3) compared to a median score of 2 (1–5) in those with DVT (*p* <0.0001) (Fig. 1b). The characteristics of the cohort are provided in Table 2.

Further analysis revealed that patients with Wells score ≤ 1 had a relative risk (RR) of developing DVT of 0.075 [95 % confidence interval (CI): 0.03–0.19], while the RR of patients with Wells score of 2, 3, and 4 were 13.3 (95 % CI: 5.5–33.3), 13.9 (95 % CI: 6.5–29.8) and, 18.5 (95 % CI: 11.5–29.8) respectively. There was a strong linear correlation between Wells score and incidence of DVT with Pearson coefficient $r = 0.94$ (95 % CI: 0.64–0.99; $R^2 = 0.88$; $p = 0.0016$) (Fig. 2a). In patients classified as low probability by their score (cut-off scores of 1), the Wells score was able to rule out the presence of DVT with a sensitivity of 100 % (95 % CI: 100–100 %) as well as a negative predictive value (NPV) of 100 % (95 % CI: 100–100 %) (Table 3).

Table 2 Patients' characteristics of the cohort

Parameter	All Patients	No DVT	DVT	*P* Value
Age in years (median/range)	54 (18–96)	54 (18–96)	54 (18–88)	0.99
Sex (male/female)	66 %/34 %	67 %/33 %	56 %/44 %	0.313[a]
LOS in days (mean ± SD)	13.5 (±10.5)	13.0 (±10)	21.1 (±13)	0.001
ICU stay in days (mean ± SD)	6.0 (±7.5)	5.7 (±7.1)	10.6 (±1)	0.007
ISS (median/range)	17 (1–66)	17 (1–66)	17 (5–54)	0.557[b]
Wells score (median/range)	1 (1–5)	1 (1–3)	2 (1–5)	<0.0001[b]

[a]Chi-Square test

[b]Mann-Whitney *U* test, rest compared using *t*-test; DVT: deep vein thrombosis; LOS: length of stay; SD: standard deviation; ICU: intensive care unit; ISS: injury severity score

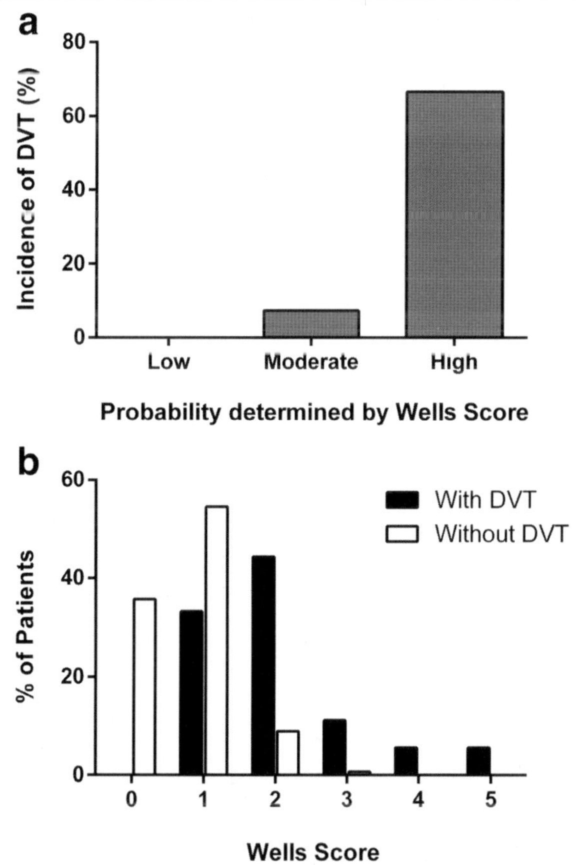

Fig. 1 Incidence of DVT by probability estimation on the Wells scoring system: low, moderate, and high. Incidence increases with increasing risk. **a** Distribution of Wells scores in patients with and without DVT on Venous duplex surveillance (VDS). **b** Median Wells score of patients with DVT was significantly higher than the median Wells score of patients without DVT (2 vs. 1, *p* <0.0001)

In patients classified as moderate or higher probability for DVT (cut-off scores of 2), the Wells score was able to detect patients at risk of developing DVT with a specificity of 90 % (95 % CI: 87–94 %), sensitivity of 67 % (95 % CI: 45–88 %), positive predictive value of 31 % (95 % CI: 16–45 %) and NPV of 98 % (95 % CI: 96–99 %) (Table 4).

Efficacy of risk stratification based on Wells score was analyzed by receiver operating characteristic (ROC) curve analysis, which demonstrated that this scoring and stratification system accurately identifies patients with a greater likelihood of developing DVT after sustaining acute trauma. The area under ROC curve (AUROCC) was 0.859 (95 % CI: 0.77–0.95; *p* <0.0001) (Fig. 2b).

Discussion

This study examined the utility of the Wells score for predicting DVT in patients who were admitted to the trauma service from January 2012 to July 2013 and underwent VDS. Wells score has been in use for more than a decade and has a predictive value in determining DVT risk in hospitalized patients [1, 9, 13, 14], but its efficacy specifically in trauma patients has not been studied. We have shown that patients after sustaining acute injuries can be categorized as low probability and moderate-high probability for developing DVT using the Wells scoring system and the incidence of DVT

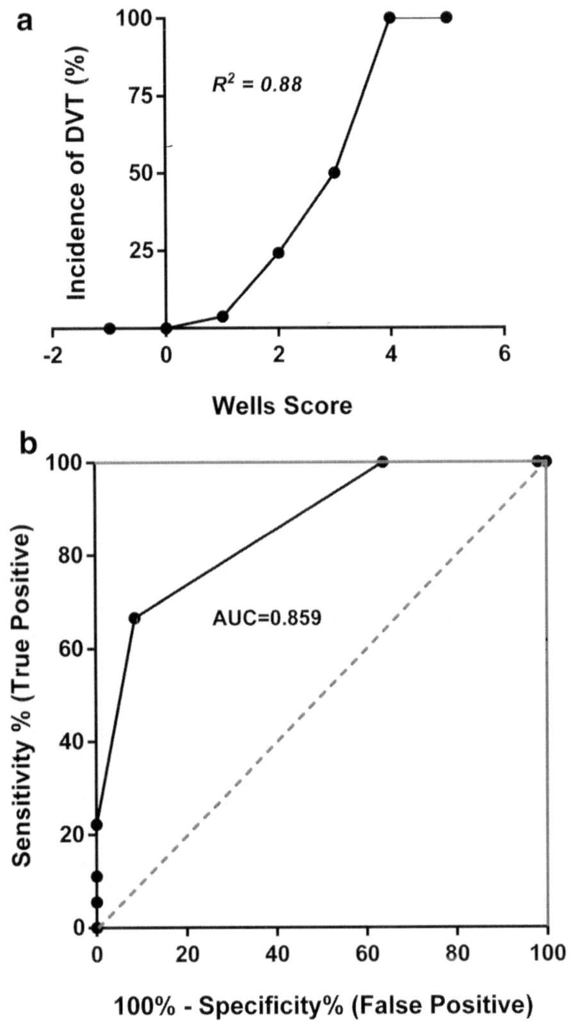

Fig. 2 Correlation between Wells score and incidence of DVT with coefficient of determination ($R^2 = 0.88$, $p = 0.0016$) demonstrating a strong linear correlation. **a** Receiver operating characteristic (ROC) curve demonstrating the performance of Wells score in predicting likelihood of DVT. **b** Area under the ROC curve (AUROCC) value shows that high Wells scoring system is efficient in identifying the patients at risk for developing DVT based on their estimated probability after trauma

Table 3 Statistical measures of performance of Wells score in predicting DVT in patients with cut off scores of 1

Parameter	Value	95 % CI
Sensitivity	100 %	100–100 %
Specificity	36 %	30–41 %
PPV	9 %	5–13 %
NPV	100 %	100–100 %

DVT deep vein thrombosis, *CI* confidence interval, *PPV* positive predictive value, *NPV* negative predictive value

Table 4 Statistical measures of performance of Wells score in predicting DVT in patients with cut off scores of 2

Parameter	Value	95 % CI
Sensitivity	67 %	45–88 %
Specificity	90 %	87–94 %
PPV	31 %	16–45 %
NPV	98 %	96–99 %

DVT deep vein thrombosis, *CI* confidence interval, *PPV* positive predictive value, *NPV* negative predictive value

increases with the increasing score. The Wells score linearly correlated with the incidence of DVT in these patients.

Routine surveillance VDS is widely used in many trauma centers for the diagnosis of DVT, however, there is a lack of standardized DVT screening system introducing a surveillance bias [8, 15] in reporting the incidence of DVT. There is also some controversy concerning the appropriate use of VDS with some studies citing the high cost of VDS with relatively low yield of clinical findings [7]. In our study, we found that a Wells score of <1 effectively ruled out the possibility of DVT with a sensitivity and NPV of 100 %, which may eliminate the need of routine VDS in fairly large cohort of patients (33.5 %). Although the scoring was very sensitive in predicting the development of DVT, its specificity was decreased in moderate and high probability patients. This may be due to the use of strict and aggressive thromboprophylaxis protocol by trauma services, which leads to a decrease in overall rate of DVT. The retrospective design of the study precluded the 'nonintervention' control arm, but the ROC curve analysis with AUROCC of 0.859 (traditional academic point system rating: good) illustrated that Wells score is able to accurately stratify the trauma patients in different DVT risk categories. A Wells score of <1 very efficiently rules out the possibility of DVT with a NPV of 100 %, thus making it an effective pretest scoring system, while a Wells score of >2 rules in a possibility of DVT with a specificity of 90 %. This risk scoring system can allow judicious use of VDS and enhanced patient-directed care with reduced costs and morbidity.

There are other VTE risk assessment models that have been created specifically for trauma patients, namely the Trauma Embolic Scoring System (TESS) [16] and the Risk Assessment Profile (RAP) [17]. Although these models have been shown to be useful risk assessment tools [16, 18], they fail to accurately stratify a significant number of patients [19, 20]. This failure probably stems from few inherent limitations of these models. The cut off threshold for defining "low risk" in these models allows at least two (or more) variables to be present in trauma patients whereas presence of even one variable

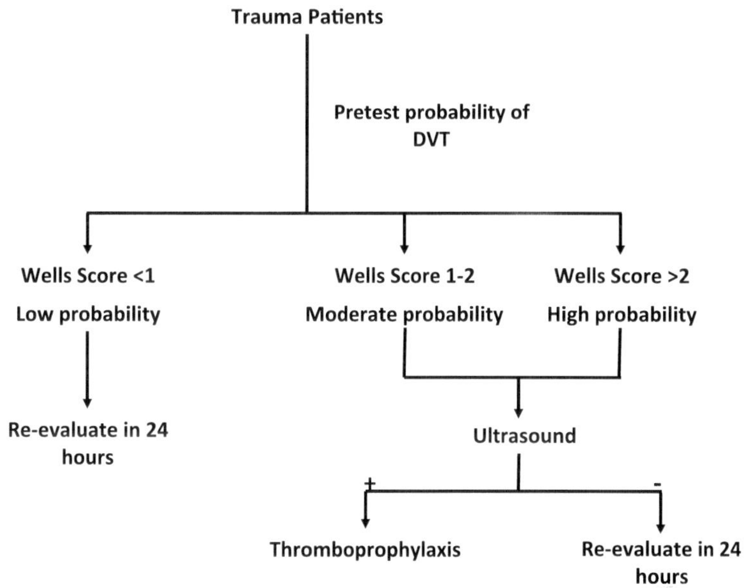

Fig. 3 Flowchart of the protocol demonstrating potential use of Wells criteria for DVT surveillance and risk stratification in trauma patients

(Score ≥1) in the Wells scoring system qualifies a patient for further DVT surveillance. Secondly, TESS does not take into account some of the variables associated with a hypercoagulable state, while RAP uses complex array of parameters, some of which may not be feasible to measure accurately in an acute trauma setting [20]. We believe these limitations are circumvented up to an extent in Wells scoring system, which is both easy to use and takes into account risk factors predisposing to a hypercoagulable state.

There are some limitations to the current study. The Wells score accuracy may have been affected if the patients' history and symptoms were not recorded accurately. As with the validation of all other scoring systems, this study of validation of Wells score is retrospective and a prospective analysis to further validate our findings will help establish the efficacy of this scoring system.

Conclusion

A Wells score of <1 in the trauma population can reliably rule out DVT and thus avoid further workup. As the Wells score increases, the risk of DVT increases linearly with it, establishing it as a valid pretest tool for risk stratification. Patients sustaining traumatic injuries can be stratified using Wells score into low, moderate and high probability of DVT, as shown in Fig. 3.

Abbreviations

AUROCC, area under receiver operating curve; CI, confidence interval; DVT, deep vein thrombosis; ICU, intensive care unit; ISS, injury severity score; LOS, length of stay; NPV, negative predictive value; NTDB, National Trauma Data Base; PE, pulmonary embolism; PPV, positive predictive value; RAP, risk assessment profile; ROC, receiver operating characteristic; TESS, Trauma Embolic Scoring System; VDS, venous duplex scanning; VTE, venous thromboembolism

Acknowledgements

We thank Mrs. Carol Ann Dickinson, Ms. Christine Vincent and Devika Kir for assistance in writing, language editing and proofreading the manuscript.

Funding

No funding sources to disclose.

Authors' contributions

SM: Analysis and interpretation of data, drafting and revision of article, final approval of work; RD: Concept and design of work, analysis and interpretation of data, drafting of article, critical review and final approval of work; KG: Acquisition of data, critical revision of work, final approval of work; PR: Contributions to conception of study, acquisition of data, critical review of work, final approval of work; EI: Substantial contributions to conception and design, critical revision of work, final approval of work; MB: Substantial contributions to conception, critical revision of work, final approval of work; KB: Substantial contributions to conception, critical revision of work, final approval of work; GB: Substantial contributions to conception and design of work, analysis and interpretation of data, critical revision of article, final approval of work.

Competing interest

The authors have declared that no conflict of interests exists.

Disclosure statement

The authors have nothing to disclose.

References

1. Bendinelli C, Balogh Z. Postinjury thromboprophylaxis. Curr Opin Crit Care. 2008;14:673–8.
2. Dunbar NM, Chandler WL. Thrombin generation in trauma patients. Transfusion. 2009;49:2652–60.
3. Rogers FB. Venous thromboembolism in trauma patients: a review. Surgery. 2001;130:1–12.
4. Toker S, Hak DJ, Morgan SJ. Deep vein thrombosis prophylaxis in trauma patients. Thrombosis. 2011;2011:505373.
5. Brohi K, Cohen MJ, Ganter MT, Schultz MJ, Levi M, Mackersie RC, Pittet JF. Acute coagulopathy of trauma: hypoperfusion induces systemic anticoagulation and hyperfibrinolysis. J Trauma. 2008;64:1211–7.
6. Selby R, Geerts W, Ofosu FA, Craven S, Dewar L, Phillips A, Szalai JP. Hypercoagulability after trauma: hemostatic changes and relationship to venous thromboembolism. Thromb Res. 2009;124:281–7.
7. Cipolle MD, Wojcik R, Seislove E, Wasser TE, Pasquale MD. The role of surveillance duplex scanning in preventing venous thromboembolism in trauma patients. J Trauma. 2002;52:453–62.
8. Haut ER, Schneider EB, Patel A, Streiff MB, Haider AH, Stevens KA, Chang DC, Neal ML, Hoeft C, Nathens AB, et al. Duplex ultrasound screening for deep vein thrombosis in asymptomatic trauma patients: a survey of individual trauma surgeon opinions and current trauma center practices. J Trauma. 2011;70:27–33.
9. Spain DA, Richardson JD, Polk Jr HC, Bergamini TM, Wilson MA, Miller FB. Venous thromboembolism in the high-risk trauma patient: do risks justify aggressive screening and prophylaxis? J Trauma. 1997;42:463–7.
10. Lee CH, Hankey GJ, Ho WK, Eikelboom JW. Venous thromboembolism: diagnosis and management of pulmonary embolism. Med J Aust. 2005;182:569–74.
11. Wells PS, Ginsberg JS, Anderson DR, Kearon C, Gent M, Turpie AG, Bormanis J, Weitz J, Chamberlain M, Bowie D, et al. Use of a clinical model for safe management of patients with suspected pulmonary embolism. Ann Intern Med. 1998;129:997–1005.
12. Le Gal G, Righini M, Roy PM, Sanchez O, Aujesky D, Bounameaux H, Perrier A. Prediction of pulmonary embolism in the emergency department: the revised Geneva score. Ann Intern Med. 2006;144:165–71.
13. Wells PS, Anderson DR, Rodger M, Forgie M, Kearon C, Dreyer J, Kovacs G, Mitchell M, Lewandowski B, Kovacs MJ. Evaluation of D-dimer in the diagnosis of suspected deep-vein thrombosis. N Engl J Med. 2003;349:1227–35.
14. Paffrath T, Wafaisade A, Lefering R, Simanski C, Bouillon B, Spanholtz T, Wutzler S, Maegele M, Trauma Registry of DGU. Venous thromboembolism after severe trauma: incidence, risk factors and outcome. Injury. 2010;41:97–101.
15. Pierce CA, Haut ER, Kardooni S, Chang DC, Efron DT, Haider A, Pronovost PJ, Cornwell EE 3rd. Surveillance bias and deep vein thrombosis in the national trauma data bank: the more we look, the more we find. J Trauma. 2008;64:932–6.
16. Rogers FB, Shackford SR, Horst MA, Miller JA, Wu D, Bradburn E, Rogers A, Krasne M. Determining venous thromboembolic risk assessment for patients with trauma: the Trauma Embolic Scoring System. J Trauma Acute Care Surg. 2012;73:511–5.
17. Greenfield LJ, Proctor MC, Rodriguez JL, Luchette FA, Cipolle MD, Cho J. Posttrauma thromboembolism prophylaxis. J Trauma. 1997;42:100–3.
18. Hegsted D, Gritsiouk Y, Schlesinger P, Gardiner S, Gubler KD. Utility of the risk assessment profile for risk stratification of venous thrombotic events for trauma patients. Am J Surg. 2013;205:517–20.
19. Acuna DL, Berg GM, Harrison BL, Wray T, Dorsch D, Sook C. Assessing the use of venous thromboembolism risk assessment profiles in the trauma population: is it necessary? Am Surg. 2011;77:783–9.
20. Zander AL, Van Gent JM, Olson EJ, Shackford SR, Badiee J, Dunne CE, Sise CB, Sise MJ. Venous thromboembolic risk assessment models should not solely guide prophylaxis and surveillance in trauma patients. J Trauma Acute Care Surg. 2015;79:194–8.

16

The selection of diagnostic modalities in the management of pelvic fracture patients requiring transfers

Chih-Yuan Fu[†], Shang-Ju Yang[†], Chien-Hung Liao[*], Being-Chuan Lin, Shih-Ching Kang, Shang-Yu Wang and Yu-Pao Hsu

Abstract

Introduction: Pelvic fractures can result in life-threatening hemorrhages. Therefore, pelvic fracture patients must usually be transferred to a trauma center for additional management. We attempted to analyze transferred pelvic fracture patients to determine which diagnostic modalities to use in different treatment settings.

Materials and methods: From May 1, 2008, to February 28, 2014, patients with pelvic fractures who were transferred from other local hospitals within 24 hours after the trauma were enrolled. We compared the pre-transfer conditions and pelvic X-ray results from the local hospitals between the group of patients that underwent further angioembolization at the trauma center and the group that did not. The role of computed tomography (CT) in the decision-making process (i.e., regarding additional angioembolization) at the different institutions was discussed.

Results: In total, 751 patients were enrolled in the current study. Of the patients who received further angioembolization at the trauma center, 77.6 % (121/156) had sacro-iliac (SI) joint disruption on their pre-transfer pelvic X-ray; this rate was significantly higher than that of the patients who did not undergo further embolization (77.6 % vs. 25.5 %, $p < 0.001$). There was no significant difference in the use of pre-transfer CT scans at the local hospitals between the patients who underwent angioembolization and those who did not (53.8 % vs. 50.3 %, $p = 0.472$). Furthermore, of these patients, there was no significant difference in the length of emergency department stay (from arrival to angioembolization) at the trauma center among the patients who underwent pre-transfer CT scans and those who did not (97.4 ± 69.3 minutes vs. 108.6 ± 21.8 minutes, $p = 0.461$).

Conclusion: When managing patients with pelvic fractures, the more attention should be paid to those with SI joint disruption on pelvic X-ray. Because these patients are more likely to require further angioembolization, they should be transferred earlier. Additional CT may be performed after the patient's transfer to the trauma center to determine subsequent treatment.

Keywords: Pelvic X-ray, Pelvic fracture, Transfer, Sacroiliac joint disruption

Introduction

Pelvic fractures can result in life-threatening retroperitoneal hemorrhages [1, 2]. The source of the hemorrhage can be divided into three categories: bleeding from the arteries, bleeding from the venous plexus, and bleeding from the cancellous bone itself. These fractures are often associated with a high mortality rate and with chest, abdominal and pelvic-organ injuries [1–3]. The management of patients with pelvic fracture may require angioembolization for hemostasis, an operation room to treat the associated injuries and an intensive care unit (ICU) for close observation [4–6]. Therefore, these patients are usually transferred from a local hospital to a trauma center for further treatment because of the discrepancies between the institutions' facilities.

During the management of patients with pelvic fractures at local hospitals, the early identification of

* Correspondence: gymetliao@gmail.com
[†]Equal contributors
Department of Trauma and Emergency Surgery, Chang Gung Memorial Hospital, Chang Gung University, 5, Fu-Hsing Street, Kwei Shan Township, Taoyuan, Taiwan

patients who require further treatment and the early transfer of these patients to the trauma center may be critical. The decision to transfer a patient has historically been based on evaluations with primary tools. Thus, the physicians faced the dilemma of whether to transfer a patient based on limited information. In the evaluation of blunt-trauma patients, primary pelvic X-ray has been usually accepted as an early diagnostic tool and is recommended by the Advanced Trauma Life Support protocol. [7] The pattern of pelvic fracture and the stability of the pelvis can be primarily evaluated with a pelvic X-ray, which remains an essential component of initial fracture and stability screening at many institutions. In the current study, we analyzed these transferred patients to delineate the role of primary pelvic X-rays at local hospitals. In addition, we attempted to identify easily accessible primary pelvic X-ray findings that indicate a need for further treatment according to the primary evaluations in the local hospitals. Furthermore, the selection of the diagnostic modalities used at institutions for patients with pelvic fractures was also discussed.

Materials and methods

From May 01, 2008, to February 28, 2014, we retrospectively reviewed the trauma registry and the medical records of trauma patients at our institution. Our institution is a government accredited tertiary care center that serves as a major trauma referral center for adjacent counties (over 20 local hospitals). The 64-slice multi-detector computed tomography (CT) scanner is used in our emergency department (ED) as a standard diagnostic tool for trauma patients. Furthermore, in-house attending physicians (trauma surgeons, orthopedic surgeons and interventional radiologists) and appropriate facilities are available to manage patients with pelvic fractures. The operating and angiography rooms are available 24 hours per day, and an angioembolization can be performed within one hour. The hybrid operating room is equipped for unstable patients who require both surgery and angiographic examination.

In our institution, pelvic fracture patients are sent to the angiography room for further intervention based on positive CT scan results (contrast extravasation or large retroperitoneal hematoma). However, there were some rare patients with unstable hemodynamics who did not respond to resuscitation. In the management of such unstable patients, the decision to undergo further hemostasis procedures was based on the results of a primary survey without CT scanning. The patients were sent to the operating room immediately if sonography revealed an intra-abdominal hemorrhage. In contrast, the patients with concomitant pelvic fracture and unstable hemodynamics were sent to the angiography room when other sources of hemorrhage were excluded by primary methods (physical examination, plain film or sonography). In addition, the patients who did not undergo a hemostasis procedure received conservative treatment and close observation in the ward or the ICU. A pelvic circumferential compression device was applied in some cases according to the clinical need and professional judgment [8].

The inclusion criteria for the current study were (1) patients aged 18 years or older, (2) patients who were diagnosed with a pelvic fracture (seen on the pre-transfer pelvic X-ray) before transfer, (3) patients who were transferred from other local hospitals within 24 h after the trauma. Pregnant patients, patients with concomitant injuries that required emergency surgery (e.g., thoracotomy, laparotomy) and patients who died in the ED without further treatment or evaluation were excluded from current study. These enrolled patients were generally evaluated and managed as described in Figure 1. Some patients underwent a primary evaluation at the local hospitals with pelvic X-ray, and some underwent abdominal/pelvic CT. After they were transferred to the trauma center, these patients were evaluated again. A definitive

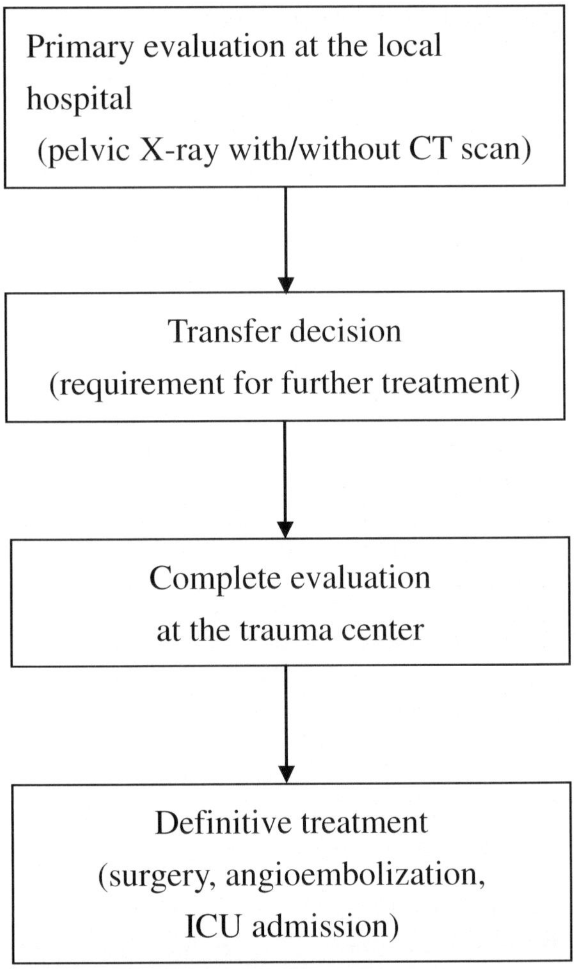

Figure 1 The algorithm for managing transferred patients

treatment decision was then made according to the information obtained from the evaluations at the local hospital, the trauma center or both.

In the present study, we investigated and compared the pre-transfer conditions of the patients who received further angioembolization after being transferred to our trauma center with the condition of those who did not receive further angioembolization. The demographic characteristics, pre-transfer pelvic X-ray results at the local hospitals, Abbreviated Injury Scale (AIS) scores for the pelvis, Injury Severity Scale (ISS) scores, number of blood transfusions, further treatments at the trauma center and outcomes of both groups of patients were routinely recorded. The role of SI joint disruption findings on the pre-transfer pelvic X-ray in the decision to transfer and the need for further angioembolization were analyzed. These two groups of patients were also compared to evaluate the role of CT scans at different institutions in subsequent management and the advantage/disadvantage of pre-transfer CT scanning for the patients who underwent further angioembolization at the trauma center. Furthermore, the difference in the length of ED stay (at the local hospitals or the trauma center) between the patients who underwent pre-transfer CT scans and those who did not was evaluated for the patients who underwent further angioembolization at the trauma center.

In this study, the patients' images were reviewed retrospectively and blindly by both trauma surgeons and radiologists (all board-certified). The pelvic fracture classification and the patency of the sacroiliac (SI) joint were analyzed. The Young-Burgess classification system was used to evaluate the pelvic fracture patterns. Lateral compression type III, anteroposterior compression types II and III, vertical shearing, and combined-type fractures were defined as unstable, whereas other patterns were considered stable [9, 10]. All of the data are presented as the percentages of patients or as the means with standard deviations. Numerical data were compared using the Wilcoxon two-sample exact test, and nominal data were compared using Fisher's exact test. All statistical analyses were performed using the SPSS computer software package (version 13.0, Chicago, IL, USA). A value of $p < 0.05$ was considered statistically significant.

Results

During the 70-month study period, 1,174 patients were admitted to our institution with pelvic fractures. In total, 751 patients (64.0 %, 751/1174) were transferred from other local hospitals for additional evaluation and management. Their demographic information is listed in Table 1. The mean patient age was 42.3 ± 19.8 years. Of these patients, 487 were male (64.8 %) and 264 were female (35.2 %).

Table 1 Demographics of the transferred patients with pelvic fractures in current study

Variables	All transferred patients (N = 751)
Demographics	
Age	42.3 ± 19.8
Sex (N)	
Male	487 (64.8 %)
Female	264 (35.2 %)
Care level designation of the referring hospitals (number of beds)	
<250	318 (42.3 %)
251-499	389 (51.8 %)
>500	44 (5.9 %)
AIS of torso injuries (scale)	
AIS of the head	3.1 ± 1.1
AIS of the chest	1.4 ± 1.3
AIS of the abdomen	2.5 ± 2.6
AIS of the pelvis	2.7 ± 1.9
ISS (score)	15.6 ± 12.5
ISS <16 (N)	508 (67.7 %)
ISS 16–25 (N)	197 (26.2 %)
ISS >25 (N)	46 (6.1 %)
Y & B classification (N)	
APC	119 (15.8 %)
LC	599 (79.8 %)
VS	19 (2.5 %)
Combination	14 (1.9 %)
Stability of pelvis (N)	
Stable	458 (61.0 %)
Unstable	293 (39.0 %)
SI joint disruption on pre-transfer pelvic X-ray (N)	
Yes	273 (36.4 %)
No	478 (63.6 %)
Post-transfer condition	
SBP on arrival (mmHg)	122.4 ± 81.0
Blood transfusion (ml)	675.4 ± 577.9
ICU admission (N)	
Yes	208 (27.7 %)
No	543 (72.3 %)
Angioembolization (N)	
Yes	156 (20.8 %)
No	595 (79.2 %)
Outcome	
Survival	737 (98.1 %)
Mortality	14 (1.9 %)

Y & B classification = Young & Burgess classification
Values are reported as the mean ± SD

In the present study, 20.8 % (156/751) of the patients received further angioembolization after being transferred to the trauma center, and the other 595 (79.2 %, 595/751) patients received conservative treatment without angioembolization. The patients who received further angioembolization at the trauma center had significantly higher AIS scores for the pelvis (3.9 ± 0.8 vs. 2.4 ± 2.0, $p = 0.015$) and ISS scores (28.8 ± 16.1 vs. 12.2 ± 7.4, $p < 0.001$) than the patients who did not undergo further angioembolization. Furthermore, comparisons of the pre-transfer conditions revealed that the patients who received further angioembolization had significantly more blood transfused (1583.3 ± 877.0 ml vs. 437.4 ± 316.9 ml, $p < 0.001$) and a lower systolic blood pressure (SBP; 94.1 ± 35.6 mmHg vs. 129.8 ± 84.5 mmHg, $p = 0.004$) compared with the patients who did not receive the further angioembolization (Table 2).

The pre-transfer pelvic X-rays showed that 273 (36.4 %, 273/751) patients had SI joint disruption, and 478 (63.6 %, 478/751) patients did not. However, of the patients without SI joint disruption on the pre-transfer pelvic X-ray (N = 478), only seven had an SI joint disruption that was eventually diagnosed with a later CT scan. Furthermore, among the patients who received further angioembolization at the trauma center (N = 156), 77.6 % (121/156) showed SI joint disruption on their pre-transfer pelvic X-ray; this value was significantly higher than for the patients who did not receive angioembolization (77.6 % vs. 25.5 %, $p < 0.001$; Table 2). In other words, the sensitivity and specificity of SI joint disruption findings on pre-transfer pelvic X-rays for evaluating the need for further angioembolization were 77.6 % (121/156) and 74.5 % (443/595), respectively.

Table 2 also shows the rate of CT scan use at the local hospitals or the trauma center for the transferred patients with pelvic fractures who received further angioembolization at the trauma center and for those who did not. There was no significant difference in the rate of pre-transfer CT scan use at the local hospitals between these two patient groups (53.8 % vs. 50.3 %, $p = 0.472$). However, the patients who underwent further angioembolization at the trauma center had significantly

Table 2 Comparisons of the demographics and pre-transfer conditions between the transferred patients with pelvic fractures who underwent further angioembolization at the trauma center and those who did not

Variables	Transferred patients with pelvic fractures		*p*-value
	Angioembolization (+) (*N* = 156)	Angioembolization (−) (*N* = 595)	
Demographics			
Age	41.3 ± 20.4	42.6 ± 23.1	1.000†
Sex (N)			1.000‡
Male	101 (64.7 %)	386 (64.9 %)	
Female	55 (35.3 %)	209 (35.1 %)	
AIS of the pelvis (scale)	3.9 ± 0.8	2.4 ± 2.0	0.015†
ISS (score)	28.8 ± 16.1	12.2 ± 7.4	<0.001†
Pre-transfer conditions (local hospitals)			
SI joint disruption on pelvic X-ray (N)			<0.001‡
Yes	121 (77.6 %)	152 (25.5 %)	
No	35 (22.4 %)	443 (74.5 %)	
SBP (mmHg)	94.1 ± 35.6	129.8 ± 84.5	<0.001†
Blood transfusion (ml)	1583.3 ± 877.0	437.4 ± 316.9	<0.001†
Role of CT scan			
Pre-transfer CT scans (local hospital)			0.472‡
Yes	84 (53.8 %)	299 (50.3 %)	
No	72 (46.2 %)	296 (49.7 %)	
Post-transfer CT scans (trauma center)			<0.001‡
Yes	92 (59.0 %)	122 (20.5 %)	
No	64 (41.0 %)	473 (79.5 %)	

Values are reported as the mean ± SD
†Wilcoxon rank-sum test
‡Fisher's exact test

higher rates of post-transfer CT scans (59.0 % vs. 20.5 %, $p < 0.001$). Among the patients who underwent further angioembolization at the trauma center (N = 156), those who underwent pre-transfer CT had a significantly longer length of ED stay at the local hospitals (6.8 ± 2.4 h vs. 3.6 ± 3.3 h, $p = 0.018$). In contrast, there was no significant difference in the length of ED stay at the trauma center between the patients who underwent pre-transfer CT and those who did not (97.4 ± 69.3 min vs. 108.6 ± 21.8 min, $p = 0.461$; Table 3).

Table 4 shows the distribution of the patients who underwent further angioembolization at the trauma center according to the institution at which the CT was performed. Of these 156 patients, seven (4.5 %) did not undergo CT at either the local hospitals or the trauma center. In total, 47 patients (30.1 %) underwent CT only at the local hospitals, and 65 (41.7 %) underwent CT only at the trauma center. CT was performed at both the local hospitals and the trauma center for 37 (23.7 %) patients.

Discussion

During a pelvic fracture evaluation, it is usually necessary to transfer the patient to a trauma center for additional evaluation and management if he/she first seen at a local hospital with limited resources. Therefore, the appropriate diagnostic modalities should be carefully selected according to the facilities and resources available at the different levels of institutions.

In the current study, the comparison of the findings on pre-transfer pelvic X-rays taken at the local hospitals revealed that the patients who received further angioembolization at the trauma center had a significantly higher probability of SI joint disruptions on pelvic X-ray compared with the patients who did not receive further angioembolization. (77.6 % vs. 25.5 %, $p < 0.001$; Table 1) For pelvic ring fractures, the literature is quite clear about the importance of posterior injuries (especially SI joint injuries) as a major factor affecting the outcomes [11, 12]. Furthermore, pelvic fractures with SI joint disruption are classified as unstable according to Tile's systems [13]. Therefore, the SI joint disruption serves as a sign of high-energy impaction that can cause severe injuries and is associated with a high probability that angioembolization will be necessary [14, 15]. The physicians who evaluated these patients at the local hospitals were not familiar with the classification system used for pelvic fractures and were not able to apply it; however, SI joint disruption can be easily observed on a simple plain film of the pelvis. Although it is difficult to predict the need for further angioembolization according to an SI joint disruption on X-ray alone (sensitivity: 77.6 %, specificity: 74.5 %), these patients can be transferred to a trauma center for further evaluation.

In contrast, an increasing number of reports indicate the necessity and importance of CT for evaluating pelvic fracture patients [16, 17]. CT can allow the evaluation of injuries to the intra-abdominal and retroperitoneal organs. Additionally, hemorrhages can be evaluated using the enhanced contrast feature, and the need for further angioembolization can be determined (e.g., in cases of contrast extravasation or large retroperitoneal hematoma) [16–18]. However, there are discrepancies in the staffing and the availability of certain equipment at various institutions. Although CT can provide valuable information, it is not always available at the local hospitals. Furthermore, although hemorrhages were diagnosed with CT at the local hospitals, patients still required transfers to the trauma center for further angioembolization or ICU admission. It has been reported that rapid transport combined with the assessment

Table 3 Comparisons between the angioembolization patients who underwent a pre-transfer CT scan and those who did not

Variables	*N* = 156		*p*-value
	Pre-transfer CT scan (+) (*N* = 84)	Pre-transfer CT scan (−) (*N* = 72)	
Age	48.2 ± 31.5	33.3 ± 33.3	0.033†
Sex (N)			0.066‡
Male	60 (71.4 %)	41 (56.9 %)	
Female	24 (28.6 %)	31 (43.1 %)	
CT at trauma center			<0.001‡
Yes	32 (38.1 %)	60 (83.3 %)	
No	52 (61.9 %)	12 (16.7 %)	
Length of ED stay			
Local hospital (from arrival to transfer; hours)	6.8 ± 2.4	3.6 ± 3.3	0.018†
Trauma center (from arrival to angioembolization; minutes)	97.4 ± 69.3	108.6 ± 21.8	0.461†

Values are reported as the mean ± SD
†Wilcoxon rank-sum test
‡Fisher's exact test

Table 4 Distribution of the transferred patients with pelvic fractures who received further angioembolization in the trauma center according to the institution(s) at which the CT scan was performed

Pre-transfer CT scan at the local hospital	Post-transfer CT scan at the trauma center	Patient number (N, %)
-	-	7 (4.5 %)
+	-	47 (30.1 %)
-	+	65 (41.7 %)
+	+	37 (23.7 %)

and management of life threatening injuries reduces morbidity and mortality [19–21]. This "scoop and run" strategy emphasizes fast transfer and a short period of on-site management [22, 23].

In the current study, pre-transfer CT was performed in over half of all transferred patients (51.0 %, 383/751); however, there was no significant difference in the rate of pre-transfer CT scan use between the patients underwent further angioembolization for hemostasis at the trauma center and those who did not (53.8 % vs. 50.3 %, $p =$ 0.472). Instead, the patients who underwent angioembolization for hemostasis had significantly higher rates of post-transfer CT use compared with the patients who did not undergo angioembolization (59.0 % vs. 20.5 %, $p <$ 0.001; Table 2). In other words, pre-transfer CT scans could not provide sufficient information to determine the need for further angioembolization, whereas the post-transfer CT played a significant role in determining the need for further angioembolization. Furthermore, in the patients who underwent angioembolization for hemostasis, the length of ED stay at the local hospitals, which could not provide subsequent hemostatic procedures, was significantly longer compared with that of the patients who did not undergo pre-transfer CT (6.8 ± 2.4 h vs. 3.6 ± 3.3 h, $p =$ 0.018). In contrast, when these patients were transferred to the trauma center, the difference in the length of ED stay between these two patient groups was not significant (97.4 ± 69.3 min vs. 108.6 ± 21.8 min, $p = 0.461$; Table 3). These results indicate that the pre-transfer CT scan could not provide sufficient information to determine the need for further angioembolization and may delay the timing of the transfer. In contrast, with the use of a multi-slice CT scanner in an area with integrated resuscitation and imaging, the CT examination in the trauma center could be performed rapidly while the patient received continuous resuscitation. Therefore, a time-consuming CT scan at a local hospital may not be beneficial for such patients and may not affect the decision to transfer. In contrast, without information from a pre-transfer CT, transferred patients can still be evaluated with rapid CT at the trauma center without delaying the subsequent angioembolization. Thus, the abovementioned results indicate that the primary pelvic X-ray at the local hospitals could be used as a screening tool to determine which patients require transfers. After the primary evaluation and resuscitation, unnecessary examinations are not suggested for the patients who require transfer. Instead, detailed examinations can be performed after the patients are transferred to the trauma center.

In the current study, only seven patients (4.5 %) underwent angioembolization for hemostasis without undergoing a CT examination at the local hospitals or the trauma center. In these cases, persistent hypotension without response to resuscitation was recorded. The patients had no obvious external hemorrhage (of wound or cranio-facial origin) or cavitary hemorrhage (according to chest X-ray or sonography). Therefore, the hypotension may have been caused by a pelvic fracture-related retroperitoneal hemorrhage, which cannot be detected with sonography. Angioembolization could be recommended based on the patient's hemodynamic instability and pelvic X-ray results. Our previous reports also indicated that pelvic X-ray is valuable for critical patients with an obviously high probability of having a retroperitoneal hemorrhage [24]. Among the patients who underwent angioembolization for hemostasis, 53.8 % (84/156) underwent pre-transfer CT. However, only 56.0 % (47/84) underwent angioembolization on the basis of the pre-transfer CT without undergoing further studies at the trauma center, while 44.0 % (37/84) underwent repeat CTs after being transferred to the trauma center, likely because of the poor quality of the images taken at the local hospital, an inadequate examination (e.g., a non-contrast-enhanced CT scan that could not evaluate the hemorrhage), deteriorated condition after transfer, or incompatibility of the reading system (e.g., the reading software or the device used to store the images). Therefore, CTs at local hospitals are not recommended for patients with pelvic fractures who are scheduled to undergo a transfer. The definitive treatment can be based on post-transfer examinations.

In the current study, patients who were transferred from local hospitals were included in the analysis. These patients may be more critical than the general population. Therefore, the percentage of patients with unstable pelvic fractures or a need for angioembolization was greater than that reported in the published literature [25, 26]. We believe there must have been a few relatively stable patients who were not transferred to our trauma center and therefore were not enrolled in this study. Furthermore, it is difficult to predict patient outcomes or the subsequent clinical pathway on the basis of primary pelvic X-ray results alone because they only provide limited information. Our conclusions may be limited by possible selection bias.

Conclusions

When managing patients with pelvic fractures, greater attention should be paid to patients with SI joint disruption on pelvic X-ray. Because these patients have a greater likelihood of requiring further angioembolization, earlier transfer is recommended for them. Additional CT to guide decisions about subsequent treatment may be performed after the patient is transferred to the trauma center.

Competing interests

The authors declare that they have no competing interests.

Authors' contributions

C-YF and S-JY drafted the manuscript. S-YW participated in the design of the study and performed the statistical analysis. C-HL conceived of the study, participated in its design and coordination and helped to draft the manuscript. B-CL, S-CK and Y-PH helped with the patient data collection. The authors have no commercial associations or sources of support that might pose a conflict of interest. All of the authors read and approved the final manuscript.

Acknowledgement

The authors thank the members of trauma registration team of Chang Gung Memorial Hospital for their assistance with patient data collection and statistical analysis.

References

1. Heetveld MJ, Harris I, Schlaphoff G, Balogh Z, D'Amours SK, Sugrue M. Hemodynamically unstable pelvic fractures: recent care and new guidelines. World J Surg. 2004;28:904–9.
2. Mauffrey C, Cuellar 3rd DO, Pieracci F, Hak DJ, Hammerberg EM, Stahel PF, et al. Strategies for the management of haemorrhage following pelvic fractures and associated trauma-induced coagulopathy. Bone Joint J. 2014;96-B(9):1143–54.
3. Vallier HA, Cureton BA, Ekstein C, Oldenburg FP, Wilber JH. Early definitive stabilization of unstable pelvis and acetabulum fractures reduces morbidity. J Trauma. 2010;69:677–84.
4. Marzi I, Lustenberger T. Management of bleeding pelvic fractures. Scand J Surg. 2014;103:104–11.
5. Fu CY, Liao CA, Liao CH, Kang SC, Wang SY, Hsu YP, et al. Intra-abdominal injury is easily overlooked in the patients with concomitant unstable hemodynamics and pelvic fractures. Am J Emerg Med. 2014;32:553–7.
6. Burkhardt M, Kristen A, Culemann U, Koehler D, Histing T, Holstein JH, et al. Pelvic fracture in multiple trauma: are we still up-to-date with massive fluid resuscitation? Injury. 2014;45 Suppl 3:S70–5.
7. Advanced Trauma Life Support. Committee on Trauma. 9th ed. Chicago, IL: American College of Surgeons; 2012.
8. Tan EC, van Stigt SF, van Vugt AB. Effect of a new pelvic stabilizer (T-POD®) on reduction of pelvic volume and haemodynamic stability in nstable pelvic fractures. Injury. 2010;41:1239–43.
9. Young JW, Burgess AR, Brumback RJ, Poka A. Pelvic fractures: value of plain radiography in early assessment and management. Radiology. 1986;160:445–51.
10. Burgess AR, Eastridge BJ, Young WR, Ellison TS, Ellison Jr PS, Poka A, et al. Pelvic ring disruptions: effective classification system and treatment protocols. J Trauma. 1990;30:848–56.
11. Stahel PF, Mauffrey C, Smith WR, McKean J, Hao J, Burlew CC, et al. External fixation for acute pelvic ring injuries: decision making and technical options. J Trauma Acute Care Surg. 2013;75:882–7.
12. Eastridge BJ, Starr A, Minei JP, O'Keefe GE, Scalea TM. The importance of fracture pattern in guiding therapeutic decision-making in patients with hemorrhagic shock and pelvic ring disruptions. J Trauma. 2002;53:446–50. discussion 450–1.
13. Pennal GF, Tile M, Waddell JP, Garside H. Pelvic disruption: assessment and classification. Clin Orthop Relat Res. 1980;151:12–21.
14. Salim A, Teixeira PG, DuBose J, Ottochian M, Inaba K, Margulies DR, et al. Predictors of positive angiography in pelvic fractures: a prospective study. J Am Coll Surg. 2008;207:656–62.
15. Sen RK, Veerappa LA. Outcome analysis of pelvic ring fractures. Indian J Orthop. 2010;44:79–83.
16. Bozeman MC, Cannon RM, Trombold JM, Smith JW, Franklin GA, Miller FB, et al. Use of computed tomography findings and contrast extravasation in predicting the need for embolization with pelvic fractures. Am Surg. 2012;78:825–30.
17. Brasel KJ, Pham K, Yang H, Christensen R, Weigelt JA. Significance of contrast extravasation in patients with pelvic fracture. J Trauma. 2007;62:1149–52.
18. Dormagen JB, Tötterman A, Røise O, Sandvik L, Kløw NE. Efficacy of plain radiography and computer tomography in localizing the site of pelvic arterial bleeding in trauma patients. Acta Radiol. 2010;51:107–16.
19. MacKenzie EJ, Rivara FP, Jurkovich GJ, Nathens AB, Frey KP, Egleston BL, et al. A national evaluation of the effect of trauma-center care on mortality. N Engl J Med. 2006;354:366–78.
20. Nathens AB, Jurkovich GJ, Rivara FP, Maier RV. Effectiveness of state trauma systems in reducing injury-related mortality: a national evaluation. J Trauma. 2000;48:25–30.
21. Liberman M, Mulder D, Sampalis J. Advanced or basic life support for trauma: meta-analysis and critical review of the literature. J Trauma. 2000;49:584–99.
22. Nirula R, Maier R, Moore E, Sperry J, Gentilello L. Scoop and run to the trauma center or stay and play at the local hospital: hospital transfer's effect on mortality. J Trauma. 2010;69:595–9.
23. Seamon MJ, Fisher CA, Gaughan J, Lloyd M, Bradley KM, Santora TA, et al. Prehospital procedures before emergency department thoracotomy: "scoop and run" saves lives. J Trauma. 2007;63:113–20.
24. Fu CY, Wang YC, Wu SC, Chen RJ, Hsieh CH, Huang HC, et al. Angioembolization provides benefits in patients with concomitant unstable pelvic fracture and unstable hemodynamics. Am J Emerg Med. 2012;30:207–13.
25. Deakin DE, Boulton C, Moran CG. Mortality and causes of death among patients with isolated limb and pelvic fractures. Injury. 2007;38:312–7.
26. Yoon W, Kim JK, Jeong YY, Seo JJ, Park JG, Kang HK. Pelvic arterial hemorrhage in patients with pelvic fractures: detection with contrast-enhanced CT. Radiographics. 2004;24:1591–605.

17

In-hospital costs of an admission for adhesive small bowel obstruction

Pepijn Krielen[†], Barend A. van den Beukel[†], Martijn W. J. Stommel, Harry van Goor, Chema Strik and Richard P. G. ten Broek[*]

Abstract

Background: Previous research on the costs of treatment for ASBO is outdated and often based on reimbursements, rather than true healthcare provider costs of the admission and related interventions. An accurate estimate of the true costs of treatment is necessary to understand the healthcare burden and to model cost-efficacy of adhesion strategies. The aim of this study was to provide an accurate cost estimate of the in-hospital costs for treatment of adhesive small bowel obstruction (ASBO) using micro-costing methods.

Methods: Consecutive patients admitted for ASBO to the Radboud University Medical Center from November 2013 to November 2015 were included. An episode of ASBO was defined as an admission for SBO with operative confirmation of adhesions or after radiological exclusion of other causes for SBO. For the purpose of generalization we used the costs of medication and interventions as provided by the Dutch Healthcare Authority and only if these were not available local hospital costs. We evaluated costs separately for operative and non-operative treatment for ASBO.

Results: During the study period 39 admissions for ASBO were eligible for analysis. An operative treatment was required in 19 patients (48.7 %). Mean hospital stay for ASBO with operative treatment was 16.0 ± 11 days versus 4.0 ± 2.0 days for non-operative treatment ($P = 0.003$). A total of 12 patients developed complications, 2 in the non-operative group (10 %) and 10 in the operative group (52.6 %; $P = 0.004$). Overall costs for an admission for ASBO with operative treatment were €16 305 (SD €2 513), and for non-operative treatment € 2 277 (SD € 265) ($p = <0.001$). The highest expenditure with operative treatment for ASBO was made for ward stay (mean €7 856, SD €6 882), OR time (mean €2 6845, SD €1 434), ICU stay (mean €2 183, SD €4 305) and (parenteral) feeding costs (mean €1797, SD €2070). A table with correction coefficient to correct for differences in price levels for goods and services between different countries has been added.

Conclusion: The in-hospital costs of an admission for ASBO are higher than previously thought. These costs can be used to guide hospital reimbursement policy and for the development of a cost-effective model for the use of adhesion barriers.

Keywords: Colorectal surgery, SBO, Surgery, Adhesions

Background

Adhesive small bowel obstruction (ASBO) is the most common pathology of the small bowel, and frequently results in surgical emergencies [1]. In a national audit in the UK small bowel obstructions accounted for 51 % of all emergency laparotomies [2]. In the United States both adhesiolysis and small bowel resection appeared in the top seven of emergency general surgeries, that count for 80 % of morbidity and death related to emergency surgery [3]. The supplementary data from this report confirmed that small bowel obstruction was the most common diagnosis in both procedures [3]. Part of the huge burden small bowel obstructions cause to patients and the healthcare system might be preventable [4, 5].

Post-operative adhesions are the cause of small bowel obstruction in 60 % of cases [6]. Application of an adhesion barrier during the index operation can reduce the risk of adhesion formation and subsequent clinical

* Correspondence: Richard.tenBroek@RadboudUMC.nl
[†]Equal contributors
Department of Surgery, Radboud University Medical Center, P.O. Box 9101, 6500, HB, Nijmegen, The Netherlands

complications of adhesions [4]. In a meta-analyses of randomized controlled trials, application of a hyaluronate carboxymethylcellulose barrier reduced the risk of reoperations for ASBO after colorectal surgery with RR 0·49, 95 % CI 0·28–0·88 [4]. Despite the evidence for efficacy these barriers are seldom applied [7]. A reason why barriers are often not applied is that policy makers question their cost-effective and consider routine application too expensive [8, 9].

Remarkably, there is little data on the financial implications of adhesion-related complication such as ASBO that can guide policymakers in developing guidance for reimbursement, management, and prevention of this condition. The studies that modelled cost-effectiveness of adhesion barriers have used incomplete estimates or the negotiated reimbursement prices for treatment of ASBO, rather than true healthcare provider costs [7, 8, 10]. By using such incomplete estimates and reimbursement prices the conclusions about cost-effectiveness of barriers might be falsified. Moreover, concerns have been raised that reimbursement prices indeed are too low, resulting in a net loss for hospitals treating patients with ASBO [11].

In a recent study, the hospital costs of patients undergoing an emergency laparotomy in general were estimated at €15 500 per patient, which is on average €7 000 more than its reimbursement [11]. The estimate was based on operating room time, ICU and hospital stay, and did not take diagnostic or medication costs into account. Thus, it may still underestimate the actual healthcare provider costs. The costs of emergency laparotomies were also not specified for ASBO in this study [11]. More accurate and up to date data is necessary to provide a better guide to reimbursement policies, adhesion prevention, and unveil opportunities for cost reduction.

In the present study we modelled the costs of an admission for ASBO based on accurate data that in addition to the operating room times, ICU and ward stay comprised full detailed information on all relevant interventions made during the admission, including medication, parenteral feeding, imaging studies, and laboratory studies.

Methods

All consecutive patients admitted with ASBO to the Radboudumc between November 2013 and November 2015 were eligible for inclusion. A waiver for ethical approval was obtained by local institutional review board after review of the protocol. To identify cases, the hospitals' discharge registry was searched for patients with a reimbursement code for small bowel obstruction. The Radboudumc is a university teaching hospital in Nijmegen, the Netherlands, with complete electronic patient files. Electronic patient files of the identified records were reviewed for an admission for ASBO during the study period. ASBO was defined as an episode with operative confirmation of adhesions, or in the non-operative group as an episode of post-operative SBO in which other potential causes of bowel obstruction were excluded by appropriate means. Patients who were treated non-operatively received tube decompression and no oral feeding. Operative treatment of ASBO consisted of an explorative laparotomy with cleaving of adhesions and if necessary partial resection of small bowel. None of the patients had laparoscopic cleaving of adhesions. Complications were defined according to the criteria of the International Classification of Diseases, Tenth Revision, the National Nosocomial Infections Surveillance System, the Center for Disease Control and Prevention, or according to the decision of the senior medical staff of the department. Complications were categorized according to the Clavien-Dindo classification [12]. All complications categorized as Clavien- Dindo grade II or higher were reported.

Costs

The total costs of the admission were divided in nine categories: operation (materials and occupancy of operating room), medication, radiology, laboratory, microbiology, ward stay, ICU days, feeding, and blood products administered during admission. All data needed for an accurate estimate of admission costs were derived from the electronic patients file. A standardized price list from the Dutch Healthcare Authority was used for the calculation of costs for occupancy of operating room, medication, radiology, laboratory, microbiology, ward stay, ICU stay, feeding and blood products [13]. No standardized price list was available for materials used during the operation. Therefore we used local prices for operation materials instead.

The price for occupancy of the operating room was based on the total anaesthesia time, and a standardized price of €16,70 per minute. Medication costs comprised the costs of all medications prescribed during the admission. The costs of medication were updated per April 2016 [14]. Costs for radiology, laboratory, microbiology were all calculated in accordance to the table provided by the Dutch healthcare authority [13]. The prices for ICU, ward stay, feeding and blood products were based on the 2015 version of the manual for costs research [15]. The costs of a day on the ICU were determined at €2015 per day. The costs of ward stay were determined at €435 per day. The prices for ward stay and ICU comprise honorarium for medical specialists, the costs for a resident managing the ward, nursing personnel, consumable goods, housing and overhead. The ICU price also counted for expenditures on respiratory support [15].

Oral feeding was also counted for in the price of ward stay. Additional expenditures for other types of feeding, such as parenteral feeding, were calculated separately and presented under the feeding category.

The average costs of operation materials were €155 if no bowel resection was performed and €436 if bowel resection was performed. The difference in price of materials was mainly attributable to the use of stapling devices.

A table of correction coefficients was added to allow for quick comparison of costs between different countries [16]. These correction coefficients are published by the European Union's statistics department (EUROSTAT) and can be used to quickly adjust prices for the differences in price levels of goods and services between countries. Thus, these coefficient provide a rough estimate of the prices for treatment of ASBO in other countries than the Netherlands. For convenience the coefficients as published by EUROSTAT were adjusted setting the Dutch price levels as the reference standard.

Data and statistical analysis

Baseline data consisted of patients age, sex, Charlson comorbidty index, ASA classification and the number of previous abdominal operations. Comparison was made between patients undergoing operative treatment and non- operative treatment using a Chi-square, Fisher's exact test, independent t-test or Mann-Whitney U test where appropriate. Continuous variables are presented as means with standard deviation, or medians with interquartile range (25–75) if non-normal distribution. Dichotomous or categorical variables are presented as absolute numbers and percentages. $P < 0.05$ was considered significant. All analyses were performed using SPSS version 23°0 (Armonk, NY: IBM Corp).

Results

From the hospital registry we identified 185 cases with a code of SBO. We excluded 49 patients because they were not admitted but only seen on the outpatient clinic. A total of 97 admitted patients were excluded, 29 patients were diagnosed with Hirschprung's disease, 16 patients had a tumor, 23 had other specified cause for bowel obstruction, and in 21 patients an adhesive aetiology was unsure. Thirty-nine patients had a total of 46 admissions for ASBO during the study period. We excluded 7 admissions because patients were transferred to other hospitals for further treatment of ABSO. A total of 39 admissions of ASBO during the study period were included in the analysis (Fig. 1). Operative treatment of ASBO was required in 19 admissions (48.7 %), 20 patients were managed non- operatively (51.3 %). Indications for operative treatment was failure of non-operative management in 14 patients (73.7 %), suspected strangulation in 4 patients (21,0 %), and 1 patient had a diagnostic laparotomy (5,2 %).

Patient characteristics are shown in Table 1. There were no significant differences between groups in terms of age, sex, number of previous operations, comorbidity index, or ASA classification. Of 19 operated patients, 9 were operated within the first 24 h. Median time from admission till operation was 2 days (IQR 1–4 days). One patient was operated after 16 days. This patient had developed an adhesive small bowel obstruction after a previous appendectomy, during late pregnancy. She was treated with parenteral feeding and had explorative laparotomy delayed to be combined with caesarean section at 32 weeks of gestational age. Her bowel obstruction quickly resolved after laparotomy, and mother and child were discharged in good condition 4 days after surgery.

Operative treatment of ASBO led to a mean hospital stay of 16.0 days (SD 11.0 days) while non- operative treatment of ASBO led to a mean hospital stay of 4.0 days (SD 2.0 days $p = 0.003$). A total of 12 patients developed complications, two in the non- operative group (10.0 %) and 10 in the operatively treated group (52.6 %; $P = 0.004$). Complications in the non- operative group were pneumonia ($n = 1$), and *de novo* atrial fibrillation ($n = 1$). One patient in the operative group developed a staphylococcal sepsis, for which prolonged ICU admission was indicated. Other complications in the operative group comprised pneumonia ($n = 2$), wound infection ($n = 2$), intra-abdominal abscess formation ($n = 1$), *de novo* atrial fibrillation ($n = 1$), urinary tract infection ($n = 1$), bacteremia ($n = 1$), and delirium ($n = 1$). Two operative patients had a second-look laparotomy. In the first patient almost the entire small bowel was entrapped in the adhesions and appeared ischemic at the initial explorative laparotomy. Because there was doubt about the reversibility of this bowel ischemia a second look laparotomy was performed the next day, at which the bowel had normal appearance and peristalsis. The second patient underwent a second look laparotomy to inspect the anastomosis made following bowel resection at initial laparotomy. The indication for this second look was made after the patients became septic on the ICU and an anastomotic leakage was expected based on clinical evaluation. At second look on day 3 a sufficient anastomosis without signs of leakage was found. Origin of sepsis remained unsure, but a pulmonary origin was suspected after negative second look. The patient fully recovered with intravenous antibiotic treatment.

Costs

Mean hospital stay for ASBO with operative treatment was 16.0 ± 11 days versus 4.0 ± 2.0 days for non-operative

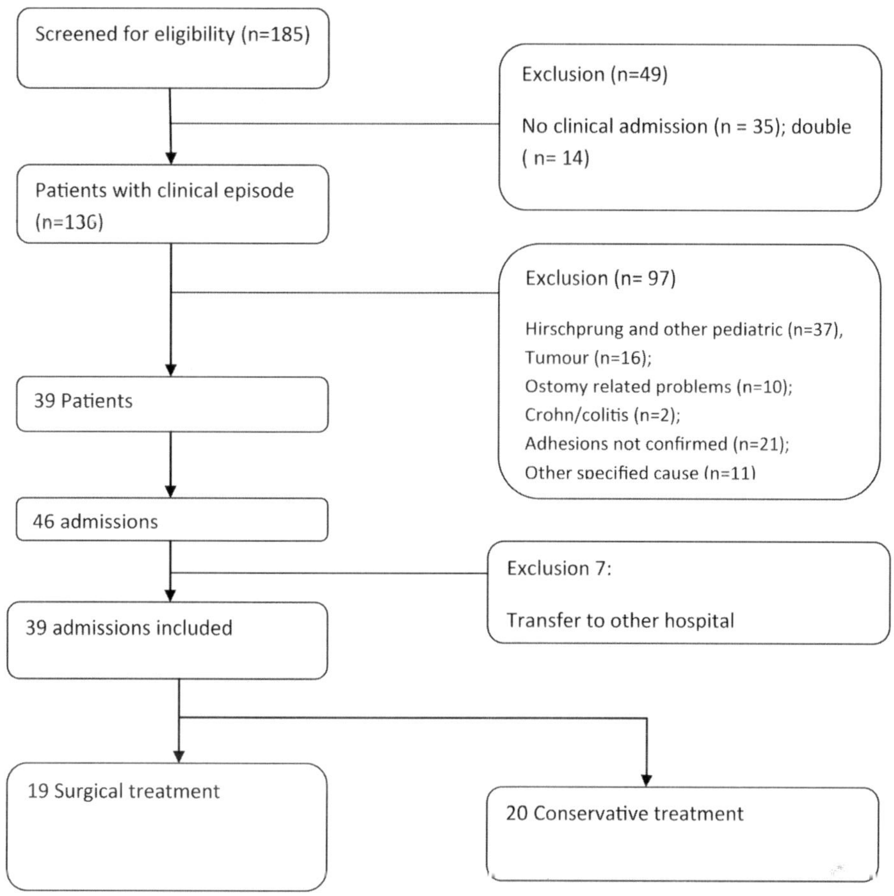

Fig. 1 Flow chart of patients included in the study

treatment ($P = 0.003$), resulting in a mean overall costs of €16 305 (SD €2 513) and 2 277 (SD €265) respectively. Mean costs were significantly different between both groups ($P < 0.005$). Costs of the different components are shown in Table 2. For both treatment strategies, ward and ICU stay was the largest component of costs (Fig. 2). The costs for operative treatment was €14 315 (SD €3 352) in uncomplicated cases and €18 095 (SD €3 776) in complicated cases, the difference was not significant. Four of the patients in the operative treatment group underwent bowel resection during laparotomy (21.5 %). Mean costs were significantly different between operative treatment with or without bowel resection, €25 395 versus €13 058 respectively. The additional operative costs for second look laparotomy in two patients were € 601 and €1 319 respectively.

Table 1 Baseline patient characteristics

	Conservative treatment ($n = 20$)	Operative treatment ($n = 19$)	P-value
Age	63.6 ± 15.7	63.4 ± 14.6	0.962
Female	12 (60.0 %)	14 (73.7 %)	0.365
Previous abdominal operations[a]	2 (IQR 2-3)	1 (IQR 1-3)	0.111
Charlson Score	3.3 ± 2.4	3.6 ± 1.7	0.568
ASA score			
- Class 2	17 (85.0 %)	16 (84.2 %)	0.946
- Class 3	3 (15.0 %)	3 (15.8 %)	
Origin			
- Home	19 (95.0 %)	19 (100.0 %)	0.336
- Nursing home	1 (5.0 %)	0 (0.0 %)	

Values are presented as mean ± standard deviation or N (percentage)
[a] median + inter quartile range

Correction coefficients

An overview of correction coefficients is presented in Table 3. The correction coefficients give a global impression of differences in price levels between countries, and were standardized to the Dutch price levels. For example the correction coefficient for the United Kingdom is 1.29. This means that prices for goods and services in the United Kingdom are generally 1.29 times higher than the costs for the same goods and services in the Netherlands. The price for a non- operative treatment

Table 2 Comparison of costs for operative vs. non-operative treatment for ASO

	Operative		Non operative		*P*-value
	Mean	SD	Mean	SD	
Operation – anesthesia time	€ 2 684.71	€ 1 434.29	NA	NA	
Operation – materials	€ 259.90	€148.74	NA	NA	
Medication	€ 634.13	€ 816.08	€ 99.34	€ 93.17	0.011
Feeding	€ 1 797.37	€ 2 069.71	€ 91.65	€ 288.56	0.002
Blood products	€ 31.74	€ 100.79	€ 0	€ 0	
Radiology	€ 510.00	€ 467.70	€ 154.92	€ 159.88	0.003
Laboratory	€ 324.49	€ 223.20	€ 69.82	€ 38.94	0.00
Microbiology	€ 69.70	€ 98.10	€ 11.06	€ 37.34	0.023
Ward	€ 7 855.74	€ 6 881.54	€ 1 850.47	€ 913.92	0.001
ICU	€ 2 183.00	€ 4 304.93	€ 0	€ 0	
Total	€ 16 304.92	€ 2 513.07	€ 2 277.27	€ 265.34	<0.001

for ASBO in the United Kingdom are roughly estimated at 1.29*€ 2 227 = €2 872.

Discussion

Adhesive small bowel is associated with high morbidity and costs. The average costs for a non- operative episode were over €2 000 and for a surgical episode over €16 000. The majority of costs were related to ward and ICU stay.

The costs for operative treatment of ASBO determined in this study were comparable to the €15 500 Shapter et al. reported in their estimation of the costs for an unspecified emergency laparotomy [11]. In their study, the costs for an emergency laparotomy were estimated from only the ICU stay, hospital stay, and duration of the operation. In our study these three parameters made up for only 77 % of total hospital costs in operative cases, indicating that Shapter's estimate is too low. Local differences in price levels between the United Kingdom and the Netherlands might account for the discrepancy, implicating that true costs in the United Kingdom are higher. Indeed the correction coefficient for the United Kingdom was 1.29, indicating that goods and services are generally more expensive in the United Kingdom as compared to the Netherlands. The most important additional expenditure in operative patients is the costs for parenteral feeding. Parenteral feeding made up for 11 % of total healthcare costs in our group. The costs for operative treatment of ASBO are much higher than reimbursements for emergency laparotomies found by Shapter et al., implicating that hospitals in the United Kingdom bear a financial loss for treating patients with ASBO [11].

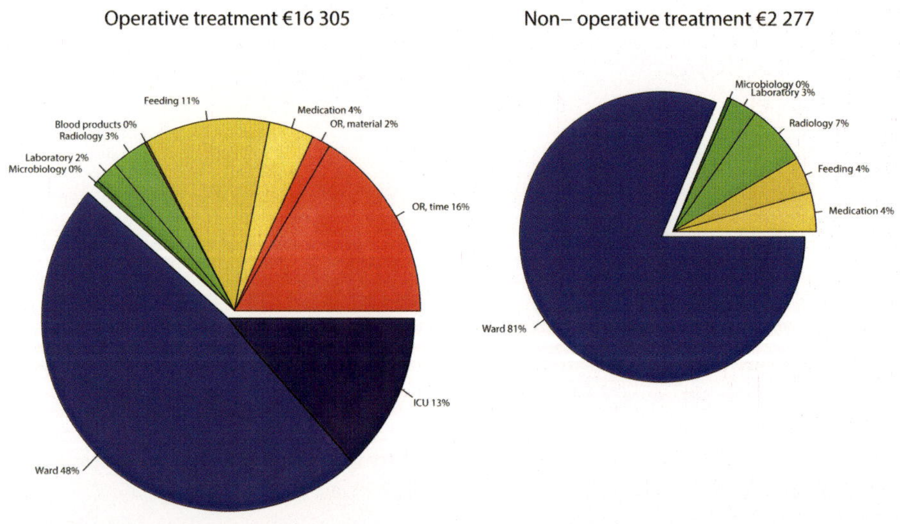

Fig. 2 Pie charts of treatment costs for ASBO

Table 3 Correction coefficients for differences in prizes of goods and surfaces

Country	Correlation coefficient
Netherlands	1.00
Australia	0.96
Austria	0.98
Belgium	0.96
Bulgaria	0.51
Canada	0.99
Croatia	0.67
Cyprus	0.80
Czech Republic	0.65
Denmark	1.24
Estonia	0.76
Finland	1.09
France	1.00
Germany	0.92
Greece	0.76
Hungary	0.60
Ireland	1.03
Israel	1.04
Italy	0.93
Latvia	0.69
Lithuania	0.64
Luxembourg	0.96
Malta	0.82
Poland	0.61
Portugal	0.77
Romania	0.56
Slovakia	0.67
Slovenia	0.75
Spain	0.86
Sweden	1.12
United Kingdom	1.29
Unites States	1.05

Source: Eurostat (http://ec.europa.eu/eurostat/web/civil-servants-remuneration/correction-coefficients) The correlation coefficients give a general estimate for the differences in price level in different countries

Correction coefficients can be used to calculate a quick estimate of the costs in a different country. However, a more precise estimate would require to recalculate the prices from the different components as listed in Table 2. An important limitation to the correction coefficients is that they are not specific for healthcare services [16]. Attempts to create more specific coefficients for healthcare have been complicated by the fact that for most condition not only the price levels of goods and services vary between countries, but also the treatment protocols itself [17]. However, we believe that it is reasonable to suggest that differences in ASBO treatment decreasing over recent years by the use of international guidelines. Adherence to the international Bologna guidelines for treatment of ASBO in this study was high [1]. As a rule, a non- operative treatment was initially instigated, unless there were signs of strangulation or ischemia. Most operative patients underwent surgery within 3 days as suggested by these guidelines.

The cost estimates in our study are useful to guide reimbursement policies and model cost-effectiveness of adhesion barriers, Because the study had high adherence to the international guidelines and the morbidity found was comparable to that reported in literature [6, 18, 19, 11]. However, the study had low power to assess the impact of factors such as complications on costs, because of the relative low sample size and retrospective nature of the study.

The relative small sample size is explained by the methodology used in this study. We included only recently admitted patients from our own institution with high ascertainment of adhesive etiology to enable the micro-costing method. Micro-costing is the gold standard for accurately defining healthcare provider costs, but seldom applied because of the large quantity of data that needs to be collected from each patient [15]. In our institution all patient data, including medication, radiology orders etc. are entered into the electronic patient file, which enabled this highly accurate method of cost estimation. For the same reasons the number of patients undergoing operative treatment was relative high in our cohort. In previous literature, non- operative treatment is successful in more than 70 % of patients with ASBO [20, 21]. We only included patients with high ascertainment of adhesive aetiology and in many of the non- operative cases the presence of adhesions could not be proved. We included only patients with high ascertainment of ASBO in this study because costs rather than treatment result was the primary endpoint. Without additional imaging or a history of previous episodes of ASBO, adhesions count for only 60 % of all cases of post-operative bowel obstruction [6]. The other 40 % might have somewhat different clinical course and costs.

We also excluded a larger number of paediatric patients with Hirschsprung's disease. Our Institution is also a referall central for paediatric surgery. Because Hirschsprung's disease has no separate reimbursement code in the Dutch reimbursement system, it often received the same code as used for bowel obstruction [22].

Our results show that the largest part of the expenditures in treatment of ASBO are related to the duration of hospital stay. Several studies have reported a reduced length of stay and lower incidence of postoperative ileus when adhesiolysis is performed through laparoscopy instead of laparotomy [23–25]. However, no randomized trials have been performed. In general, it will be more difficult to perform laparoscopic surgery on patients with multiple operations in history and when the bowel is very distended, increasing the risk of bowel injuries [26]. In the study of Wullstein et al. incidence of bowel injuries was higher during laparoscopic surgery for ASBO compared to open, despite a possible favourable selection in laparoscopic cases [24]. Thus, the results that laparoscopic surgery for ASBO reduces hospital stay and subsequent costs should be interpreted with caution.

The results of our study have important implications for policies regarding reimbursements. Reimbursement for operative cases of ASBO is generally too low [11]. The costs that we found for operatively treated episodes of ASBO were also much higher than the estimate Wilson applied in a cost-effectiveness model for adhesion barriers [8]. With the higher costs we found for operative cases of ASBO, it becomes more likely that adhesion barriers are cost effective in high risk procedures such as colorectal surgery. Adhesion barriers are proven to be effective in reducing the risk of reoperation for ASBO in randomized controlled trials [4, 5, 27, 28]. Moreover, a complete evaluation of cost-effectiveness of adhesion barriers should also count for other complications of adhesions, such as complications associated with adhesiolysis during repeat abdominal surgery, infertility treatments and chronic abdominal pain [8, 10].

Conclusion

The costs of an admission for ASBO are higher than what is reported in the previous literature. Our results can be used to guide reimbursement policy and the development of a cost-effectiveness model for the use of adhesion barriers.

Acknowledgements
Not applicable.

Funding
None.

Authors' contributions
PK– Study design, collection of data, statistical analysis, drafted manuscript, final approval of manuscript. BB – Study, design, collection of data, statistical analysis, drafted manuscript, final approval of manuscript. MS – Study design, interpretation of data, critically reviewed manuscript, final approval of manuscript. HG - Study design, interpretation of data, critically reviewed manuscript, final approval of manuscript. CS - Study design, supervision of statistical analysis, interpretation of data, critically reviewed manuscript, final approval of manuscript. RB – Study design, creation of data collection tool, supervision of statistical analysis, interpretation of data, critically reviewed manuscript, final approval of manuscript.

Competing interests
The authors declare that they have no competing interests.

References

1. Catena F, Ansaloni L, Di Saverio S, Pinna AD. World Society of Emergency Surgery. P.O.P.A. study: prevention of postoperative abdominal adhesions by icodextrin 4 % solution after laparotomy for adhesive small bowel obstruction. A prospective randomized controlled trial. J Gastrointest Surg. 2012;16(2):382–8.
2. NELA Project Team. The Second Patient Report of the National Emergency Laparotomy Audit (NELA). London: The Royal College of Anaesthetists; 2016.
3. Scott JW, Olufajo OA, Brat GA, Rose JA, Zogg CK, Haider AH, et al. Use of National Burden to Define Operative Emergency General Surgery. JAMA Surg. 2016;151(6):e160480.
4 Ten Broek RP, Stommel MW, Strik C, van Laarhoven CJ, Keus F, van Goor H. Benefits and harms of adhesion barriers for abdominal surgery: a systematic review and meta-analysis. Lancet. 2014;383(9911):48–59.
5 Fazio VW, Cohen Z, Fleshman JW, Van GH, Bauer JJ, Wolff BG, et al. Reduction in adhesive small-bowel obstruction by Seprafilm adhesion barrier after intestinal resection. Dis Colon Rectum. 2006;49(1):1–11.
6 Ten Broek RP, Issa Y, van Santbrink EJ, Bouvy ND, Kruitwagen RF, Jeekel J, et al. Burden of adhesions in abdominal and pelvic surgery: systematic review and met-analysis. BMJ. 2013;347:f5588.
7 Schreinemacher MH, Ten Broek RP, Bakkum EA, van Goor H, Bouvy ND. Adhesion awareness: a national survey of surgeons. World J Surg. 2010;34(12):2805–12.
8 Wilson MS. Practicalities and costs of adhesions. Colorectal Dis. 2007;9 Suppl 2:60–5.
9 Trew G, Cooke ID, Lower AM, McVeigh E. Post-operative abdominal adhesions-awareness of UK gynaecologists-a survey of members of the Royal College of Obstetricians and Gynaecologists. Gynecol Surg. 2009;6(1):25–37.
10 Ten Broek RP, Bakkum EA, Laarhoven CJ, van Goor H. Epidemiology and Prevention of Postsurgical Adhesions Revisited. Ann Surg. 2016;263(1):12–9.
11 Shapter SL, Paul MJ, White SM. Incidence and estimated annual cost of emergency laparotomy in England: is there a major funding shortfall? Anaesthesia. 2012;67(5):474–8.
12 Dindo D, Demartines N, Clavien PA. Classification of surgical complications: a new proposal with evaluation in a cohort of 6336 patients and results of a survey. Ann Surg. 2004;240(2):205–13.
13 Dutch healthcare authority. https://www.nza.nl/. 2016. Accessed 1 Apr 2016.
14 medicijnkosten.nl. http://www.medicijnkosten.nl/. 2016. Accessed 1 May 2016.
15 Hakkaart-van Roijen L, van der Linden N, Bouwmans C, Kanters T, Tan SS. [Kostenhandleiding: Methodologie van kostenonderzoek en referentieprijzen voor economische evaluaties in de gezondheidszorg]. Zorg instituut Nederland; 2015.
16 Correction Coefficients. http://ec.europa.eu/eurostat/web/civil-servants-remuneration/correction-coefficients. 2016. Accessed 15 Sept 2016.
17 Busse R, Schreyogg J, Smith PC. Variability in healthcare treatment costs amongst nine EU countries - results from the HealthBASKET project. Health Econ. 2008;17(1 Suppl):S1–8.
18 Di SS, Coccolini F, Galati M, Smerieri N, Biffl WL, Ansaloni L, et al. Bologna guidelines for diagnosis and management of adhesive small bowel obstruction (ASBO): 2013 update of the evidence-based guidelines from the world society of emergency surgery ASBO working group. World J Emerg Surg. 2013;8(1):42.
19 Foster NM, McGory ML, Zingmond DS, Ko CY. Small bowel obstruction: a population-based appraisal. J Am Coll Surg. 2006;203(2):170–6.
20 Shih SC, Jeng KS, Lin SC, Kao CR, Chou SY, Wang HY, et al. Adhesive small bowel obstruction: how long can patients tolerate conservative treatment? World J Gastroenterol. 2003;9(3):603–5.
21 Chen SC, Yen ZS, Lee CC, Liu YP, Chen WJ, Lai HS, et al. Nonsurgical management of partial adhesive small-bowel obstruction with oral therapy: a randomized controlled trial. CMAJ. 2005;173(10):1165–9.
22 [DBC zorgproducten]. Dutch Healthcare Institute 2016;Available from: URL: http://dbc-zorgproducten-tarieven.nza.nl/nzaZpTarief/ZoekfunctieDot.aspx. Accessed 1 May 2016.
23 Sajid MS, Khawaja AH, Sains P, Singh KK, Baig MK. A systematic review comparing laparoscopic vs open adhesiolysis in patients with adhesional small bowel obstruction. Am J Surg. 2016;212(1):138–50.

24 Wullstein C, Gross E. Laparoscopic compared with conventional treatment of acute adhesive small bowel obstruction. Br J Surg. 2003;90(9):1147–51.
25 Davies SW, Gillen JR, Guidry CA, Newhook TE, Pope NH, Hranjec T, et al. A comparative analysis between laparoscopic and open adhesiolysis at a tertiary care center. Am Surg. 2014;80(3):261–9.
26 Ten Broek RP, Strik C, van Goor H. Preoperative nomogram to predict risk of bowel injury during adhesiolysis. Br J Surg. 2014;101(6):720–7.
27 Kusunoki M, Ikeuchi H, Yanagi H, Noda M, Tonouchi H, Mohri Y, et al. Bioresorbable hyaluronate-carboxymethylcellulose membrane (Seprafilm) in surgery for rectal carcinoma: a prospective randomized clinical trial. Surg Today. 2005;35(11):940–5.
28 Park CM, Lee WY, Cho YB, Yun HR, Lee WS, Yun SH, et al. Sodium hyaluronate-based bioresorbable membrane (Seprafilm) reduced early postoperative intestinal obstruction after lower abdominal surgery for colorectal cancer: the preliminary report. Int J Colorectal Dis. 2009;24(3):305–10.

Clinical prediction score for superficial surgical site infection after appendectomy in adults with complicated appendicitis

Pinit Noorit[1], Boonying Siribumrungwong[2] and Ammarin Thakkinstian[3*]

Abstract

Background: Superficial surgical site infection (SSI) is common after appendectomy. This study aims to determine a clinical prediction score for SSI after appendectomy in complicated appendicitis.

Methods: Data from randomized controlled trial of delayed versus primary wound closures in complicated appendicitis was used. Nineteen patient- and operative-related predictors were selected in the logit model. Clinical prediction score was then constructed using coefficients of significant predictors. Risk stratification was done by receiver operating characteristic (ROC) curve analysis. Bootstrap technique was used to internal validate the score.

Results: Among 607 patients, the SSI incidence was 8.7% (95% CI 6.4, 11.2). Four predictors were significantly associated with SSI, i.e., presence of diabetes, incisional length > 7 cm, fecal contamination, and operative time > 75 min with the odds ratio of 2.6 (95% CI 1.2, 5.9), 2.8 (1.5, 5.4), 3.6 (1.9, 6.8), and 3.4 (1.8, 6.5), respectively. Clinical prediction score ranged from 0 to 4.5 with its discrimination concordance (C) statistic of 0.74 (95% CI 0.66, 0.81). Risk stratification classified patients into very low, low, moderate, and high risk groups for SSI when none, one, two, and more than two risk factors were presented with positive likelihood ratio of 1.00, 1.45, 3.32, and 9.28, respectively. A bootstrap demonstrated well calibration and thus good internal validation.

Conclusions: Diabetes, incisional length, fecal contamination, and operative time could be used to predict SSI with acceptable discrimination. This clinical risk prediction should be useful in prediction of SSI. However, external validation should be performed.

Keywords: Appendicitis, Surgical site infection, Wound infection, Risk factors, Prediction scores

Background

Superficial surgical site infection (SSI) is common after appendectomy especially in complicated appendicitis (i.e., gangrenous and ruptured) with incidence of 9 to 53% [1, 2]. It increases pain, length of stay, and costs [3]. Risk factors associated with SSI are classified into patient-related, operative-related, and microbe-related factors. It can also be considered according to time of operation as preoperative, intraoperative, and postoperative [4–6].

Accurate prediction of SSI is helpful for management, set up surveillance protocol, and risk stratification for further clinical trial [7]. Risk prediction of SSI after appendectomy had been developed by the National Healthcare Safety Network [8]. The results demonstrated that emergency procedure, gender, hospital bed size > 500, and contaminated wound classification were significant with concordance statistic of 0.70. However, it is difficult to apply into clinical practice due to lack of risk stratification. Other prediction scores of SSI in other contaminated abdominal surgery were available with acceptable discriminative performances [4, 9], but they included heterogeneous groups of patients (i.e., pancreatic, hepatobiliary, and colorectal surgery), which could not be applied to complicated appendicitis [4, 10, 11]. Therefore,

* Correspondence: Ammarin.tha@mahidol.ac.th
[3]Section for Clinical Epidemiology and Biostatistics, Faculty of Medicine, Ramathibodi Hospital, Mahidol University, Rama VI road, Rachatevi, Bangkok 10400, Thailand
Full list of author information is available at the end of the article

this study was conducted to identify risk factors and created clinical prediction score with risk stratification for SSI in complicated appendicitis.

Methods

Study design

This study was a part of a randomized controlled trial (RCT) comparing SSI between delayed and primary wound closure in complicated appendicitis [12]. Patients were recruited from two university hospitals (i.e., Ramathibodi and Thammasat University Hospitals) and four regional hospitals (i.e., Lampang Hospital from the North, Chonburi hospital from the Eastern, Surin form the North-eastern, and Pathumthani hospital from the Central). Preoperative inclusion criteria were adult patients, aged ≥ 18 years, who had appendectomy via right lower quadrant abdominal incision. The intraoperative eligible criteria were complicated appendicitis (i.e., gangrenous and rupture). Definition of gangrenous appendicitis was inflamed appendix with necrotic wall (dark, grayish color); ruptured appendicitis was defined as presence of a hole in the appendix, intraoperative rupture, or presence of frank pus. Exclusion criteria were obesity (body mass index (BMI) ≥ 40 kg/m^2), autoimmune disease, end-stage renal/liver disease, or human immunodeficiency virus. Preoperative and postoperative intravenous antibiotics covering gram-negative and facultative/anaerobic bacilli had been regularly prescribed in all patients until their body temperature (BT) < 37.8 °C for 24 to 48 h, then switched to oral antibiotics for 7 to 10 days as specified in the RCT protocol [12]. The study was reported according to the Transparent Reporting of a Multivariable Prediction Model for Individual Prognosis or Diagnosis (TRIPOD) statement [7]. The original study was approved by the Ethics committee of Ramathibodi Hospital and the collaborating hospitals, in addition to Chonburi hospital for the current study.

Outcome and predictors

SSI was defined following the Center of Disease Control (CDC) criteria as infection within 30 days that involved skin and subcutaneous tissue, with any of the following: purulent drainage, positive culture of organism isolated from fluid or tissue, or any of the following symptoms/signs: pain or tenderness, localized swelling, redness/heat, or the wound was opened by physician without a positive culture [13]. SSI was assessed before discharging home, at 1-week and 1-month follow-up.

Predictors included in the analysis were patient-related and operative-related factors. Patient-related factors were age, gender, BMI, active smoking, American Society of Anesthesiologists' (ASA) classification, diabetes, hypertension, duration of symptom before admission, presence of fever at admission (BT ≥ 37.8 °C), white blood cell count, and anemia (hemoglobin ≤ 10 g/dL). Operative-related factors included wound length, subcutaneous fat thickness, type of appendicitis (gangrenous or ruptured), wound contamination with exudative fluid, frank pus, fecal contamination (presence of fecolith or wound contamination with fecal material), presence of phlegmon, operative time, and use of closed suction drain.

Sample size

As for a rule of thumb of simulation study, at least 10–20 of interested events (i.e., SSI) were required per one predictor in the final model to prevent model optimism [14]. Our data contained 48 SSIs [12]; thus, the final model should include not more than five predictors.

Statistical analysis

Baseline characteristics of the patients were described. Predictors were compared between SSI and non-SSI using chi-square (or exact test) and Student's *t* test (or Mann-Whitney *U* test) for categorical and continuous data, respectively. Variables with p value less than 0.10 would be included in multivariable analysis. For adjusting purpose, type of wound closure (i.e., delayed primary or primary closure) was included in the multivariable analysis. Forward stepwise logistic regression was applied to identify predictors that significantly associated with SSI (p value < 0.05) and thus should be kept in a final parsimonious model.

The coefficients of significant predictors in the parsimonious model were then used to generate risk scores. Then, area under the curve (or concordance (C) statistics) along with its 95% confidence interval (CI) was estimated to quantify discrimination performance. Calibration of the model was assessed using Hosmer-Lemeshow goodness of fit test. Sensitivity, specificity, and positive likelihood ratio (LR) were also estimated. Cutoff point for risk stratification was calibrated according to the LR performance. Post-test probability was finally estimated according to the stratified risk groups.

An internal validation of the risk prediction score was assessed using a bootstrap with 1000 replications [15]. For calibration, the Somer'D coefficient which is an estimate of the correlation between the observed and predicted values of SSI was estimated for all bootstrap data (called D_{boot}) and derived (original) data (called D_{org}). A bias was then estimated by subtracting the D_{org} with the mean D_{boot}, lower value reflected less bias and thus better calibration. In addition, the original C statistic was compared to an average C statistic from the bootstraps for discrimination performance. All analysis was performed using STATA version 15.0.

Results

A total of 607 patients were enrolled from November 2012 to February 2016. Mean age was 45 (standard deviation (SD) 18) years, and 53% of patients were male. Four hundred and nine (76%) had ruptured whereas 148 (24%) had gangrenous appendicitis. A total of 52 patients had SSIs with incidence of 8.7% (95% CI 6.4, 11.0). One patient developed organ space SSI with auto-drainage through incision and was successfully treated non-operatively. Some variables were missing leaving 543 cases with 48 SSIs for the main analysis.

Model development and validation

Univariable analysis was performed to assess association between each risk factor and SSI, see Table 1. For ease of application, continuous variables were categorized into two groups based on 75 percentiles except operative time that was categorized according to National Nosocomial Infections Surveillance (NNIS) [16]. The cut points were 25.7 kg/m^2, 48 h, 7 cm, 4.5 cm, and 75 min for BMI, duration symptoms, incisional length, subcutaneous fat thickness, and operative time, respectively. Among 19 predictors, eight had $p < 0.10$ including BMI, diabetes, duration of symptoms, appendicitis classification, incisional length, subcutaneous fat thickness, fecal contamination, and length of operative time. Stepwise logistic regression identified four predictors in the parsimonious model, i.e., presence of diabetes, incisional length, fecal contamination, and operative time > 75 min, see Table 2. The risk prediction equation was written as

$$\ln\left[\frac{P}{1-P}\right] = -3.70 + 0.96 * (diabetes) + 1.22 * (operative\ time) + 1.27 * (fecal\ contamination) + 1.03 * (incisional\ length)$$

The C statistics of this model was 0.74 (95% CI 0.66, 0.81) indicating acceptable discrimination of SSI from non-SSI. Hosmer-Lemeshow goodness of fit test was applied and demonstrated good calibration of the model (chi-square = 4.42, p value = 0.491), see Additional File 1: Table S1. Coefficients of significant predictors were used to calculate prediction score. Diabetes and incision length were weighted 1; operative time and fecal contamination were weighted 1.2 and 1.3, respectively. Adding them up resulted in risk score ranged from 0 to 4.5, see Table 2. Cutoff points were identified based on positive LR of each distinct score from ROC curve analysis. The score was classified as 0, 1–1.3, 2–2.5, and > 2.5 for very low, low, moderate, and high risk groups, respectively. Sensitivity, specificity, positive LR, and posttest probabilities were demonstrated in Table 3. Fagan's nomogram was constructed, and posttest probabilities were calculated based on incidence of SSI in this study which was 8.7% (95% CI 6.4, 11.0), see Fig. 1 [12]. Patients had probabilities of SSI of 12.2 (95% CI 9.0, 15.5), 24.0 (95% CI 18.5, 29.5), and 46.9 (95% CI 38.8, 53.9) for low, moderate, and high risk groups, respectively.

A bootstrap with 1000 replications was performed to assess internal validation, which yielded estimated D_{org} and D_{boot} coefficients of 0.476 and 0.500 (95% CI 0.496, 0.506) for the derivative and bootstrap models, respectively. The average bias was only – 0.025 (95% CI – 0.030, – 0.019), suggesting good calibration. The bootstrap C statistics was 0.750 (95% CI 0.748, 0.753), with a bias of – 0.012 (95% CI – 0.015, – 0.010).

Discussion

Our study demonstrated that presence of diabetes, incisional length > 7 cm, fecal contamination, and operative time > 75 min were significantly associated with superficial SSI after open appendectomy via right lower quadrant abdominal incision in complicated appendicitis. A risk prediction score was then constructed with good performances, i.e., well calibrated and good discrimination with C statistic of 0.74 (95% CI 0.66, 0.81). The score was classified into four groups: very low, low, moderate, and high risk with positive LR of 1.453, 3.315, and 9.281 for the latter three groups, respectively.

All predictors included in the model were consistently demonstrated to be associated with SSI in other studies (i.e., diabetes [17, 18], incisional length [19], fecal contamination [18, 19], and operative time [9, 20]). Both preoperative and intraoperative factors play roles in SSI. Higher BMI [21, 22] and subcutaneous fat thickness [23] had been shown to be associated with SSI in other studies but they were not and thus excluded from the model during a selection process in this study.

About 11.8% of total patients whose data were missing were dropped out during development of risk prediction model. Characteristics of patients between complete and incomplete data were explored, distributions of BMI, diabetes, hypertension, and operative time were quite different, but only BMI was significant, see Additional file 2: Table S2. Multiple imputation by chain equations with 10 imputations was attempted to fill in missing data. The final risk prediction model was constructed, and their coefficients were not much different comparing with using only complete data, see Additional file 3: Table S3. Bias from using only complete data should be less likely.

Laparoscopic appendectomy has been associated with less incidence of SSI than open surgery and has replaced

Table 1 Risk factors associated with superficial surgical site infection in complicated appendicitis

Risk factors	No SSI	SSI	*P* value
Patient-related			
Gender, number (%)			
Male	291 (90.9)	29 (9.1)	0.773
Female	255 (91.7)	23 (8.3)	
Age, year, mean (SD)	45.5 (0.78)	44.4 (2.31)	0.674
BMI, kg/m^2, mean (SD)	23.3 (0.19)	24.5 (0.48)	0.023
Smoking, number (%)			
Yes	85 (90.4)	9 (9.6)	0.693
No	460 (91.2)	43 (8.6)	
ASA classification, number (%)			
Class I	319 (92.7)	25 (7.3)	0.290
Class II	151 (88.8)	19 (11.2)	
Class III	65 (90.1)	7 (9.7)	
Class IV	5 (83.3)	1 (16.7)	
Diabetes, number (%)			
Yes	40 (78.4)	11 (21.6)	0.001
No	502 (92.5)	41 (7.5)	
Hypertension, number (%)			
Yes	104 (91.2)	10 (8.8)	0.989
No	439 (91.3)	42 (8.7)	
Duration of symptoms, hours, median (IQR)	24 (14, 48)	24 (24, 48)	0.055
Presence of fever (≥ 37.8 °C), number (%)			
Yes	284 (92.2)	24 (7.8)	0.389
No	258 (90.2)	28 (9.8)	
White blood cell count, cell/mm^3, mean (SD)	15,563 (4998)	16,658 (4551)	0.130
Hct < 30%, number (%)			
Yes	25 (92.6)	2 (7.4%)	0.821
No	517 (91.3)	49 (8.7%)	
Operative-related			
Appendicitis severity classification, number (%)			
Gangrene	141 (97.2)	4 (2.8)	0.004
Ruptured	405 (89.4)	48 (10.6)	
	No SSI	SSI	*P* value
Wound			
Incisional length, cm, mean (SD)	5.6 (2.24)	6.9 (2.62)	< 0.001
Subcutaneous fat thickness, cm, mean (SD)	3.0 (2.00)	3.7 (2.20)	0.033
Visible wound contamination, number (%)			
Exudative fluid			
Yes	147 (88.6)	19 (11.6)	0.139
No	399 (92.4)	33 (7.6)	
Purulent fluid			
Yes	202 (90.2)	22 (9.8)	0.450
No	344 (92.0)	30 (8.0)	
Fecal contamination, number (%)			
Yes	143 (85.1)	25 (14.9)	0.001
No	378 (93.8)	25 (6.2)	
Operative time (minutes), number (%)			
≤ 75	129 (83.8)	25 (16.2)	< 0.001
> 75	412 (93.9)	27 (6.2)	
Used of closed suction drain, number (%)			
Yes	109 (93.2)	8 (6.8)	0.413
No	433 (90.8)	44 (9.2)	

ASA American Society of Anesthesiologists, *BMI* body mass index, *SD* standard deviation, *SSI* superficial surgical site infection

open appendectomy in some countries [24]. However, it required much experienced with high cost. Therefore, it is still less performed in developing country than developed country, and open appendectomy is still the standard of care [25].

Clinical application

Applying our model is simplified by counting number of four risk factors (i.e., diabetes, operative time > 75 min, fecal contamination, and incision length > 7 cm). According to the risk stratification scores, patient with 0, 1, 2, and > 2 risk factors will be respectively classified into very low, low, moderate, and high risk groups with positive LR for low, moderate, and high scores of 1.4, 3.3,

Table 2 Risk factors of superficial surgical site infection: a multiple logistic regression

Variables	Coefficient	SE	*P* value	OR (95% CI)	Score
Diabetes					
Yes	0.96	0.42	0.021	2.6 (1.2, 5.9)	1
No					0
Operative time					
≤ 75 min	1.22	0.33	< 0.001	3.4 (1.8, 6.5)	1.2
> 75 min					0
Fecal contamination					
Yes	1.27	0.33	< 0.001	3.6 (1.9, 6.8)	1.3
No					0
Incisional length					
≤ 7 cm	1.03	0.33	0.002	2.8 (1.5, 5.4)	1
> 7 cm					0
Total					0–4.5

CI confidence interval, *SE* standard error, *OR* odds ratio

Table 3 Risk stratification of prediction values of scoring system

Risk classification	Scores	Outcome		Sensitivity (%)	Specificity (%)	Correctly classify (%)	LR+[a]	Posttest probability (95% CI)[b]
		SSI	No SSI					
Low	1–1.3	21	411	85.4	41.2	8.84	1.453	12.2 (9.0, 15.5)
Moderate	2–2.5	18	74	56.3	83.0	80.7	3.315	24.0 (18.5, 29.5)
High	> 2.5	9	10	18.8	98.0	91.0	9.281	46.9 (38.8, 53.9)

Coefficient of constant term in the final model (− 3.70) was omitted for easier understanding and interpretation
[a]Compared to patients with very low risk (score = 0)
[b]Based on pretest probability, incidence of SSI, of 8.7%
CI confidence interval, *LR* likelihood ratio, *SSI* superficial surgical site infection

and 9.2, in which positive LR of 5 to 10 could moderately shift pre- to posttest probability as for EBM working group recommendation [26]. To calculate posttest probabilities of SSI, Fagan's nomogram could be used or to estimate posttest probability of SSI occurrence according to risk prediction score [27]. For instance, if patient has history of diabetes, operative time > 75 mins, and fecal contamination, she/he will be classified as high risk group (three factors); posttest probability of SSI for this patient is about 46%. If patient does not have history of diabetes, but has fecal contamination and incision length > 7 cm, this patient will be classified as moderate risk and thus her/his posttest probability is about 20–30%.

The results from previous randomized controlled trial [12] demonstrated that delayed primary wound closure had no benefit over primary wound closure in normal risk patients and primary wound closure should be done with risk of SSI of 8.7% (95% CI 6.4, 11.2). We further suggested closing the wound primarily in the low risk group with risk of SSI of 12.3 (95% CI 9.0, 15.5). However, in moderate and high risk groups, primarily closing the wound should be done with caution. Other wound interventions such as wound edge protectors [28], subcutaneous wound drainage [29], or daily wound probing [30] should be considered to apply.

Early detection and treatment of SSI is also important to reduce impact of SSI to a patient, which includes pain, isolation, insecurity, and costs [31]. Knowing risk of SSI can help physician educate, inform, and arrange appropriate infection surveillance protocol. Patients should be advised about symptoms and signs of SSI

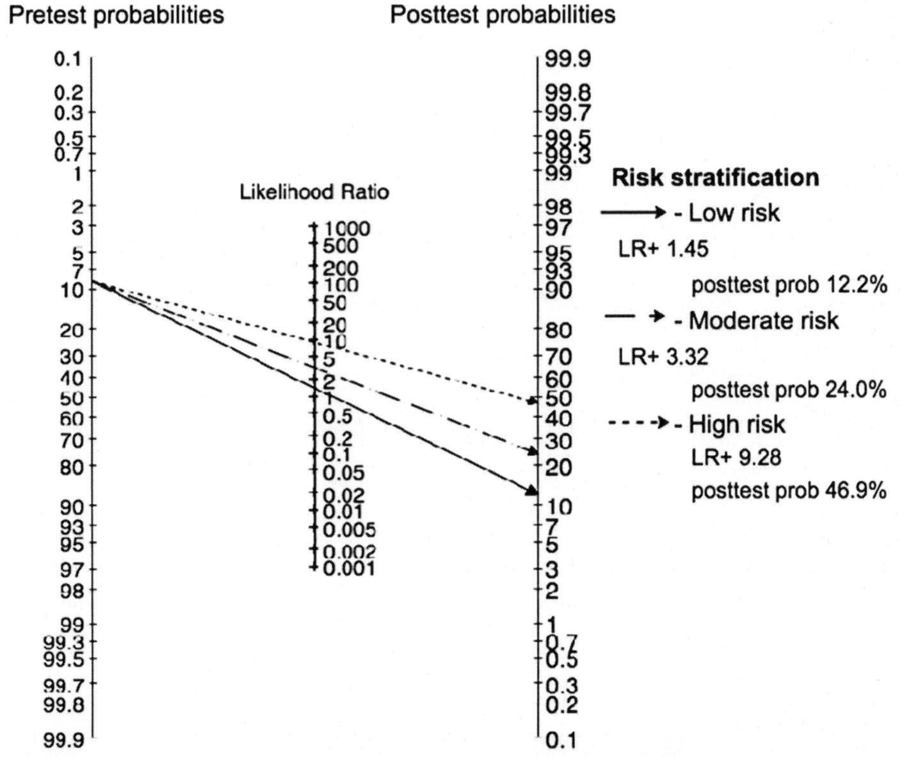

Fig. 1 Fagan's plot for risk prediction score for superficial surgical site infection in complicated appendicitis

before discharging home. Patient information sheets or self-assessment questionnaires may be useful [32].

The model was derived with standard methodological analysis including 4 markedly significant variables. Risk stratification was also easy to apply by just counting occurring variables at the end of operation. The internal validation also demonstrated good discrimination and calibration. The final prediction model contained 4 variables that should not result in model optimism with 48 events of SSI as for recommendation by TRIPOD [7]. An internal validation was performed using a bootstrapping technique, which was more appropriated than splitting data when a number of event of interest was small [7]. However, external validation and impact of applying the model to outcomes should be done in the future [33].

Conclusions

The risk prediction score of SSI has been developed containing diabetes, operative time, fecal contamination, and incisional length. The score internally performed well with good calibration and discrimination. This can be ease of use in clinical practice. However, the score should also be further externally validated.

Additional files

Additional file 1: Table S1. Hosmer Lemeshow goodness of fit. Table describing details of Hosmer-Lemeshow goodness of fit. (DOCX 17 kb)

Additional file 2: Table S2. Describe distribution of variables between complete and incomplete data. Baseline characteristics comparison between cases with complete and incomplete data. (DOCX 21 kb)

Additional file 3: Table S3. Risk factors of superficial surgical site infection based on imputed data. Significant variables with their estimated coefficiencies in the final parsimonious model estimated from imputed data. (DOCX 16 kb)

Abbreviations

ASA: American Society of Anesthesiologists; BMI: Body mass index; BT: Body temperature; C: Concordance; CDC: Center of Disease Control; CI: Confidence interval; LR: Likelihood ratio; NNIS: National Nosocomial Infections Surveillance; ROC: Receiver operating characteristic; SD: Standard deviation; SSI: Superficial surgical site infection; TRIPOD: Transparent Reporting of a Multivariable Prediction Model for Individual Prognosis or Diagnosis

Funding

This study was granted by the Health Systems Research Institute, Thailand (grant number 59 062). The funding was for conducting a randomized controlled trial of comparing SSI between delayed and primary wound closure.

Authors' contributions

PN generated the research question, checked and cleaned the data, and analyzed and wrote the manuscript. BY and AT analyzed the data and commented on the manuscript. All authors read and approved the final manuscript

Competing interests

The authors declare that they have no competing interests.

Author details

[1]Department of Surgery, Chonburi hospital, Chonburi, Thailand. [2]Department of Surgery, Faculty of Medicine, Thammasat University Hospital, Pathum thani, Thailand. [3]Section for Clinical Epidemiology and Biostatistics, Faculty of Medicine, Ramathibodi Hospital, Mahidol University, Rama VI road, Rachatevi, Bangkok 10400, Thailand.

References

1. Siribumrungwong B, Srikuea K, Thakkinstian A. Comparison of superficial surgical site infection between delayed primary and primary wound closures in ruptured appendicitis. Asian J Surg. 2014;37:120–4.
2. Siribumrungwong B, Noorit P, Wilasrusmee C, Thakkinstian A. A systematic review and meta-analysis of randomised controlled trials of delayed primary wound closure in contaminated abdominal wounds. World J Emerg Surg. 2014;9:49.
3. Sullivan E, Gupta A, Cook CH. Cost and consequences of surgical site infections: a call to arms. Surg Infect. 2017;18:451–4.
4. Ejaz A, Schmidt C, Johnston FM, Frank SM, Pawlik TM. Risk factors and prediction model for inpatient surgical site infection after major abdominal surgery. J Surg Res. 2017;217:153–9.
5. Pedroso-Fernandez Y, Aguirre-Jaime A, Ramos MJ, Hernandez M, Cuervo M, Bravo A, Carrillo A. Prediction of surgical site infection after colorectal surgery. Am J Infect Control. 2016;44:450–4.
6. Alavi K, Sturrock PR, Sweeney WB, Maykel JA, Cervera Servin JA, Tseng J, Cook EF. A simple risk score for predicting surgical site infections in inflammatory bowel disease. Dis Colon rectum. 2010;53:1480–6.
7. Collins GS, Reitsma JB, Altman DG, Moons KG. Transparent Reporting of a multivariable prediction model for Individual Prognosis Or Diagnosis (TRIPOD): the TRIPOD Statement. Br J Surg. 2015;102:148–58.
8. Mu Y, Edwards JR, Horan TC, Berrios Torres SI, Fridkin SK. Improving risk-adjusted measures of surgical site infection for the national healthcare safety network. Infect Control Hosp Epidemiol. 2011;32:970–86.
9. de Oliveira AC, Ciosak SI, Ferraz EM, Grinbaum RS. Surgical site infection in patients submitted to digestive surgery: risk prediction and the NNIS risk index. Am J Infect Control. 2006;34:201–7.
10. Neumayer L, Hosokawa P, Itani K, El-Tamer M, Henderson WG, Khuri SF. Multivariable predictors of postoperative surgical site infection after general and vascular surgery: results from the patient safety in surgery study. J Am Coll Surg. 2007;204:1178–87.
11. van Walraven C, Musselman R. The Surgical Site Infection Risk Score (SSIRS): a model to predict the risk of surgical site infections. PLoS One. 2013;8:e67167.
12. Siribumrungwong B, Chantip A, Noorit P, Wilasrusmee C, Ungpinitpong W, Chotiya P, Leerapan B, Woratanarat P, McEvoy M, Attia J, Thakkinstian A. Comparison of superficial surgical site infection between delayed primary versus primary wound closure in complicated appendicitis: a randomized controlled trial. Ann Surg. 2018; 267(4):631–37.
13. Horan TC, Andrus M, Dudeck MA. CDC/NHSN surveillance definition of health care-associated infection and criteria for specific types of infections in the acute care setting. Am J Infect Control. 2008;36:309–32.
14. Courvoisier DS, Combescure C, Agoritsas T, Gayet-Ageron A, Perneger TV. Performance of logistic regression modeling: beyond the number of events per variable, the role of data structure. J Clin Epidemiol. 2011;64:993–1000.
15. Harrell FE Jr, Lee KL, Mark DB. Multivariable prognostic models: issues in developing models, evaluating assumptions and adequacy, and measuring and reducing errors. Stat Med. 1996;15:361–87.
16. System NNIS. National Nosocomial Infections Surveillance (NNIS) System Report, data summary from January 1992 through June 2004, issued October 2004. Am J Infect Control. 2004;32:470–85.
17. Martin ET, Kaye KS, Knott C, Nguyen H, Santarossa M, Evans R, Bertran E, Jaber L. Diabetes and risk of surgical site infection: a systematic review and meta-analysis. Infect Control Hosp Epidemiol. 2016;37:88–99.
18. Reichman DE, Greenberg JA. Reducing surgical site infections: a review. Rev Obstet Gynecol. 2009;2:212–21.
19. Itatsu K, Sugawara G, Kaneoka Y, Kato T, Takeuchi E, Kanai M, Hasegawa H, Arai T, Yokoyama Y, Nagino M. Risk factors for incisional surgical site

infections in elective surgery for colorectal cancer: focus on intraoperative meticulous wound management. Surg Today. 2014;44:1242–52.
20. Imai E, Ueda M, Kanao K, Miyaki K, Kubota T, Kitajima M. Surgical site infection surveillance after open gastrectomy and risk factors for surgical site infection. J Infect Chemother. 2005;11:141–5.
21. Waisbren E, Rosen H, Bader AM, Lipsitz SR, Rogers SO Jr, Eriksson E. Percent body fat and prediction of surgical site infection. J Am Coll Surg. 2010;210:381–9.
22. Tserenpuntsag B, Haley V, Van Antwerpen C, Doughty D, Gase KA, Hazamy PA, Tsivitis M. Surgical site infection risk factors identified for patients undergoing colon procedures, New York State 2009–2010. Infect Control Hosp Epidemiol. 2014;35:1006–12.
23. Fujii T, Tsutsumi S, Matsumoto A, Fukasawa T, Tabe Y, Yajima R, Asao T, Kuwano H. Thickness of subcutaneous fat as a strong risk factor for wound infections in elective colorectal surgery: impact of prediction using preoperative CT. Dig Surg. 2010;27:331–5.
24. Jaschinski T, Mosch C, Eikermann M, Neugebauer EA. Laparoscopic versus open appendectomy in patients with suspected appendicitis: a systematic review of meta-analyses of randomised controlled trials. BMC Gastroenterol. 2015;15:48.
25. Camilleri-Brennan J, Drake T, Spence R, Bhangu A, Harrison E. Management and outcomes from appendectomy: an international, prospective, multicentre study. S Afr J Surg. 2017;55:86–7.
26. Jaeschke RGG, Lijmer J. Diagnostic tests. In: Users' guides to the medical literature: a manual for evidence-based clinical practice. Chicago: United States of America; 2008.
27. Safari S, Baratloo A, Elfil M, Negida A. Evidence based emergency medicine; part 4: pre-test and post-test probabilities and Fagan's nomogram. Emerg (Tehran). 2016;4:48–51.
28. Sajid MS, Rathore MA, Sains P, Singh KK. A systematic review of clinical effectiveness of wound edge protector devices in reducing surgical site infections in patients undergoing abdominal surgery. Updat Surg. 2017;69:21–8.
29. Manzoor B, Heywood N, Sharma A. Review of subcutaneous wound drainage in reducing surgical site infections after laparotomy. Surg Res Pract. 2015;2015:715803.
30. Towfigh S, Clarke T, Yacoub W, Pooli AH, Mason RJ, Katkhouda N, Berne TV. Significant reduction of wound infections with daily probing of contaminated wounds: a prospective randomized clinical trial. Arch Surg. 2011;146:448–52.
31. Andersson AE, Bergh I, Karlsson J, Nilsson K. Patients' experiences of acquiring a deep surgical site infection: an interview study. Am J Infect Control. 2010;38:711–7.
32. Pham JC, Ashton MJ, Kimata C, Lin DM, Nakamoto BK. Surgical site infection: comparing surgeon versus patient self-report. J Surg Res. 2016;202:95–102.
33. Steyerberg EW, Moons KG, van der Windt DA, Hayden JA, Perel P, Schroter S, Riley RD, Hemingway H, Altman DG. Prognosis Research Strategy (PROGRESS) 3: prognostic model research. PLoS Med. 2013;10:e1001381.

Delta neutrophil index as an early predictor of acute appendicitis and acute complicated appendicitis in adults

Dong Hyuk Shin[1†], Young Suk Cho[2†], Gyu Chong Cho[2], Hee Cheol Ahn[3], Seung Min Park[3], Seung Wook Lim[3], Young Taeck Oh[3,4], Ji Woong Cho[5], Sang O. Park[6] and Young Hwan Lee[3,4*]

Abstract

Background: This retrospective study aimed to evaluate the ability of the delta neutrophil index (DNI) to predict histologically normal appendicitis preoperatively and to differentiate between simple and complicated appendicitis.

Methods: The data from 650 patients were divided into positive and negative appendectomy groups (histologically normal appendicitis). The patients in the acute appendicitis group were further sub-divided into simple and complicated appendicitis groups.

Results: The DNI was significantly higher in the positive group than in the negative appendectomy group (0.4 vs. −0.4, $p < 0.001$) as well as in the complicated group compared with that in the simple appendicitis group (1.2 vs. 0.3, $p < 0.001$). The DNI independently predicted a positive appendectomy and an acute complicated appendicitis in multivariate logistic regression analysis [odds ratio (OR) 2.62, 95% confidence interval (CI) (1.11~6.16), $p = 0.028$ and odds ratio (OR) 4.10, 95% confidence interval (CI) (2.94~5.80), $p < 0.001$]. The optimum cut-off for a positive appendectomy and acute complicated appendicitis were 0.2 [area under curve (AUC) 0.709] and 0.6 (AUC 0.727).

Conclusions: We suggest that obtaining a preoperative DNI is a useful parameter to aid in the diagnosis of histologically normal appendicitis and to differentiate between simple and complicated appendicitis.

Keywords: Appendicitis, Complicated appendicitis, Delta neutrophil index

Background

Acute appendicitis is the most common cause of acute abdominal pain requiring urgent surgical intervention in an emergency department (ED) [1, 2]. Increasing time periods between symptom onset and surgical treatment is a risk factor for a ruptured appendix [3]. Successful treatment depends on early diagnosis and prompt intervention.

Several blood tests are used to aid diagnosis of acute appendicitis. Approximately 80% of patients are known to have leukocytosis in acute appendicitis [4]. However, an elevated white blood cell (WBC) count has a low predictive value because the WBC is also elevated in up to 70% of patients with other causes of right lower abdominal quadrant pain [5]. Elevated C-reactive protein (CRP) levels are common in acute appendicitis, but studies disagree on its sensitivity and specificity [6]. A more recently suggested laboratory evaluation is the determination of the neutrophil-to-lymphocyte and platelet-to-lymphocyte ratios. However, their sensitivity and specificity is not more sensitive or specific than that of the WBC or CRP [7, 8].

Immature granulocytes are an indicator of increased myeloid cell production and are known to increase in infectious or inflammation conditions [9–14]. The delta neutrophil index (DNI) measures the fraction of immature granulocytes in the circulation and has recently been introduced as a new inflammatory marker [15–17]. The DNI is assessed by an automated blood cell analyzer, and tests required for the DNI can be performed simultaneously with the routine complete blood

* Correspondence: hwaniyo@naver.com
[†]Equal contributors
[3]Department of Emergency Medicine, Sacred Heart Hospital, Hallym University School of Medicine, Anyang, Republic of Korea
[4]Department of Emergency Medicine, College of Medicine, Kangwon National University, Chuncheon, Gangwon 200-701, Republic of Korea
Full list of author information is available at the end of the article

Table 1 Demographic characteristics and hematologic markers between the negative and positive appendectomy groups

	Negative appendectomy (35)	Positive appendectomy (615)	*p*
Age (years)	27 (19~40)	35 (23~48)	0.046
Male, *n* (%)	13 (37.1)	320 (52.0)	0.086
WBC (cells/mL)	10,000 (7110~12,750)	12,740 (9850~15,500)	<0.001
NLR	3.3 (1.8~5.6)	6.7 (4~10.8)	<0.001
LMR	4.7 (3.6~5.9)	3.1 (2.1~4.6)	<0.001
PLR	118.5 (90.9~173.7)	153.1 (112.1~215.5)	0.003
DNI (%)	−0.4 (−2.1~0.2)	0.4 (−0.6~1.4)	<0.001
CRP (mg/dL)	2.89 (1.03~32.30)	7.28 (1.88~31.00)	0.121
GPS score	1 (1~1)	1 (1~1)	0.122

WBC white blood cell, *NLR* neutrophil-to-lymphocyte ratio, *LMR* lymphocyte-to-monocyte ratio, *PLR* platelet-to-lymphocyte ratio, *DNI* delta neutrophil index, *CRP* C-reactive protein, *GPS score* Glasgow prognostic score

count (CBC) testing [9]. Recent studies have examined its ability to predict infectious conditions [9, 10, 18, 19]. In this study, we investigated the usefulness of the DNI as an early predictor of acute appendicitis and acute complicated appendicitis in adults.

Methods

This retrospective observational study was performed on adults (≥19 years old) who underwent surgical treatment in suspicion of acute appendicitis from January 2015 to January 2016. Patients were enrolled from two tertiary teaching hospitals. We first selected all subjects above 19 years of age who had visited an ED and had received a surgical appendectomy during our study period, and then, we excluded them using exclusion criteria. The exclusion criteria were as follows: (1) age under 19 years old, (2) pregnant, (3) patients who did not undergo their initial blood test at the ED, (4) patients with a known immunologic deficiency state or hematologic disorders, and (5) patients who were being treated with a bone marrow suppressive agent. We then divided the final subjects into positive and negative appendectomy groups. Among the positive appendectomy group, subjects were further sub-divided into non-complicated (simple acute appendicitis) group and complicated (perforation, abscess, and localized or generalized peritonitis) group based on the surgical and histological findings. The initial biochemical markers obtained at the ED were compared between the positive appendectomy vs. the negative appendectomy groups and the non-complicated appendicitis vs. complicated appendicitis groups.

All of the blood test results used in this study were the first blood tests performed at the ED. For the complete blood cell count (CBC), the Unicel DxH^{TM} 800 Cellular Analysis System (Beckman Coulter, USA) was used. Leukocytosis and leukopenia were defined as a WBC ≥9.8 (×10^9)/L and a WBC <4.3 (×10^9)/L according to our hospital's laboratory medicine department's reference value, respectively. The neutrophil-to-lymphocyte ratio (NLR), lymphocyte-to-monocyte ratio (LMR), and platelet-to-lymphocyte ratio (PLR) were calculated by the ratios of the neutrophil count to lymphocyte count, lymphocyte count to monocyte count, and platelet count to lymphocyte count, respectively. C-reactive protein (CRP) was measured by a TBA 120FR Chemistry Analyzer (Tokyo, Japan), and the minimum reported value was 0.05 mg/dL. The DNI was obtained automatically by the ADVIA 2120i Hematology Analyzer (Tarrytown, NY, USA).

This study was conducted after approval from the Institutional Review Board (IRB) at our hospital. Written informed consent was exempted by the IRB. We conducted the study in accordance with the Declaration of Helsinki [20, 21]. To protect personal information, patient name, hospital number, date of birth, and social security number were deleted after assigning a serial number.

Statistical analysis

The continuous variables with a normal distribution were presented as the mean and standard deviation (SD) and for those without a normal distribution were presented as medians and interquartile ranges (IQRs). The categorical variables were described with frequency (%).

Table 2 Multivariate logistic regression analysis of parameters for predicting a positive appendectomy

	Odds ratio	95% CI	*p*
Age	3.11	1.06~9.14	0.039
WBC (cells/mL)	2.64	1.15~6.01	0.021
NLR	1.53	0.49~4.72	0.461
LMR	0.60	0.23~1.59	0.305
PLR	1.75	0.57~5.33	0.327
DNI (%)	2.62	1.11~6.16	0.028

WBC white blood cell, *NLR* neutrophil-to-lymphocyte ratio, *PLR* platelet-to-lymphocyte ratio, *DNI* delta neutrophil index

Table 3 Receiver operating characteristics analysis of parameters for the prediction of a positive appendectomy

	AUC (95% CI)	Criterion	Sensitivity (95% CI)	Specificity (95% CI)	p
Age	0.592 (0.540–0.644)	>44	31.5 (27.9–35.4)	88.6 (73.3–96.8)	<0.001
WBC (cells/mL)	0.682 (0.422–0.817)	>10,500	70.9 (67.1–74.5)	65.7 (47.8–80.9)	<0.001
NLR	0.723 (0.687–0.757)	>5.7	57.2 (53.2–61.2)	80.0 (63.1–91.6)	<0.001
LMR	0.696 (0.659–0.731)	≤3.57	57.6 (53.5–61.5)	77.1 (59.9–89.6)	<0.001
PLR	0.648 (0.610–0.685)	>178.61	38.1 (34.2–42.0)	85.7 (69.7–95.2)	0.003
DNI (%)	0.709 (0.672–0.744)	>0.2	59.8 (55.8–63.7)	77.1 (59.9–89.6)	<0.001

We compared the continuous variables by using the Mann-Whitney test and the categorical variables by the chi-square or the Fisher's exact test, according to the expected frequency. Parameters showing significant differences between the two groups were further analyzed by multivariate logistic regression and by the receiver operating characteristics (ROC) to verify the usefulness as an independent predictor. After finding the best cut-off value, the sensitivity and specificity of that cut-off value was calculated. We used SPSS ver. 21.0 and MedCalc version 12.4 for our statistical analysis, and the statistical significance was based on a p value less than 0.05.

Results

Characteristics of the study subjects

Six hundred fifty patients who underwent a surgical appendectomy were included during the study period. Three hundred thirty three patients were males (51.2%), and the overall mean age was 33 years old. There were 35 patients in the negative appendectomy group and 615 patients in the positive appendectomy group. In the subgroups, there were 438 patients in the non-complicated appendicitis group and 177 patients in the complicated appendicitis group. The median age of the negative appendectomy group was significantly younger than that of the positive appendectomy group (27 vs. 35, $p = 0.046$). The proportion of females was higher in the negative appendectomy group than in the positive appendectomy group (62.9 vs. 48.0%, $p = 0.086$), although this difference was not statistically significant (Table 1).

DNI to predict acute appendicitis

The median DNI values in the negative appendectomy group and the positive appendectomy group were −0.4 (−2.1~−0.2) and 0.4 (−0.6~1.4), respectively, and there was a significant difference in the DNI values between the groups (<0.001) (Table 1). Variables with a statistically significant difference between the groups were included for multivariate logistic analysis. In the multivariate logistic regression analysis, the DNI independently predicted a positive appendectomy [odds ratio (OR) 2.62, 95% confidence interval (CI) (1.11~6.16), $p = 0.028$] (Table 2). The area under curve (AUC) for the ability of the DNI to predict the presence of acute appendicitis was 0.709. The optimum cut-off for the initial DNI was 0.2, giving a sensitivity of 59.8% and specificity of 77.1% (Table 3).

DNI to predict acute complicated appendicitis

The median DNI values in the non-complicated group and the complicated group were 0.3 (−1.2~1.0) and 1.2 (0.3~2.7), respectively, and there was a significant difference in the DNI values between the groups (<0.001) (Table 4). Variables with a statistically significant difference between the groups were included in a multivariate logistic analysis. In the multivariate logistic regression analysis, the DNI independently predicted acute complicated appendicitis [odds ratio (OR) 4.10, 95% confidence interval (CI) (2.94~5.80), $p < 0.001$] (Table 5). The AUC for the ability of the DNI to predict the presence of an acute complicated appendicitis was 0.727. The optimum cut-off for the initial DNI was 0.6, giving a sensitivity of 65.0% and specificity of 71.0% (Table 6).

Discussion

In this study, we determined that the DNI was significantly higher in the acute appendicitis group than in the negative appendectomy group, and the DNI was an independent predictor of acute appendicitis in adults. The predictive value of the DNI for acute appendicitis was

Table 4 Demographic characteristics and hematologic markers between the non-complicated and complicated appendicitis groups

	Non-complicated (438)	Complicated (177)	p
Age (years)	34 (23~45)	39 (26~56)	<0.001
Male, n (%)	235 (53.7)	85 (48.0)	0.210
WBC (cells/mL)	12,700 (9795~15,500)	12,910 (9965~15,520)	0.510
NLR	6.6 (3.8~10.8)	7.1 (4.5~11.1)	0.190
LMR	3.2 (2.1~4.7)	2.9 (2.1~4.3)	0.350
PLR	153.2 (111.6~212.2)	152.2 (115~221.8)	0.690
DNI (%)	0.3 (−1.2~1.0)	1.2 (0.3~2.7)	<0.001
CRP (mg/dL)	5.85 (1.81~22.14)	95.78 (33.96~154.75)	<0.001
GPS score	1 (1~1)	1 (1~1)	<0.001

WBC white blood cell, *NLR* neutrophil-to-lymphocyte ratio, *LMR* lymphocyte-to-monocyte ratio, *PLR* platelet-to-lymphocyte ratio, *DNI* delta neutrophil index, *CRP* C-reactive protein, *GPS score* Glasgow prognostic score

Table 5 Multivariate logistic regression analysis of clinical parameters for predicting complicated appendicitis

	Odds ratio	95% CI	*p*
Age	2.07	2.94~5.80	0.002
DNI (%)	4.10	2.94~5.80	<0.001
CRP (mg/dL)	23.16	0.49~4.58	<0.001
GPS score	0.50	0.23~1.55	0.420

DNI delta neutrophil index, *CRP* C-reactive protein, *GPS score* Glasgow prognostic score

fair (AUC 0.709) and similar to that of NLR (AUC 0.723). Additionally, the DNI was significantly higher in the acute complicated appendicitis group than in the acute simple appendicitis group, and the DNI was an independent predictor of acute complicated appendicitis in adults. The predictive value of DNI for acute complicated appendicitis was fair (AUC 0.727) and lower than that of CRP (AUC 0.842). Since the DNI can easily be performed in the ED along with the routine CBC, it can help clinicians determine between acute appendicitis and acute complicated appendicitis in the early phase of the diagnostic process.

Other hematological parameters such as the WBC, NLR, LMR, and PLR were also significantly different between the negative and positive appendectomy groups. Interestingly, although the CRP was higher in the positive appendectomy group, the difference was not statistically significant ($p = 0.121$). The WBC was an independent variable in the multivariate analysis, but the ability to predict acute appendicitis was not reliable (AUC 0.682). The NLR showed a slightly larger AUC than DNI (0.723 vs. 0.709) but was not an independent variable in the multivariate analysis. The DNI was the only parameter with statistical significance in the multivariate analysis and AUC > 0.70 analysis. The DNI may be a better biomarker than other previously known markers, such as WBC, NLR, LMR, and PLR.

In comparison between acute simple and complicated appendicitis, only DNI and CRP were significantly different between the groups. The WBC, NLR, LMR, and PLR were not different between the simple and complicated appendicitis groups. This finding may be in-line with the fact that, in some patients, the WBC initially decreases in the circulation after appendiceal perforation [22]. Both the DNI and CRP were an independent predictor and had an AUC >0.70. Concerning CRP, it has no value in predicting acute appendicitis, but it is the most reliable biochemical marker in predicting the complications in this study result. Our study result is similar to that of a previous study, which reported that early CRP levels were not different between a normal appendix and acute appendicitis but were significantly different between simple appendicitis and perforated appendicitis [23]. It appears that CPR takes time to rise after inflammation and, therefore, has limited value in the early phase of the diagnostic process. CRP should be a more valuable predictor for complicated appendicitis than an early simple appendicitis. On the other hand, DNI is both useful in the early prediction of acute appendicitis and prediction of complicated appendicitis.

Although direct comparison is not possible in this study, the diagnostic efficiency of DNI for acute appendicitis may not be inferior to that of more complex scoring systems such as Alvarado score, Appendicitis Inflammatory Response (AIR) score, Raja Isteri Pengiran Aank Saleha Appendicitis (RIPASA) score, or Adult Appendicitis Score (AAS). The World Society of Emergency Surgery (WSES) Jerusalem guidelines stated that the Alvarado score (with a cut-off score <5) is sensitive to exclude acute appendicitis, but not sufficiently specific in diagnosing acute appendicitis and an ideal diagnostic scoring system remains an area for future research [24]. Di Saverio et al. argued that the group of "not likely appendicitis" may be too broad and need further distinction in this subgroup [25]. Kim et al. also reported consistent risk of missing cases of true acute appendicitis (32.4%) for a cut-off of Alvarado score ≥4 [26]. Although, the DNI is not a perfect diagnostic parameter for acute appendicitis (sensitivity of 60% and specificity of 77% with the cut-off value of >0.2) like various scoring systems, the DNI is much easier to obtain along with the routine CBC, so it is likely to be more applicable in clinical practice.

Another interesting finding concerning the demographic data is that negative appendectomies occurred more commonly in young female patients. This may be attributed to gynecological diseases mimicking AA. Conversely, the median age was older in acute complicated appendicitis than in acute simple appendicitis. This finding is in-line with the fact that perforation is more common in elderly than younger patients [27, 28].

Table 6 Receiver operating characteristics analysis of parameters for the prediction of complicated appendicitis

	AUC (95% CI)	Criterion	Sensitivity (95% CI)	Specificity (95% CI)	*p*
Age	0.591 (0.683–0.770)	>51	35.0 (28–42.5)	84.1 (80.3–87.4)	<0.001
DNI (%)	0.727 (0.683–0.770)	>0.6	65.0 (57.5–72)	71.0 (66.5–75.2)	<0.001
CRP (mg/dL)	0.842 (0.790–0.886)	>28.48	80.0 (59.3–93.2)	81.3 (75.4–86.3)	<0.001
GPS score	0.539 (0.490–0.588)	>0	99.0 (96–99.9)	7.3	<0.001

DNI delta neutrophil index, *CRP* C-reactive protein, *GPS score* Glasgow prognostic score

Fifty-one-year-old was the optimal cut-off value in predicting complicated appendicitis, but age was not valuable as a predictor (AUC 0.591).

Our study has several limitations. First, this retrospective study was carried out without estimating an adequate sample size for adequate power. The number of subjects within the negative appendectomy group was very small (35) compared to the positive appendectomy group (615). Second, the symptom onset to blood test time interval was not considered in this study. Lastly, we do not exactly understand or have studied the pathophysiological mechanism of an increase in the DNI. However, we think this issue is beyond the scope of this clinical study.

Conclusion

According to the results of our study, a DNI of >0.2 seems to be a reliable parameter to obtain a more accurate diagnosis of an acute appendicitis, and a DNI of >0.6 may help differentiate complicated from non-complicated appendicitis. The ability of the DNI to predict the presence of an acute appendicitis or a complicated appendicitis is only fair, and a DNI ≤0.2 does not exclude acute appendicitis nor does a DNI ≤0.6 exclude acute complicated appendicitis. However, if the patient is clinically suspected of an acute appendicitis and the DNI is more than 0.2, a prompt confirmatory study such as CT or an MRI should be considered early in the course of the diagnostic process.

Abbreviations

AA: Acute appendicitis; AUC: Area under the ROC curve; CBC: Complete blood cell count; CI: Confidence interval; CRP: C-reactive protein; CT: Computed tomography; DNI: Delta neutrophil index; ED: Emergency department; IQRs: Interquartile ranges; IRB: Institutional Review Board; LMR: Lymphocyte-to-monocyte ratio; MRI: Magnetic resonance imaging; NLR: Neutrophil-to-lymphocyte ratio; OR: Odds ratio; PLR: Platelet-to-lymphocyte ratio; ROC: Receiver operating characteristics; SD: Standard deviation; WBC: White blood cell

Acknowledgments

Not applicable.

Funding

No funding to declare.

Authors' contributions

GCC and YHL designed and conducted the research/study. YTO, SOP and SWL collected and analyzed the data. DHS and YSC wrote the manuscript. SMP, HCA, and JWC critically revised for important intellectual contents. YHL approved the final version. All authors have read and approved the final manuscript.

Competing interests

The authors declare that they have no competing interests.

Author details

[1]Department of Emergency Medicine, Kangbuk Samsung Hospital, Sungkyunkwan University School of Medicine, Seoul, Republic of Korea. [2]Department of Emergency Medicine, School of Medicine, Kangdong Sacred Heart Hospital, Hallym University, Seoul, Republic of Korea. [3]Department of Emergency Medicine, Sacred Heart Hospital, Hallym University School of Medicine, Anyang, Republic of Korea. [4]Department of Emergency Medicine, College of Medicine, Kangwon National University, Chuncheon, Gangwon 200-701, Republic of Korea. [5]Department of Surgery, Kangnam Sacred Heart Hospital, Hallym University Medical Center, Hallym University College of Medicine, Seoul, Republic of Korea. [6]Department of Emergency Medicine, School of Medicine, Konkuk University Konkuk University Medical Center, Seoul, Republic of Korea.

References

1. Gaitini D, Beck-Razi N, Mor-Yosef D, Fischer D, Ben Itzhak O, Krausz MM, Engel A. Diagnosing acute appendicitis in adults: accuracy of color Doppler sonography and MDCT compared with surgery and clinical follow-up. AJR Am J Roentgenol. 2008;190(5):1300–6.
2. Kearney D, Cahill RA, O'Brien E, Kirwan WO, Redmond HP. Influence of delays on perforation risk in adults with acute appendicitis. Dis Colon Rectum. 2008;51(12):1823–7.
3. Papandria D, Goldstein SD, Rhee D, Salazar JH, Arlikar J, Gorgy A, Ortega G, Zhang Y, Abdullah F. Risk of perforation increases with delay in recognition and surgery for acute appendicitis. J Surg Res. 2013;184(2):723–9.
4. Elangovan S. Clinical and laboratory findings in acute appendicitis in the elderly. J Am Board Fam Pract. 1996;9(2):75–8.
5. Calder JD, Gajraj H. Recent advances in the diagnosis and treatment of acute appendicitis. Br J Hosp Med. 1995;54(4):129–33.
6. Hallan S, Asberg A. The accuracy of C-reactive protein in diagnosing acute appendicitis—a meta-analysis. Scand J Clin Lab Invest. 1997;57(5):373–80.
7. Kahramanca S, Ozgehan G, Seker D, Gokce EI, Seker G, Tunc G, Kucukpinar T, Kargici H. Neutrophil-to-lymphocyte ratio as a predictor of acute appendicitis. Ulusal Travma Ve Acil Cerrahi Dergisi. 2014;20(1):19–22.
8. Yazar FM, Bakacak M, Emre A, Urfalioglu A, Serin S, Cengiz E, Bulbuloglu E. Predictive role of neutrophil to lymphocyte and platelet-to-lymphocyte ratios for diagnosis of acute appendicitis during pregnancy. Kaohsiung J Med Sci. 2015;31(11):591–6.
9. Nahm CH, Choi JW, Lee J. Delta neutrophil index in automated immature granulocyte counts for assessing disease severity of patients with sepsis. Ann Clin Lab Sci. 2008;38(3):241–6.
10. Seok Y, Choi JR, Kim J, Kim YK, Lee J, Song J, Kim SJ, Lee KA. Delta neutrophil index: a promising diagnostic and prognostic marker for sepsis. Shock. 2012;37(3):242–6.
11. Kim HW, Ku S, Jeong SJ, Jin SJ, Han SH, Choi JY, Kim JM, Song YG. Delta neutrophil index: could it predict mortality in patients with bacteraemia? Scand J Infect Dis. 2012;44(7):475–80.
12. Park BH, Kang YA, Park MS, Jung WJ, Lee SH, Lee SK, Kim SY, Kim SK, Chang J, Jung JY, et al. Delta neutrophil index as an early marker of disease severity in critically ill patients with sepsis. BMC Infect Dis. 2011;11:299.
13. Cornbleet PJ. Clinical utility of the band count. Clin Lab Med. 2002;22(1):101–36.
14. Seebach JD, Morant R, Ruegg R, Seifert B, Fehr J. The diagnostic value of the neutrophil left shift in predicting inflammatory and infectious disease. Am J Clin Pathol. 1997;107(5):582–91.
15. Kratz A, Maloum K, O'Malley C, Zini G, Rocco V, Zelmanovic D, Kling G. Enumeration of nucleated red blood cells with the ADVIA 2120 hematology system: an international multicenter clinical trial. Lab Hematol. 2006;12(2):63–70.
16. Harris N, Jou JM, Devoto G, Lotz J, Pappas J, Wranovics D, Wilkinson M, Fletcher SR, Kratz A. Performance evaluation of the ADVIA 2120 hematology analyzer: an international multicenter clinical trial. Lab Hematol. 2005;11(1):62–70.
17. Harris N, Kunicka J, Kratz A. The ADVIA 2120 hematology system: flow cytometry-based analysis of blood and body fluids in the routine hematology laboratory. Lab Hematol. 2005;11(1):47–61.
18. Ansari-Lari MA, Kickler TS, Borowitz MJ. Immature granulocyte measurement using the Sysmex XE-2100. Relationship to infection and sepsis. Am J Clin Pathol. 2003;120(5):795–9.
19. Nigro KG, O'Riordan M, Molloy EJ, Walsh MC, Sandhaus LM. Performance of an automated immature granulocyte count as a predictor of neonatal sepsis. Am J Clin Pathol. 2005;123(4):618–24.

20. Goodyear MD, Krleza-Jeric K, Lemmens T. The Declaration of Helsinki. BMJ. 2007;335(7621):624–5.
21. World Medical Association Declaration of Helsinki. Recommendations guiding physicians in biomedical research involving human subjects. Cardiovasc Res. 1997;35(1):2–3.
22. Graffeo CS, Counselman FL. Appendicitis. Emerg Med Clin North Am. 1996;14(4):653–71.
23. Wu HP, Lin CY, Chang CF, Chang YJ, Huang CY. Predictive value of C-reactive protein at different cutoff levels in acute appendicitis. Am J Emerg Med. 2005;23(4):449–53.
24. Di Saverio S, Birindelli A, Kelly MD, Catena F, Weber DG, Sartelli M, Sugrue M, De Moya M, Gomes CA, Bhangu A, et al. WSES Jerusalem guidelines for diagnosis and treatment of acute appendicitis. World J Emerg Surg. 2016;11:34.
25. Di Saverio S, Birindelli A, Piccinini A, Catena F, Biscardi A, Tugnoli G. How reliable is Alvarado score and its subgroups in ruling out acute appendicitis and suggesting the opportunity of nonoperative management or surgery? Ann Surg. 2017;265(6):E84–5.
26. Kim K, Rhee JE, Lee CC, Kim KS, Shin JH, Kwak MJ, Kim JH, Suh GJ, Hahn SK, Singer AJ. Impact of helical computed tomography in clinically evident appendicitis. Emerg Med J. 2008;25(8):477–81.
27. Hardin Jr DM. Acute appendicitis: review and update. Am Fam Physician. 1999;60(7):2027–34.
28. Yamini D, Vargas H, Bongard F, Klein S, Stamos MJ. Perforated appendicitis: is it truly a surgical urgency? Am Surg. 1998;64(10):970–9.

Thoracic trauma severity contributes to differences in intensive care therapy and mortality of severely injured patients: analysis based on the TraumaRegister DGU®

Jörg Bayer[1*], Rolf Lefering[2], Sylvia Reinhardt[3], Jan Kühle[1], Jörn Zwingmann[1], Norbert P. Südkamp[1], Thorsten Hammer[1] and TraumaRegister DGU[4]

Abstract

Background: Thoracic trauma is a relevant source of comorbidity throughout multiply-injured patient care. We aim to determine a measurable influence of chest trauma's severity on early resuscitation, intensive care therapy, and mortality in severely injured patients.

Methods: Patients documented between 2002 and 2012 in the TraumaRegister DGU®, aged ≥ 16 years, Injury severity score (ISS) ≥ 16 are analyzed. Isolated brain injury and severe head injury led to exclusion. Subgroups are formed using the Abbreviated Injury Scale$_{Thorax}$.

Results: Twenty-two thousand five hundred sixty-five patients were predominantly male (74%) with mean age of 45.7 years (SD 19.3), blunt trauma (95%), mean ISS 25.6 (SD 9.6). Overall mean intubation period was 5.6 days (SD 10.7). Surviving patients were discharged from the ICU after a mean of about 5 days following extubation. Thoracic trauma severity (AIS$_{Thorax}$ ≥ 4) and fractures to the thoracic cage significantly prolonged the ventilation period. Additionally, fractures extended the ICU stay significantly. Suffering from more than one thoracic injury was associated with a mean of 1–2 days longer intubation period and longer ICU stay. Highest rates of sepsis, respiratory, and multiple organ failure occurred in patients with critical compared to lesser thoracic trauma severity.

Conclusion: Thoracic trauma severity in multiply-injured patients has a measurable impact on rates of respiratory and multiple organ failure, sepsis, mortality, time of mechanical ventilation, and ICU stay.

Keywords: Severely injured, Polytrauma, Thoracic trauma, Chest injury, Organ failure, Mortality

Background

Chest trauma ranks as the most important injury in severely injured patients, and about 50% of those with multiple trauma suffer from an associated chest injury [1, 2]. Injury to the thorax may affect the thoracic wall (e.g., rib, sternum fracture) as well as thoracic organs (e.g., lung, heart, vessels) to a different extent. Only a minority of patients with thoracic trauma tends to develop respiratory failure requiring intubation and ventilator support to correct hypoxia and hypercapnia [3]. On the other hand, 35 to 58% of severely injured patients require prehospital intubation, depending on the severity of concomitant chest injury [4, 5]. While severely injured patients usually require intensive care therapy irrespective of accompanying thoracic injuries, organ dysfunction and multiple organ failure (MOF) are known to develop more often in patients with severe thoracic trauma [6]. In severely injured patients, including

* Correspondence: joerg.bayer@uniklinik-freiburg.de
[1]Department of Orthopedics and Trauma Surgery, Medical Center – Albert-Ludwigs-University of Freiburg, Faculty of Medicine, Albert-Ludwigs-University of Freiburg, Hugstetter Str. 55, 79106 Freiburg, Germany
Full list of author information is available at the end of the article

those with severe traumatic brain injury (TBI), at least one organ failed in about 52%, with lung failure occurring in 26% [6]. Overall, MOF rates of 13 to 33% have been reported in severely injured patients. While lung failure rates ranged from 50 to 65% in MOF patients [6, 7], only 7% of patients without MOF suffered from lung failure [6]. Overall, MOF patients require prolonged ventilation and remain longer in the intensive care unit (ICU), thus consuming considerable health care resources [7].

Severe multiple trauma is often associated with traumatic lung injury and presents with a wide spectrum of severity [8]; the reported mortality of chest trauma can be as high as 60% [2], and 20 to 25% of deaths in severely injured patients are attributed to chest injury [9, 10].

Taking care of a severely injured patient is demanding. Differences in prehospital and early clinical trauma management have been reported that depends on the severity of an accompanying chest trauma [5]. Multiply-injured patients with blunt chest trauma require significantly longer periods of mechanical ventilation and a significantly longer stay in the ICU than trauma patients without a thoracic injury [2]. Furthermore, chest injuries predispose to pneumonia [11], adult respiratory distress syndrome (ARDS) [12], and multiple organ dysfunction syndrome (MODS) [6]. Therefore, we aimed to determine whether the chest trauma's severity in severely injured patients reveals a measurable influence on early resuscitation, intensive care therapy, and mortality.

Methods

The TraumaRegister DGU®

The TraumaRegister DGU® (TR-DGU) of the German Trauma Society (Deutsche Gesellschaft für Unfallchirurgie, DGU) was founded in 1993. The aim of this multicenter database is the anonymized and standardized documentation of severely injured patients' care.

Data are collected prospectively in four consecutive time periods from the accident site until hospital discharge: (A) pre-hospital phase, (B) emergency room and initial surgery, (C) ICU, and (D) discharge. Documentation includes detailed information on demographics, injury pattern, comorbidities, pre- and in-hospital management, course in the ICU, relevant laboratory findings including each individual's data on transfusions, and outcome. The inclusion criterion is admission to the hospital via the emergency room with subsequent ICU/ICM care or reaching the hospital with vital signs and dying before admission to the ICU.

The infrastructure for documentation, data management, and data analysis is provided by AUC—Academy for Trauma Surgery (AUC—Akademie der Unfallchirurgie GmbH), a company affiliated with the German Trauma Society. Scientific leadership is provided by the Committee on Emergency Medicine, Intensive Care and Trauma Management (Sektion NIS) of the German Trauma Society. The participating hospitals submit their anonymized data into a central database via a web-based application. The quality of the scientific data analysis is monitored by peer review procedure established by Sektion NIS.

The participating hospitals are primarily located in Germany (90%), but a rising number of hospitals in other countries are contributing data as well (at the moment from Austria, Belgium, China, Finland, Luxemburg, Slovenia, Switzerland, The Netherlands, and the United Arab Emirates). Currently, approximately 35,000 cases from more than 600 hospitals have been entered into the database per year.

Participation in TR-DGU is voluntary. For hospitals associated with TraumaNetzwerk DGU®, however, the entry of at least a basic data set is obligatory for reasons of quality assurance. Hospitals interested in trauma research must enter a standard data collection form that contains more comprehensive information (e.g., organ failure, sepsis) on the patient course compared with the basic data set.

Patients

Patients documented between 2002 and 2012 in the TR-DGU were analyzed for eligibility in this investigation. Patient selection was carried out based upon the following criteria:

(1) online documentation from European trauma centers, (2) age ≥ 16 years, (3) ISS ≥ 16, (4) exclusion of isolated brain injuries, and (5) exclusion of severe head injury defined as $AIS_{Head} \geq 4$ to prevent confounding, since severe head trauma may pose an indication for intubation itself [13].

Injuries were graded according to the 2005 version of the Abbreviated Injury Scale (AIS) [14], and the injury severity score (ISS) was calculated as described [15]. While the ISS is calculated from the three worst affected body regions as the sum of squares of the respective AIS severity levels, the New ISS (NISS) is calculated in a similar way, but instead of their location, the three worst injuries enter the equation [15, 16].

Length of mechanical ventilation in ICU was defined as the number of days spent in the ICU with endotracheal intubation or a tracheostomy and mandatory mechanical ventilation (excluding, e.g., non-invasive ventilation).

Length of hospital stay was defined as the time spent in primary care in the hospital participating in the TR-DGU.

Organ failure was assessed by the SOFA score as described previously. The SOFA score describes organ function in the respiratory, cardiovascular, renal, hematologic, hepatic, and central nervous systems [17]. Each organ system was graded to evaluate the severity of organ dysfunction or failure. Patients with organ failure entered in the TR-DGU database had to have met the SOFA score criteria for organ failure for at least 2 days. Multiple organ failure (MOF) and sepsis were assessed according to published guidelines [18]. Sepsis was defined as a systemic response to infection (presence of microorganisms). Data on respiratory failure, MOF, and sepsis were available on patients documented via the standard data collection form only.

Patient subgroups were defined according to the chest injury severity (AIS_{Thorax}). The first group consisted of patients with no relevant thoracic injuries ($AIS_{Thorax} = 0$ or 1), serving as a control group ("controls"). Group AIS-2 consisted of patients with $AIS_{Thorax} = 2$. Group AIS-3 consisted of patients with $AIS_{Thorax} = 3$. Group AIS-4 consisted of patients with $AIS_{Thorax} = 4$. Group AIS-5/6 consisted of patients with $AIS_{Thorax} = 5$ and 6, comprising the highest severity of chest trauma.

AIS_{Thorax} included all thoracic injuries coded as AIS = 4xxxxx.x [14]. Injuries to the thoracic spine were excluded, as these were coded with an AIS = 6xxxxx.x number.

Statistical analysis

Demographic and clinical characteristics comparing the aforementioned groups were evaluated using descriptive statistics. Continuous variables are presented as mean with standard deviation (SD), while categorical variables are presented as number of cases with percentages. The respective statistics refer to patients with valid data sets only. Therefore, the total number of patients or characteristics may sometimes vary.

Data for respiratory failure (ARDS), sepsis, and MOF are not part of the basic data set; therefore, not all hospitals provide this information, and patient numbers vary.

Formal statistical testing would require an initial overall test (chi-squared, analysis of variance, or Kolmogoroff-Smirnov) followed by pair-wise comparisons in case of significance. With five subgroups, the number of pair-wise tests would be ten per variable. Since the number of patients in the five subgroups ranged from 2000 to 8000, even minor differences would reach statistical significance. The 95% confidence interval in groups of 2000 cases (or more) would be about +/− 2% (or less) in case of categorical variables, and +/− 0.025*SD in case of continuous variables. For these reasons, we refrained from formal statistical testing, and our analysis is mainly descriptive.

Statistical testing for influencing factors on length of ICU stay and mechanical ventilation was performed using multiple linear regression analysis. In this analysis, the dependent variables were length of ICU stay and length of mechanical ventilation, respectively. The independent variables consisted of patient characteristics (age ≥ 60 years, gender, concomitant diseases), injury severity (ISS, $AIS_{Thorax} \geq 4$, $AIS_{Head} = 3$, $AIS_{Abdomen} \geq 3$, $AIS_{Extremity} \geq 3$), therapeutic interventions (ICU admission intubated/ventilated, blood transfusion), and type of injury to thoracic structures (vascular, lung, bone). Only surviving patients were included in this statistics. A p value of $< .05$ was considered significant.

All data were analyzed using SPSS, version 22.0 (IBM Inc., Armonk, NY, USA).

To analyze changes over time, we divided our 10-year data set into subgroups of 2 consecutive years each.

The present study is in line with the publication guidelines of the TraumaRegister DGU® and registered as TR-DGU project ID 2011–015.

Our study cohort has been described, analyzed for different characteristics, and published before [5].

Results

Data of 37,495 severely injured patients, including patients with head injuries of any severity, with an ISS ≥ 16 and aged ≥ 16 years were entered into the database. Of these, 64.3% suffered from at least moderate ($AIS_{Thorax} \geq 2$) and 26.7% from severe thoracic injury ($AIS_{Thorax} \geq 4$), respectively.

After excluding patients suffering from severe head injury ($AIS_{Head} \geq 4$), a total of 22,565 severely injured patients aged a mean 45.7 years (SD 19.3) and presented a mean ISS of 25.6 (SD 9.6) were identified for further analysis.

The standard data collection form (including data for respiratory failure, MOF, and sepsis) was filed for 16,793 (74.4%) patients, yet ~13% of these datasets were incomplete and excluded for analysis of the respective absent parameter.

Demographics

The study group's basic characteristics are summarized in Table 1. The patients suffering mainly from blunt trauma included in our study are predominantly male.

The distribution of injuries to different thoracic structures is dependent on thoracic trauma severity and is shown in Table 2. Most patients suffer from injuries to the lung, whereas injury to intrathoracic vessels is less prevalent in patients suffering from thoracic trauma ($AIS_{Thorax} \geq 2$).

Intensive Care

After primary work up in the emergency department, the rate of patients transferred directly to the Intensive Care Unit (ICU) was higher for $AIS_{Thorax} \geq 3$ (42.3– 47.8%) than $AIS_{Thorax} \leq 2$ (37.1–30.8%). The remaining patients underwent, for example, early (e.g., external fracture stabilization) or emergency (e.g., laparotomy) surgery.

The higher their AIS_{Thorax} score, the more patients who were admitted to the ICU were intubated and

Table 1 Basic characteristics: groups according to the AIS_{Thorax} (0 + 1, 2, 3, 4, and 5 + 6)

	Controls n = 4870	AIS-2 n = 1973	AIS-3 n = 8052	AIS-4 n = 5433	AIS-5/6 n = 2237
Age (years) Mean ± SD	44.2 ± 19.6	41.7 ± 18.6	45.3 ± 19.2	47.4 ± 19.0	49.3 ± 19.1
ISS Mean ± SD	21.5 ± 6.4	21.4 ± 5.9	23.5 ± 6.9	28.1 ± 9.3	39.4 ± 12.5
New ISS Mean ± SD	25.5 ± 8.3	23.5 ± 7.4	26.2 ± 7.4	33.7 ± 9.7	48.4 ± 12.6
Males	3439 71.3%	1414 72.0%	6009 75.1%	4074 75.5%	1667 75.3%
Blunt trauma	4405 93.7%	1855 97.0%	7518 96.5%	5028 95.7%	1979 92.0%

Total numbers and percentages for gender and injury mechanism
Total numbers for gender and trauma mechanism differ from the initial group

mechanically ventilated. Additionally, a one-point increase in the AIS_{Thorax} resulted in about a 1-day longer intubation period in ICU. Overall, we report a mean intubation period of 5.6 days (SD 10.7) in all our severely injured patients. Again, length of the ICU stay increased with the AIS_{Thorax} score and was a mean of 10.1 days (SD 13.4) in our overall population (Table 3).

In the subgroup of surviving patients only, the higher their AIS_{Thorax} score was, the longer the intubation period and ICU stay were. The mean duration of intubation was 5.6 days (SD 10.4) and mean length of ICU stay was 10.6 days (SD 13.2) for all groups presenting different thoracic trauma severity. Within each group, patients stayed in the ICU for a mean of approximately 5 days after extubation (Fig. 1).

In our multiple linear regression analysis for influencing factors (patient characteristics, injury severity, therapeutic interventions, and type of injury to thoracic structures) on ICU length of stay and length of mechanical ventilation, we found no effect for higher thoracic trauma severity ($AIS_{Thorax} \geq 4$) on ICU length of stay (+ 0.2 days; $p = 0.54$) but a significant effect on intubation days (+ 0.7 days; $p = 0.005$).

While vascular and lung injury did not significantly affect ICU length of stay and ventilation days, fractures significantly prolonged ICU length of stay (+ 1.7 days; $p < 0.001$) and intubation days (+ 0.9 days; $p < 0.001$).

We detected an influence from having one versus several diagnosed thoracic injuries on the duration of both mechanical ventilation and length of ICU stay, namely a one- to two-day mean increase in the duration of mechanical ventilation and ICU stay in patients suffering from multiple thoracic injuries. This was seen within each group of thoracic trauma severity (AIS_{Thorax}) ≥ 3. Again, irrespective of the counted thoracic injuries, patients remained about 5 days longer in the ICU than being mechanically ventilated (Table 4).

In patients scoring an $AIS_{Thorax} \geq 2$, one thoracic injury meant a mean 5.2 days of mechanical ventilation and 9.5 days of ICU stay versus 6.9 and 11.8 days with multiple thoracic injuries, respectively.

Table 2 Distribution of injuries to different thoracic structures in patients with at least moderate thoracic injury

	AIS-2	AIS-3	AIS-4	AIS-5/6	$AIS_{Thorax} \geq 2$
Vascular	0.2%	0.5%	4%	12.7%	542 (3.1%)
Lung	68.7%	80%	91.9%	84.5%	14,640 82.7%
Bone	39.8%	55.8%	46%	65.1%	9238 52.2%

Groups according to the AIS_{Thorax} (2, 3, 4, and 5 + 6) and all patients with $AIS_{Thorax} \geq 2$
Number of patients (with $AIS_{Thorax} \geq 2$) and percentages are given for "vascular" (intrathoracic vascular injury), "lung" (e.g., lung contusion, laceration, pneumothorax) and "bone" (rib and sternal fractures) injuries

Length of hospital stay

The length of hospital stay of all our severely injured patients decreased from a mean of 28.1 days (SD 27.2) in the controls with an $AIS_{Thorax} \leq 1$ to 23.4 days (SD 24.2) for those with AIS-5/6 (Table 3). When considering the surviving patients only, we identified no differences in length of hospital stay in conjunction with varying chest trauma severities (Fig. 2). Overall, the surviving patients, irrespective of their chest trauma severity, were hospitalized a mean of 28.8 days (SD 24.9).

While multiple chest trauma diagnoses in our severely injured patients—compared to a single diagnosis—were not associated with longer hospital stays for $AIS_{Thorax} \leq 4$, patients with an $AIS_{Thorax} \geq 5$ suffering from multiple chest trauma had an approximately 3.5 days longer mean hospital stay than patients presenting a single thoracic trauma diagnosis (20.9 versus 24.2 days).

Organ failure/mortality

Our severely injured patients revealed a higher rate of lung failure (defined as a Horowitz index ≤ 200 mmHg for at least 2 days (SOFA-Score [17]) the higher their AIS_{Thorax} was. While 13.9% of the patients with an $AIS_{Thorax} \leq 1$ suffered from acute lung failure, 40.3% of those with an $AIS_{Thorax} \geq 5$ did.

Rates of sepsis, respiratory failure, and MOF were higher in patients with greater thoracic trauma severity. The AIS-5/6 group displayed more than twice the rate of MOF, respiratory failure, and sepsis than the control subgroup (Table 5).

Early death within 24 h after admission to the hospital occurred in 6.7% of all our severely injured patients, and a total of 10.6% died during their hospital stay. When

Table 3 Influence of thoracic trauma severity on mechanical ventilation and ICU/hospital stay in all patients

	Controls	AIS-2	AIS-3	AIS-4	AIS-5/6
Mechanical ventilation/intubation	2708 (62.7%)	1199 (65.4%)	5003 (66.7%)	3525 (71.9%)	1499 (81.1%)
Length of mechanical ventilation	3.9 ± 9.9 [1]	4.6 ± 9.7 [1]	5.2 ± 9.8 [1]	7.1 ± 11.4 [2]	8.1 ± 12.9 [2]
Length of ICU stay	8.1 ± 12.7 [4]	9.3 ± 13.7 [5]	9.8 ± 12.3 [5]	11.7 ± 13.9 [7]	12.6 ± 16.4 [7]
Length of hospital stay	28.1 ± 27.2 [21]	28.4 ± 27.2 [21]	26.5 ± 24.1 [20]	25.5 ± 23.6 [20]	23.4 ± 24.2 [18]

Number of patients and percentages requiring mechanical ventilation during their ICU stay. Length of mechanical ventilation, ICU stay, and hospital stay in days (mean ± SD); [median]. Subgroups according to the AIS_{Thorax} (0 + 1, 2, 3, 4, and 5 + 6)

examining the distribution of chest trauma severity in our deceased patients, we found higher mortality in those with an $AIS_{Thorax} \geq 4$ (this applies to the early deaths as well as all deaths during hospital stay) (Table 5).

Death usually occurred while the patients were in the ICU. Late mortality, meaning death occurring later than 3 days after ICU discharge, occurred more often in patients with an $AIS_{Thorax} \leq 3$ (about 10% of patients in each group). An $AIS_{Thorax} = 4$ was associated with 5.2%, an $AIS_{Thorax} \geq 5$ with 3% of the late deaths.

Patients sustaining multiple chest injuries within one AIS_{Thorax} severity score did not reveal mortality rates different from those of patients with one thoracic trauma diagnosis.

Changes over time

The rate of severely injured patients being admitted intubated to the ICU dropped steadily over the decade we examined. While 83% of patients arrived in the ICU on mechanical ventilation between 2002 and 2003, only 59.3% were intubated between 2010 and 2012. We noted the same pattern in all groups during those years when patients are segregated according to their chest trauma severity (Fig. 3).

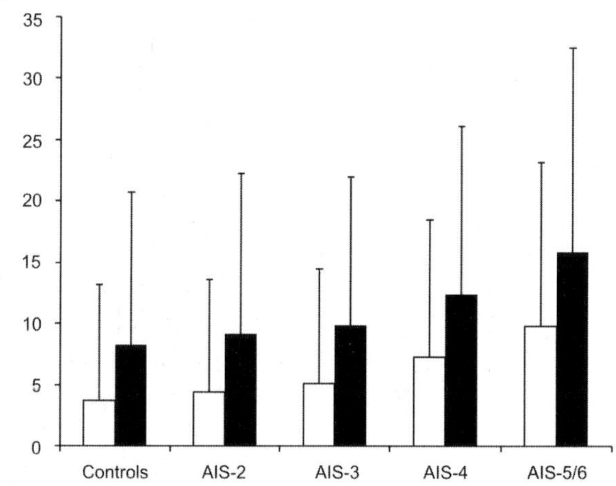

Fig. 1 Influence of thoracic trauma severity on mechanical ventilation and ICU stay in surviving patients. Length of mechanical ventilation (open boxes) and ICU stay (black columns) in days (mean value + standard deviation) for different thoracic trauma severity. Subgroups according to the AIS_{Thorax} (0 + 1, 2, 3, 4, and 5 + 6)

While the rate of acute lung failure in all groups (including the subgroups with varying chest trauma severity (data not shown)) revealed no distinct trend over the decade, mortality during hospital stay did fall from 13.5 to 10.1% for all patients from 2002 to 2012. Mortality in all groups is now lower than it was in 2002 (Fig. 4).

Discussion

We present a retrospective analysis of severely injured patients suffering from thoracic traumas of different magnitude. As in other studies [6, 13, 19–22], our population consists mainly of middle-aged males with a mean ISS ≥ 16 suffering from blunt trauma. Severe head trauma ($AIS_{Head} \geq 4$) alone can be an indication for intubation [13], and concomitant head and thoracic trauma influence each other in terms of intensive care therapy [21, 23]. Previous studies have shown that severely injured patients with head and chest injuries require prolonged intensive care stay and mechanical ventilation [23], and thoracic injury is known to be an independent risk factor for 30-day mortality and poor outcome in patients suffering traumatic brain injuries [21]. Thus, by excluding patients with severe head trauma ($AIS_{Head} \geq 4$), we minimized the risk of confounding our target parameters by such injuries' effects.

Severe multiple trauma is often associated with traumatic lung injury. While the prehospital intubation of patients with severe thoracic trauma without manifest respiratory insufficiency has been debated [13, 24], Ruchholtz et al. reported that 95% of their severely injured patients suffering from severe thoracic trauma ($AIS_{Thorax} = 4$), without prehospital intubation presented the indication for intubation over the medium term [13].

Table 4 Mechanical ventilation and length of ICU stay is dependent on the number of thoracic injuries

	AIS-2		AIS-3		AIS-4		AIS-5/6	
	One	Mul	One	Mul	One	Mul	One	Mul
Mechanical ventilation	4.7	4.2	4.7	5.8	6.4	7.5	6.2	8.6
ICU stay	9.4	8.9	8.9	10.8	10.6	12.3	9.8	13.4

Mechanical ventilation time and length of ICU stay in mean days for singular or multiple chest trauma diagnoses
Subgroups according to the AIS_{Thorax} (2, 3, 4, and 5 + 6)

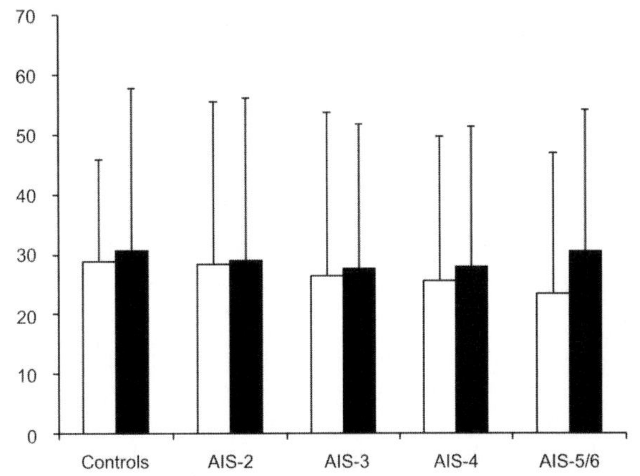

Fig. 2 Influence of thoracic trauma severity on hospital stay in all severely injured and surviving patients. Length of hospital stay in days (mean value + standard deviation) for different thoracic trauma severity in all severely injured (open boxes) and surviving patients only (black columns). Subgroups according to the AIS_{Thorax} (0 + 1, 2, 3, 4, and 5 + 6)

In our population, 62 to 81% of patients admitted to the ICU were already intubated, and most underwent interventions (e.g., surgery) prior to their admission. In line with others, we also detected higher rates of mechanical ventilation at ICU admission in conjunction with higher AIS_{Thorax} scores [22]. Our severely injured patients were mechanically ventilated for a mean 5.6 days—less time than Hildebrand et al.'s severely injured patients (mechanically ventilated for a mean 11 days) but comparable to Sauaia et al. Those two working groups also excluded severely injured patients with severe traumatic brain injury [7, 22]. Hildebrand et al. demonstrated a greater increase in mechanical-ventilation days in conjunction with each additional point in the AIS_{Thorax} than we did, but they only analyzed patients with an $AIS_{Thorax} \geq 3 \leq 5$ [22].

Our reported lengths of ICU stay falls within the range of Sauaia et al. and Fröhlich et al. regarding their populations of severely injured patients [6, 7]. Compared to Hildebrand et al., all our patients exhibit an almost 5-day shorter mean length of stay in the ICU, despite similar ISS scores and overall mortality, exclusion of severe head trauma in both studies, and our population's higher percentage of acute lung failure [22].

Interesting enough, we found no statistical significant influence of more severe thoracic trauma ($AIS_{Thorax} \geq 4$) on ICU length of stay, but a significant effect on prolonging the mechanical ventilation period. When breaking the AIS_{Thorax} down into actual injuries to thoracic structures, only fractures to the rib cage and sternum significantly prolonged the ICU stay and intubation. This is reflected in a scoring system where patients suffering from thoracic trauma are, among other parameters, assessed for the extent of rib fractures to estimate the requirement of mechanical ventilation and prolonged care [25].

We demonstrate with our severely injured patients that not only the most severe injury to the chest—which determines the AIS_{Thorax} score—was pertinent to the length of the intubation period, but also that the total number of chest injuries influenced both, length of mechanical ventilation and ICU stay. This may, again, be reflected in the recently developed scoring system to predict the outcome of patients with chest wall injuries where parameters like age, extent of pulmonary contusion, number of rib fractures, and existing bilateral rib fractures are taken into account. Patients with total scores ≥ 5 were mechanically ventilated and hospitalized for a longer period, while those with scores ≥ 7 revealed a still greater risk for mortality, ICU admission, and mechanical ventilation [25]. However, we detected no correlation between multiple injuries to the chest and increased mortality in our study.

The 10.6% overall mortality we report falls within the published range of in-hospital-mortality in a severely injured population (9 to 16.2%) [6, 19, 22]. To the best of our knowledge, AIS_{Thorax}-dependent differences in mortality have not been reported before. Interestingly, our data reveal that single and multiple injuries resulting in an $AIS_{Thorax} = 3$ and 2 did not increase mortality compared to $AIS_{Thorax} = 0$ and 1 in our severely injured patients. Perhaps lesser injuries to the chest, despite increasing the rate of acute lung failure in our population,

Table 5 Organ failure, sepsis, and mortality rates are dependent on thoracic trauma severity

	Controls	AIS-2	AIS-3	AIS-4	AIS-5/6
Multiple organ failure[a]	625 (19.3%)	268 (20.4%)	1171 (22.5%)	1107 (30.7%)	534 (42.4%)
Respiratory failure[a]	450 (13.9%)	231 (17.6%)	1130 (21.7%)	1157 (32.1%)	506 (40.3%)
Sepsis[a]	231 (7.1%)	107 (8.2%)	477 (9.1%)	411 (11.4%)	203 (16.0%)
Early mortality	254 (5.2%)	44 (2.2%)	276 (3.4%)	436 (8.0%)	491 (21.9%)
Hospital mortality	418 (8.6%)	93 (4.7%)	561 (7.0%)	687 (12.6%)	635 (28.4%)

Number of patients and percentage within the respective cohort of thoracic trauma severity are shown
Early mortality: death within 24 h after hospital admission
[a]Parameter available only for patients documented with the standard form (*n* = 16,793; missing data in 13%); therefore, total patient numbers vary

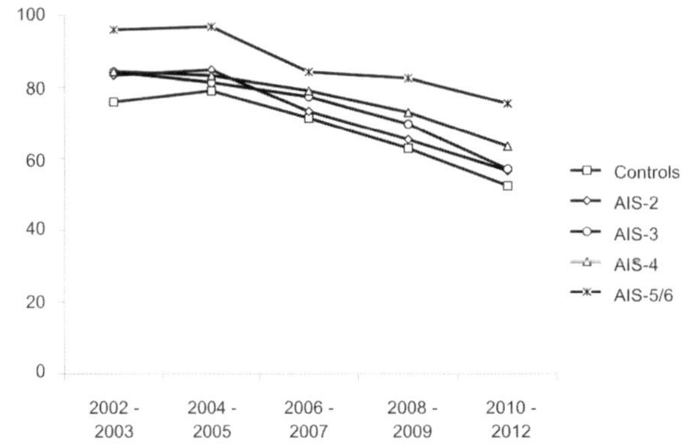

Fig. 3 Rates of mechanical ventilation in severely injured patients changed over time. Percent of mechanically ventilated severely injured patients at ICU admission over consecutive time spans. Subgroups according to the AIS_{Thorax} (0 + 1, 2, 3, 4, and 5 + 6)

do not inflict greater injury to the other organ systems, and the body can recuperate. While the 10.9 to 40.3% range of AIS_{Thorax}-dependent acute lung failure we report resembles the published incidence of 8 to 37% in trauma patients [26, 27], others have shown the associated mortality to range from 16 to 29% [26–28].

An $AIS_{Thorax} \geq 4$ may exert widespread chest-trauma effects throughout the body, thereby furthering the development of multiple organ dysfunction and failure and raising an independent risk factor for acute lung injury (ALI), ARDS, and pulmonary failure [29, 30]. Furthermore, it is well known that 80% of patients with multiple organ dysfunction syndrome (MODS) start with lung failure [23], and that severe thoracic trauma is an independent risk factor for developing MODS [6, 31]. MODS-related deaths range from 13 to 36% [6, 7, 32]. Our data support these findings, as we noted increasing rates of respiratory failure with increasing thoracic trauma severity, and demonstrate the first major rise in MOF in association with an $AIS_{Thorax} \geq 4$. In the context

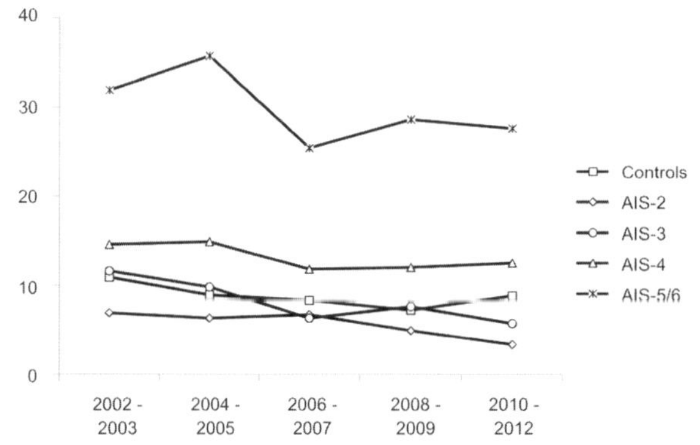

Fig. 4 Mortality in severely injured patients changed over time. Hospital mortality rates shown over consecutive time spans for different thoracic trauma severity. Subgroups according to the AIS_{Thorax} (0 + 1, 2, 3, 4, and 5 + 6)

of sepsis, our reports are comparable to published rates in severely injured patients, which range from 3.1 to 17% [33]. However, we also demonstrate that the severity of thoracic trauma is associated with increasing sepsis rates in severely injured patients.

We report different mean LOS for all severely injured patients and surviving patients only. The mean LOS for all patients is shorter than for surviving patients and shortest for all patients with AIS-5/6. This is not surprising, since per definition $AIS_{Thorax} = 6$ is a not survivable injury and many patients with $AIS_{Thorax} = 5$ will die because of the magnitude of injury. More striking is the fact that across the AIS groups in surviving patients, LOS seems not to differ. One explanation could be that patients with lower AIS_{Thorax} exhibit more serious injuries in other body regions (e.g., abdominal, extremities) responsible for longer hospitalization in these groups. This is underlined by the fact that we only found a tendency towards longer ICU stay with increasing thoracic trauma severity, and this effect was not statistically significant in our multiple linear regression analysis. Another possibility is the early discharge of patients with higher AIS_{Thorax} for respiratory weaning/respiratory rehabilitation, thus shortening the period of care in the primary care facility documenting these cases.

When considering where death occurred, most of our patients died in the ICU. However, an $AIS_{Thorax} < 4$ incurred a higher rate of deaths on regular wards than an $AIS_{Thorax} \geq 4$. We were unable to analyze the causes of death in these different groups since they are not documented in the TR-DGU's primary data set. Thus, we have too little knowledge to determine why, after being discharged from the ICU, severely injured patients, without severe head and severe thoracic trauma, had a higher rate of death than patients with severe chest trauma.

The percentage of intubated, severely injured patients admitted to the ICU has declined in recent years, independent of the severity of their thoracic trauma. This might be a reflection of prehospital behavior, where changes over the last 20 years—from routine intubation in most severely injured patients to intubation, based on clearer indications—has led to better care [34]. Moreover, in patients in whom the indication for mechanical ventilation arose because of the accompanying thoracic trauma, early non-invasive ventilation has proven to significantly reduce mortality and the intubation rate without increasing complications [35].

We publish a decline in the mortality rate of severely injured patients in recent years irrespective of the severity of the chest trauma they sustained. This observation concurs with prior data reporting an overall drop in the mortality of severely injured patients [6].

This study is limited by its retrospective nature. Hospitals participating in the TR-DGU are regularly audited, and sample tests are taken to ensure data quality. However, the validity of their documentation is not verified by external monitors as in prospective trials [36]. The present analysis is based upon a European population where the majority experienced blunt trauma, which might differ from cohorts with a higher percentage of penetrating injuries. Our interpretation of the causes of mortality is limited by referring to the TR-DGU database, since the actual cause of death is not recorded; thus, we could not ascribe higher mortality rates to either inherent thoracic (e.g., respiratory failure) or to other causes (e.g., sepsis, MOF). Additionally, we excluded patients with severe head injury ($AIS_{Head} \geq 4$) in our study to minimize confounding and, as a result, our findings cannot be readily transferred to severely injured patients sustaining additional major head trauma.

To interpret our results, one has to keep in mind that our "control group" is mainly characterized by the absence of relevant thoracic trauma ($AIS_{Thorax} \leq 1$). Thus, to generate an ISS ≥ 16 without severe injury to the head, patients needed at least one severe injury or a combination of injuries to the remaining body regions. Albeit, since we clearly focus on the influence of thoracic trauma in severely injured patients, we feel this to be an adequate "control group."

Conclusion

The extent of thoracic trauma in severely injured patients is a relevant risk factor for intensive care therapy, organ failure, sepsis, and mortality. We demonstrate that the higher the AIS_{Thorax} score, the higher the rate of intubated patients admitted to the ICU. Higher AIS_{Thorax} scores and multiple injuries to the chest correlated with longer periods of mechanical ventilation and ICU stays. Mortality in our population began to rise in conjunction with an $AIS_{Thorax} \geq 4$. Overall, while most patient deaths occurred during their ICU stay, death later than 3 days after ICU discharge occurred more often in patients with milder chest injuries ($AIS_{Thorax} \leq 3$).

Abbreviations

AIS: Abbreviated injury scale; ALI: Acute lung injury; ARDS: Adult respiratory syndrome; ICU: Intensive care unit; ISS: Injury severity score; LOS: Length of hospital stay; MODS: Multiple organ dysfunction syndrome; MOF: Multiple organ failure; NISS: New ISS; SD: Standard deviation; TBI: Traumatic brain injury; TR-DGU: The TraumaRegister DGU®

Acknowledgements

The authors thank Carole Cürten for language editing.
Participating hospitals are listed in alphabetical order under www.traumaregister-dgu.de

Funding

The article processing charge was funded by the German Research Foundation (DFG) and the Albert-Ludwigs-University Freiburg in the funding program Open Access Publishing.

Authors' contributions

JB conceived and designed the study, interpreted the data, and drafted the manuscript. RL was in charge of the statistical reports. RL, SR, JK, JZ, NS, and TH contributed to the study design, interpreted the data, and critically revised the manuscript. All authors read and approved the final manuscript.

Competing Interests

The authors declare that they have no competing interests.

Author details

[1]Department of Orthopedics and Trauma Surgery, Medical Center – Albert-Ludwigs-University of Freiburg, Faculty of Medicine, Albert-Ludwigs-University of Freiburg, Hugstetter Str. 55, 79106 Freiburg, Germany. [2]FOM - Institute for Research in Operative Medicine, University Witten/Herdecke, Faculty of Health, Ostmerheimer Str. 200, 51109 Köln, Germany. [3]Department of Orthopedics and Trauma Surgery, Oberschwabenklinik St. Elisabeth, Elisabethenstr. 15, 88212 Ravensburg, Germany. [4]Committee on Emergency Medicine, Intensive Care and Trauma Management of the German Trauma Society (Sektion NIS), Berlin, Germany.

References

1. Vecsei V, Arbes S, Aldrian S, Nau T. Chest injuries in polytrauma. Eur J Trauma. 2005;31:239–43.
2. Bardenheuer M, Obertacke U, Waydhas C, Nast-Kolb D. Epidemiology of the severely injured patient. A prospective assessment of preclinical and clinical management. AG Polytrauma of DGU. Unfallchirurg. 2000;103:355–63.
3. Huang YK, Liu KS, Lu MS, Wu MY, Tsai FC, Lin PJ. Extracorporeal life support in post-traumatic respiratory distress patients. Resuscitation. 2009;80:535–9.
4. Ruchholtz S, Lefering R, Paffrath T, Oestern HJ, Neugebauer E, Nast-Kolb D, et al. Reduction in mortality of severely injured patients in Germany. Dtsch Arztebl Int. 2008;105:225–31.
5. Bayer J, Lefering R, Reinhardt S, Kühle J, Südkamp NP, Hammer T. Severity-dependent differences in early management of thoracic trauma in severely injured patients—analysis based on the TraumaRegister DGU(R). Scand J Trauma Resusc Emerg Med. 2017;25:10.
6. Fröhlich M, Lefering R, Probst C, Paffrath T, Schneider MM, Maegele M, et al. Epidemiology and risk factors of multiple-organ failure after multiple trauma: an analysis of 31,154 patients from the TraumaRegister DGU. J Trauma Acute Care Surg. 2014;76:921–7.
7. Sauaia A, Moore EE, Johnson JL, Chin TL, Banerjee A, Sperry JL, et al. Temporal trends of postinjury multiple-organ failure: still resource intensive, morbid, and lethal. J Trauma Acute Care Surg. 2014;76:582–92.
8. Ried M, Bein T, Philipp A, Muller T, Graf B, Schmid C, et al. Extracorporeal lung support in trauma patients with severe chest injury and acute lung failure: a 10-year institutional experience. Crit Care. 2013;17:R110.
9. Gaillard M, Herve C, Mandin L, Raynaud P. Mortality prognostic factors in chest injury. J Trauma. 1990;30:93–6.
10. Inthorn D, Huf R. Thoracic trauma in multiple trauma. Anasthesiol Intensivmed Notfallmed Schmerzther. 1992;27:498–501.
11. Brasel KJ, Guse CE, Layde P, Weigelt JA. Rib fractures: relationship with pneumonia and mortality. Crit Care Med. 2006;34:1642–6.
12. Treggiari MM, Hudson LD, Martin DP, Weiss NS, Caldwell E, Rubenfeld G. Effect of acute lung injury and acute respiratory distress syndrome on outcome in critically ill trauma patients. Crit Care Med. 2004;32:327–31.
13. Ruchholtz S, Waydhas C, Ose C, Lewan U, Nast-Kolb D. Prehospital intubation in severe thoracic trauma without respiratory insufficiency: a matched-pair analysis based on the Trauma Registry of the German Trauma Society. J Trauma. 2002;52:879–86.
14. Gennarelli TA, Wodzin E. AIS 2005. Barrington, IL: Association for the Advancement of Automotive Medicine; 2005.
15. Baker SP, O'Neill B, Haddon W Jr, Long WB. The injury severity score: a method for describing patients with multiple injuries and evaluating emergency care. J Trauma. 1974;14:187–96.
16. Osler T, Baker SP, Long W. A modification of the injury severity score that both improves accuracy and simplifies scoring. J Trauma. 1997;43:922–5.

17. Vincent JL, Moreno R, Takala J, Willatts S, De Mendonca A, Bruining H, et al. The SOFA (Sepsis-related Organ Failure Assessment) score to describe organ dysfunction/failure. On behalf of the Working Group on Sepsis-Related Problems of the European Society of Intensive Care Medicine. Intensive Care Med. 1996;22:707–10.
18. American College of Chest Physicians/Society of Critical Care Medicine Consensus Conference: definitions for sepsis and organ failure and guidelines for the use of innovative therapies in sepsis. Crit Care Med 1992; 20:864-874.
19. Geiger EV, Lustenberger T, Wutzler S, Lefering R, Lehnert M, Walcher F, et al. Predictors of pulmonary failure following severe trauma: a trauma registry-based analysis. Scand J Trauma Resusc Emerg Med. 2013;21:34.
20. Di Bartolomeo S, Sanson G, Nardi G, Scian F, Michelutto V, Lattuada L. A population-based study on pneumothorax in severely traumatized patients. J Trauma. 2001;51:677–82.
21. Dai D, Yuan Q, Sun Y, Yuan F, Su Z, Ding J, et al. Impact of thoracic injury on traumatic brain injury outcome. PLoS One. 2013;8:e74204.
22. Hildebrand F, Giannoudis PV, Griensven M, Zelle B, Ulmer B, Krettek C, et al. Management of polytraumatized patients with associated blunt chest trauma: a comparison of two European countries. Injury. 2005;36:293–302.
23. Hildebrand F, van Griensven M, Garapati R, Krettek C, Pape HC. Diagnostics and scoring in blunt chest trauma. Eur J Trauma. 2002;28:157–67.
24. Trupka A, Waydhas C, Nast-Kolb D, Schweiberer L. Early intubation in severely injured patients. Eur J Emerg Med. 1994;1:1–8.
25. Pressley CM, Fry WR, Philp AS, Berry SD, Smith RS. Predicting outcome of patients with chest wall injury. Am J Surg. 2012;204:910–3.
26. Becher RD, Colonna AL, Enniss TM, Weaver AA, Crane DK, Martin RS, et al. An innovative approach to predict the development of adult respiratory distress syndrome in patients with blunt trauma. J Trauma Acute Care Surg. 2012;73:1229–35.
27. Martin M, Salim A, Murray J, Demetriades D, Belzberg H, Rhee P. The decreasing incidence and mortality of acute respiratory distress syndrome after injury: a 5-year observational study. J Trauma. 2005;59:1107–13.
28. Salim A, Martin M, Constantinou C, Sangthong B, Brown C, Kasotakis G, et al. Acute respiratory distress syndrome in the trauma intensive care unit: morbid but not mortal. Arch Surg. 2006;141:655–8.
29. Ashbaugh DG, Bigelow DB, Petty TL, Levine BE. Acute respiratory distress in adults. Lancet. 1967;2:319–23.
30. Ware LB, Matthay MA. The acute respiratory distress syndrome. N Engl J Med. 2000;342:1334–49.
31. Minei JP, Cuschieri J, Sperry J, Moore EE, West MA, Harbrecht BG, et al. The changing pattern and implications of multiple organ failure after blunt injury with hemorrhagic shock. Crit Care Med. 2012;40:1129–35.
32. Laudi S, Donaubauer B, Busch T, Kerner T, Bercker S, Bail H, et al. Low incidence of multiple organ failure after major trauma. Injury. 2007;38:1052–8.
33. Pfeifer R, Tarkin IS, Rocos B, Pape HC. Patterns of mortality and causes of death in polytrauma patients—has anything changed? Injury. 2009;40:907–11.
34. Hussmann B, Lendemans S. Pre-hospital and early in-hospital management of severe injuries: changes and trends. Injury. 2014;45:S39–42.
35. Chiumello D, Coppola S, Froio S, Gregoretti C, Consonni D. Noninvasive ventilation in chest trauma: systematic review and meta-analysis. Intensive Care Med. 2013;39:1171–80.
36. Lefering R, Paffrath T. Reality of care based on the data from the Trauma Registry of the German Society of Trauma Surgery. Unfallchirurg. 2012;115:30–2.

21

Getting the invite list right: a discussion of sepsis severity scoring systems in severe complicated intra-abdominal sepsis and randomized trial inclusion criteria

Matti Tolonen[1], Federico Coccolini[2], Luca Ansaloni[3], Massimo Sartelli[4], Derek J. Roberts[5], Jessica L. McKee[6], Ari Leppaniemi[1], Christopher J. Doig[7], Fausto Catena[8], Timothy Fabian[9], Craig N. Jenne[10], Osvaldo Chiara[11], Paul Kubes[12,13], Yoram Kluger[14], Gustavo P. Fraga[15], Bruno M. Pereira[16], Jose J. Diaz[17], Michael Sugrue[18], Ernest E. Moore[19], Jianan Ren[20], Chad G. Ball[21], Raul Coimbra[22,23], Elijah Dixon[24], Walter Biffl[25], Anthony MacLean[26], Paul B. McBeth[5,10,27], Juan G. Posadas-Calleja[10], Salomone Di Saverio[28], Jimmy Xiao[6], Andrew W. Kirkpatrick[5,10,27,29*], From the Closed Or Open after Laparotomy (COOL) for Source Control in Severe Complicated Intra-Abdominal Sepsis Investigators

Abstract

Background: Severe complicated intra-abdominal sepsis (SCIAS) is a worldwide challenge with increasing incidence. Open abdomen management with enhanced clearance of fluid and biomediators from the peritoneum is a potential therapy requiring prospective evaluation. Given the complexity of powering multi-center trials, it is essential to recruit an inception cohort sick enough to benefit from the intervention; otherwise, no effect of a potentially beneficial therapy may be apparent. An evaluation of abilities of recognized predictive systems to recognize SCIAS patients was conducted using an existing intra-abdominal sepsis (IAS) database.

Methods: All consecutive adult patients with a diffuse secondary peritonitis between 2012 and 2013 were collected from a quaternary care hospital in Finland, excluding appendicitis/cholecystitis. From this retrospectively collected database, a target population (93) of those with either ICU admission or mortality were selected. The performance metrics of the Third Consensus Definitions for Sepsis and Septic Shock based on both SOFA and quick SOFA, the World Society of Emergency Surgery Sepsis Severity Score (WSESSSS), the APACHE II score, Manheim Peritonitis Index (MPI), and the Calgary Predisposition, Infection, Response, and Organ dysfunction (CPIRO) score were all tested for their discriminant ability to identify this subgroup with SCIAS and to predict mortality.

Results: Predictive systems with an area under-the-receiving-operating characteristic (AUC) curve > 0.8 included SOFA, Sepsis-3 definitions, APACHE II, WSESSSS, and CPIRO scores with the overall best for CPIRO. The highest identification rates were SOFA score ≥ 2 (78.4%), followed by the WSESSSS score ≥ 8 (73.1%), SOFA ≥ 3 (75.2%), and APACHE II ≥ 14 (68.8%) identification. Combining the Sepsis-3 septic-shock definition and WSESSS ≥ 8 increased detection to 80%. Including CPIRO score ≥ 3 increased this to 82.8% (Sensitivity-SN; 83% Specificity-SP; 74%. Comparatively, SOFA ≥ 4 and WSESSSS ≥ 8 with or without septic-shock had 83.9% detection (SN; 84%, SP; 75%, 25% mortality).
(Continued on next page)

* Correspondence: Andrew.Kirkpatrick@albertahealthservices.ca
[5]Department of Surgery, University of Calgary, Calgary, Alberta, Canada
[10]Department of Critical Care Medicine, University of Calgary, Calgary, Alberta, Canada
Full list of author information is available at the end of the article

(Continued from previous page)

Conclusions: No one scoring system behaves perfectly, and all are largely dominated by organ dysfunction. Utilizing combinations of SOFA, CPIRO, and WSESSSS scores in addition to the Sepsis-3 septic shock definition appears to offer the widest "inclusion-criteria" to recognize patients with a high chance of mortality and ICU admission.

Keywords: Intra-abdominal sepsis, Septic shock, Risk stratification, Randomized controlled trial, Trial methodology, Organ dysfunction, Epidemiology

Background

Sepsis is a complex and increasing global health problem [1–5]. International consensus currently uses the working definition of sepsis as life-threatening organ dysfunction caused by a dysregulated host response to infection [2]. The number of cases per year is estimated as approaching 18–19 million worldwide [4–6]. In the most severe cases, mortality rates approach 30–40% when shock is present [2, 7, 8], although may be 80% in the developing world [9]. When the focus of infection is located within the abdominal cavity, a particularly severe form of sepsis may result in association with the anatomy and physiology of the abdominal cavity and the viscera within [10, 11]. Cases of intra-abdominal sepsis (IAS) may be defined as complicated when the inflammation or contamination spreads beyond a single organ [12, 13]. Complicated IAS may also be considered severe complicated IAS (SCIAS) when organ dysfunction is present with a mortality rate of 10–30% or with a mortality rate of 40–70% [14, 15] when septic shock is present [2, 7, 16, 17].

Despite advances in diagnosis, surgery, and antimicrobial therapy, mortality rates associated with CIAS and IAS remain exceedingly high [18]. Despite appropriate therapy, progress to septic shock and multiple organ dysfunction driven by inflammation is common. Delayed or inadequate source control remains an independent predictor of mortality [19, 20]. However, recognizing "failed source control" [21, 22], from a self-propagating biomediator storm is often difficult or impossible without abdominal re-exploration (relaparotomy). At present, pharmacologic approaches are not the answer. Attempting to derive pharmacologic therapies for combating post-infective inflammation has proven an expensive and frustrating process [23]. Over 100 attempts at blocking single biological response mediators have failed to address the early cytokine storm of sepsis [24, 25]. A controversial, potentially morbid, potentially life-saving technique is the adoption of an open abdomen (OA) following source control laparotomy. Uncontrolled use of the OA following sepsis is increasingly being reported as another potentially desirable option for the sickest SCIAS patents [12, 21, 22, 26–28]. However, accepting the OA is either potentially a life-saving intervention or a morbid unnecessary procedure with increased risks of complications such as enterocutaneous fistulae [29, 30]; an adequately powered prospective randomized controlled trial is urgently required.

Given the complexity of adequately powering multicenter trials, it is essential to recruit an inception cohort of patients sick enough to benefit from the intervention; otherwise, no effect of a potentially beneficial therapy may be apparent. Many scoring systems have been proposed for use in predicting clinical outcomes in the critically ill. Potential systems that have been suggested include the Acute Physiology and Chronic Health Evaluation (APACHE II) [31–34], multiple organ failure (MOF) scores [35], P-POSSUM [32, 36], Therapeutic Intervention Scoring System (TISS-28) [37, 38], and the National Early Warning Score (NEWS) definitions of sepsis [39, 40]; some are more intended for sepsis specifically such as the Sepsis Severity Score [33] and those specifically intended to consider intra-abdominal pathology such as the Mannheim Peritonitis Index [41], the World Society of Emergency Surgery Sepsis Severity Score (WSESSSS) [7], and even systems intended for pancreatitis such as the Ranson [42, 43] and Imrie [43] scores [44]. However, none is currently accepted as being ideal for predicting outcomes in SCIAS [7]. We thus conducted an evaluation of the abilities of recognized predictive systems for clinical outcomes in SCIAS to detect patients of interest using an existing IAS database.

Methods

A retrospectively collected database of SCIAS cases was created at a quaternary care hospital in Helsinki, Finland. This database enrolled all consecutive adult patients with a diffuse secondary peritonitis between 2012 and 2013, although cases of appendicitis or cholecystitis were excluded. The institutional human research review committee approved the study design, and as it was an observational retrospective cohort study, neither informed consent nor ethics committee's approval was required. An attribute of this dataset was that intraoperative evaluations for development of organ dysfunctions were performed. Although this data has been previously published [45], for the current project the original data was revisited and updated regarding to new Sepsis-3 definitions of organ dysfunction. The demographics included in this database have been previously described and were sufficient to allow calculation of the Mannheim Peritonitis Index (MPI), WSESSSS (Table 1), Calgary Predisposition, Infection, Response, and Organ Dysfunction (CPIRO) (Table 2), Acute Physiology and Chronic Health Evaluation (APACHE) II, and the consensus definitions and quick SOFA (qSOFA) score of the Sepsis-3 International Consensus Definitions. From this database, a cohort of patients who either died or were admitted to the intensive care unit were selected. Thereafter, the performance metrics of these putative predictive and scoring systems were tested (using a number of varying thresholds within each system where appropriate) for their discriminant ability to identify SCIAS and, thereafter, predict ICU admission or 30-day mortality. To assess whether utilizing combinations of scoring systems provided additive predictive power, the performance of combinations of systems was also calculated. This was done through simple mathematical addition of patient of interest recognition. Potential combinations to test were selected based on their being practically usable by on-call clinicians without retrospective data or extensive laboratory results, an acceptable AUROC (> 0.80) in our analysis reflecting a practical combination of scores in terms of highest sensitivity with a reasonable specificity. Analyses were performed using SPSS© Statistics version 22 for Mac (IBM©, Armonk, NY, USA). Sensitivity and specificity were calculated for each prognostic system. Receiving operating characteristics (ROC) curves were plotted and area under curve (AUC) calculated with 95% confidence interval (CI).

Table 1 World Society of Emergency Surgery Sepsis Severity Score for complicated intra-abdominal infections

Clinical conditions at admission	
Sepsis with organ dysfunction at admission	3 points
Septic shock (acute circulatory failure characterized by persistent arterial hypotension) requiring vasopressor agents	5 points
Setting of acquisition	
Healthcare-associated infection	2 points
Origin of intra-abdominal infection	
Colonic non-diverticular perforation peritonitis	2 points
Small bowel perforation peritonitis	3 points
Diverticular diffuse peritonitis	2 points
Post-operative diffuse peritonitis	2 points
Delay in source control	
Delayed initial intervention (pre-operative duration of peritonitis (localized or diffuse) > 24 h	3 points
Risk factor	
Age > 70	2 points
Immunosuppression (chronic glucocorticoids, immunosuppressive agents, chemotherapy, lymphatic disease, virus)	3 points

Reproduced from Sartelli et al [7]

Table 2 Calgary Predisposition, Infection, Response, and Organ Dysfunction (CPIRO)

Score	Variable	Point
Predisposition	Age > 65 years	1
	Comorbidities	1
Response	Leukopenia	1
	Hypothermia	1
Organ dysfunction	Cardiovascular dysfunction	1
	Respiratory dysfunction	1
	Renal dysfunction	1
	CNS dysfunction	1
Total		8

Table reproduced from Posadas-Calleja et al. [57]

Results

In the original data set, there were 223 patients. Of these patients, 33 (13.5%) died within 30-days and 72 (32.2%) were admitted to the ICU. The target group of interest, with either 30-day mortality or ICU admission, constituted 93 patients with a 22% mortality. The majority (88%) of this group stayed in ICU more than 3 days and had a mean highest SOFA score of 7.9 [median 8; IQR 5–10]. Accounting for those that died in ICU, the mean length of ICU stay was 7.8 days [median 5.0; IQR 3–8.75], with 90% staying 3 or more days.

Overall predictive rates were tested for different threshold values of the scoring systems: qSOFA ≥ 2; SOFA 2, 3, 4 and Sepsis-3 septic shock definition; MPI ≥ 30, 32, 34; APACHE II ≥ 12, 14, 16; WSES ≥ 8, 9, 10; CPIRO ≥ 3, 4 (Table 3). In addition, the combined predictive capability of using the scores together was also tested and are reported in Table 4. Systems with a good (AUC > 0.8) performance included the SOFA, Sepsis-3 sepsis classification, APACHE II, WSESSSS, and CPIRO scores and overall; the greatest AUC was for the CPIRO score regardless if the consideration was of patients requiring ICU admission and dying (Fig. 1) or just with mortality (Fig. 2).

While selecting all patients with diffuse secondary peritonitis would yield greater enrollment, the disease severity would include patients with lower mortality that may not benefit from OA therapy. Thus, the most efficient identification rates of the desired cohort for a single system was a SOFA score ≥ 2 with 78.4% identification, followed by SOFA ≥ 3 with 75.2%, WSESSSS score ≥ 8 with 73.1%, and the APACHE II ≥ 14 with 68.8% identification (Table 1). Combining predictive systems together improved the identification rates (Table 4). Combining the Sepsis-3 septic shock definition with the WSESSS criteria increased detection to the highest rate of 79.6%, a rate that was not

Table 3 Predictive capabilities of potential COOL study sepsis and critical illness scoring systems using Helsinki outcomes data

System	Identified	Outcome mortality	Sensitivity (%)	Specificity (%)	AUC[b]	95% CI
qSOFA ≥ 2	34 (36.6%)	13 (32%)	37	95	0.723	[0.653–0.792]
SOFA ≥ 2	72 (77.4%)	25 (27%)	77	83	0.825	[0.766–0.885]
SOFA ≥ 3	70 (75.3%)	24 (27%)	75	85		
SOFA ≥ 4	60 (64.5%)	20 (28%)	65	91		
Septic shock[a]	36 (38.7%)	15 (37%)	39	96	0.82	[0.761–0.88]
MPI ≥ 30	48 (51.6%)	21 (28%)	51	79	0.774	[0.713–0.835]
MPI ≥ 32	42 (45.2%)	18 (32%)	45	89		
MPI ≥ 34	22 (23.7%)	9 (33%)	24	96		
APACHE II ≥ 14	64 (68.8%)	24 (26%)	69	78	0.828	[0.775–0.881]
APACHE II ≥ 16	52 (55.9%)	20 (30%)	56	89		
APACHE II ≥ 18	42 (45.2%)	19 (39%)	45	95		
WSESSSS ≥ 8	68 (73.1%)	27 (27%)	73	76	0.809	[0.752–0.866]
WSESSSS ≥ 9	58 (62.4%)	24 (29%)	62	82		
WSESSSS ≥ 10	47 (50.5%)	20 (32%)	51	88		
CPIRO ≥ 3	54 (58.1%)	21 (31%)	58	90	0.856	[0.806–0.905]
CPIRO ≥ 4	28 (30.1%)	13 (42%)	30	98		

Ninety-three patients were selected out of the database based on 30-day mortality or ICU admission
[a]AUC is for sepsis classification according to Sepsis-3 consensus definitions
[b]Only one area under the curve (AUC) was calculated for each scoring system without thresholds within

changed with the further addition of patients detected by a CPIRO score of ≥ 4 (Table 1). However, when the CPIRO was utilized with a threshold of 3 or greater, for an inclusive criteria of Sepsis-3 septic shock OR WSESSS ≥ 8 or CPIRO ≥ 3, this resulted in a detection rate of the desired population of 82.8%, with a sensitivity of 83% and a 74% specificity for detection of a population with the mortality rate remaining 26%. The other highest combination of scoring systems was combining a SOFA ≥ 4 with WSESSSS ≥ 8 which had a slightly higher detection rate of 83.9%, with 84% sensitivity and 75% specificity in a population with 25% mortality. This detection was unchanged in either direction by adding the criterion of septic shock.

Discussion

The Closed or Open after Laparotomy (COOL) for Source Control in Severe Complicated Intra-abdominal Sepsis Trial (https://clinicaltrials.gov/ct2/show/NCT03163095) is a prospective multi-institutional worldwide study examining outcomes in those managed with primary fascial closure or OA in SCIAS [46]. To properly power this trial,

Table 4 Combined predictive capabilities of potential COOL study sepsis and critical illness scoring systems using Helsinki outcomes data

System	Identified	Outcome mortality	Sensitivity (%)	Specificity (%)
Septic shock OR CPIRO ≥ 3	57 (61.3%)	21 (30%)	61	90
Septic shock OR CPIRO ≥ 4	42 (45.2%)	17 (35%)	45	95
SOFA ≥ 4 OR CPIRO ≥ 3	65 (69.9%)	22 (27%)	70	87
SOFA >4 (4 OR greater here) ≥ OR WSESSSS ≥ 8	78 (83.9%)	28 (25%)	84	75
Septic shock OR WSESSSS ≥ 8	74 (79.6%)	28 (26%)	80	75
Septic shock OR CPIRO ≥ 4 OR WSES ≥ 8	74 (79.6%)	28 (26%)	80	75
Septic shock OR CPIRO ≥ 3 OR WSES ≥ 8	77 (82.8%)	29 (26%)	83	74
Septic shock OR SOFA ≥ 4	60 (76.3%)	20 (28%)	65	91
Septic shock OR SOFA ≥ 4 OR WSES ≥ 8	78 (83.92%)	28 (25%)	84	75

Ninety-three patients were selected out of the database based on 30-day mortality or ICU admission

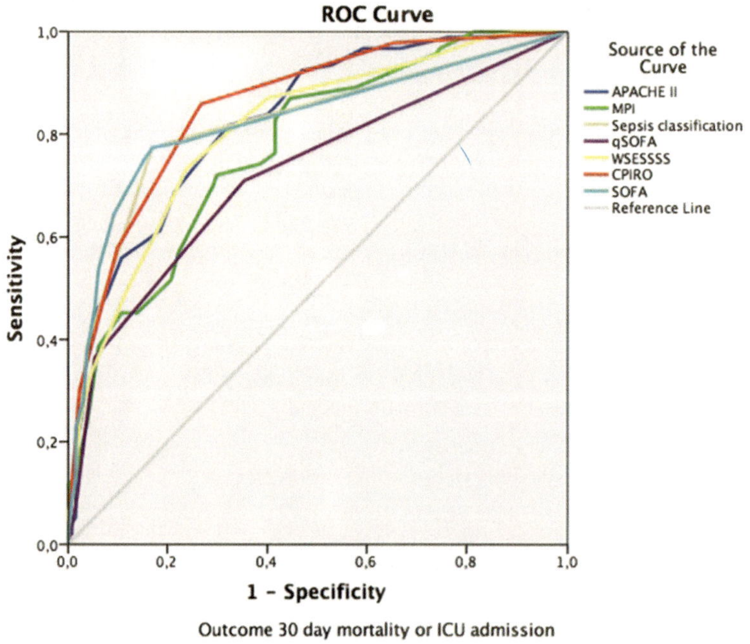

Fig. 1 Area under the receiver-operating curve (AUC) for candidate scoring systems considering recruitment population of interest with ICU Admission or mortality

it is necessary to utilize optimal and validated scoring tool(s) to identify surgical patients with SCIAS at high risk of death requiring ICU care early in their hospital course, typically prior to ICU admission. Such potential tool(s) should be easy to use and functional while still in the operating room prior to potential formal primary fascial closure. A remarkable variety of potential scoring systems for predicting outcomes in relation to septic populations have developed over time leading to a somewhat discrepant epidemiological picture that is compounded by the variety of populations and health care settings in which they have been studied. Systems have been used for

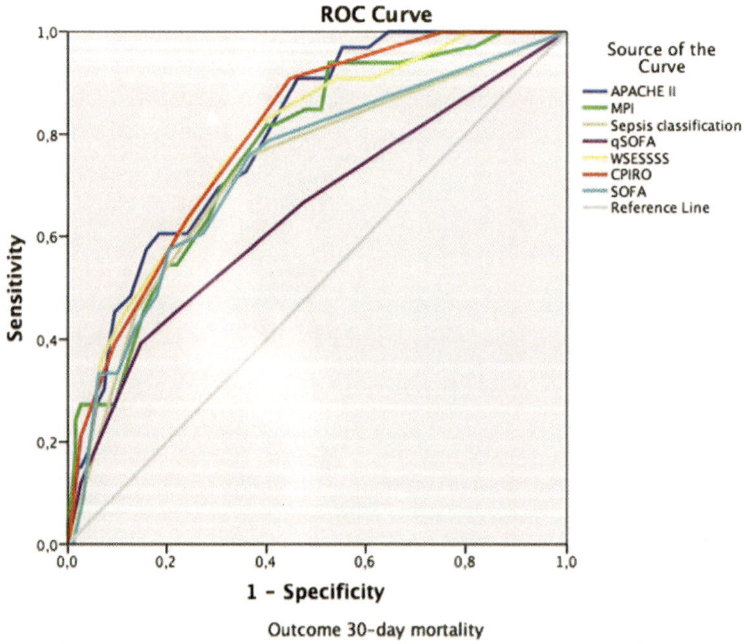

Fig. 2 Area under the receiver-operating curve (AUC) for candidate scoring systems considering recruitment population of interest with mortality only

a variety of reasons including quality assessment and audit, epidemiological reporting and comparison, study recruitment and analysis, and outcome clinical predictions [7, 28, 31–37, 39–44].

When interrogated against a cohort of SCIAS patients recruited from an advanced health-care system, each predictive model performed with different attributes. Even considering a specific scoring tool, the specific tool may have varying sensitivity and specificity for identifying patients of interest depending on the threshold value of the tool selected. Thus, no one scoring system behaved perfectly, and all appear to be largely dominated by organ dysfunction with a modest increase in detection provided by the inclusion of further patient characteristics some of which may not be readily available pre-operatively before potential surgery and admission to ICU. Nonetheless in this population, patients identified by the Sepsis-3 septic shock definition in addition to the WSESSS criteria with a score of 8 or greater had a detection rate of 80%. Adding the potential increased detection of the CPIRO score ≥ 3 increased the detection rate to 83%. Thus, the COOL investigators decision to include any of the three identifying criteria of Sepsis-3 septic shock criterion, WSESSSS ≥ 8, or CPIRO ≥ 3 seems statistically justified based on this analysis.

The strengths of the Helsinki dataset are that it involves an inception cohort exclusively of patients with IAS. A methodological concern involves the degree to which scores developed for septic patients with a wide range of precipitating causes will specifically identify patients with SCIAS. It is relevant to compare the specific experiences of the Helsinki data with evaluations in other general septic cohorts and especially cohorts of those with SCIAS. Although sepsis has been thoroughly studied in general critical care unit populations, accurate data collection has been less well studied outside of the ICU and early in intra-abdominal sepsis populations [39]. Thus, the literature does not support any one scoring or predictive systems as being established for use in SCIAS (Table 5).

For practical discussion, it will be important to detect potential enrollees on the ward and in the emergency department prior to post-surgical ICU admission. A previous determination of predictive capabilities of patients on the ward or emergency department with suspected infection examined the Sepsis-1, Sepsis-3, and NEWS definitions of sepsis [39, 40]. Szakmany and colleagues concluded that the Sepsis-3 definition identified patients with the highest risk. SOFA score and NEWS were better predictors of poor outcome, while the SOFA score appeared to be the best tool for identifying patients with high risk of death and sepsis-induced organ dysfunction [39]. Representative performance characteristics in this cohort with sepsis from all causes found that there was considerable overlap. Alternatively, application of SIRS-based criteria (Sepsis-1) did not identify 105 (27.3%) patients, all of whom had evidence of acute organ dysfunction [39]. This analysis again raised concerns about the performance of qSOFA as it only identified 13% of patients otherwise diagnosed with sepsis, missed 30% of those with organ dysfunction, and failed to predict mortality.

The COOL investigators were particularly interested in evaluations of scoring systems involving SCIAS populations. While there have been numerous scores that attempt to prognosticate outcomes for general septic populations, focused studies in CIAS are fewer. In 1997, Bosscha and colleagues, studying 50 patients, commented that there was no ideal and accepted predictive scoring system for IAS and only the MPI and APACHE II scores contributed independently to mortality prediction [44]. A comparison of the attributes of APACHE II, SAPS, sepsis score, MOF score, and TISS-28 in 145 patients with secondary peritonitis also concluded that the APACHE II and TISS-28 were significantly better than other systems and specifically criticized the power of the MPI [37]. They also specifically recommended that combining scoring systems together should be the standard classification system for grading severity of IAS [44]. Hanisch and colleagues analyzed 382 patients with "abdominal septic shock" in 2011 using the SOFA, APACHE II, SAPS, and MODS score and concluded that it was impossible to predict individual patient outcomes with any certainty and that the APACHE II performed the worst [47]. Concerns about APACHE, even the newest proprietary APACHE IV, were recently repeated by Chan and colleagues in a 2016 retrospective cohort analysis of IAS patients. They commented that the APACHE scores might not accurately predict mortality in those requiring source control laparotomies as the post-operative trajectory might be greatly modulated by the surgical procedure [48]. Concurrently, in 2014 Das and colleagues evaluated the SAPS, APACHE-II, and P-POSSUM systems to identify high risk surgical patients with intra-abdominal sepsis and planned relaparotomy [32]. Contrary to these other experiences, the APACHE II score was the best at predicting mortality in this small series of 34 patients with a 21% mortality rate [32]. However, although considered a good marker, the APACHE II utility in peritonitis has been questioned because of the conundrum of using the APACHE II to evaluate interventions despite the fact that interventions might significantly alter many of the physiological variables required for its calculation [7]. The authors of the RELAP trial [49] evaluated the APACHE II, SAPS, MPI, MODS, SOFA, and acute part of the APACHE-II score and noted that none were of clinical value to predict patients with a need for relaparotomy for IAS control and modest abilities in predicting in-hospital mortality [50].

Table 5 Previous assessments of predictive capabilities of sepsis scoring systems

Population	Inclusion criteria	Scores tested	Outcome 1	Outcome 2 (if applicable)
Ward or ED (*n* = 380) Szakmany 2017 [39]	NEWS ≥ 3		30-day mortality	Organ dysfunction
		Sepsis-1	68% SENS	
		Sepsis-3	86% SENS	
		qSOFA ≥ 2	22% SENS	26% SENS
		SOFA	0.70 AUC	86% SENS
		SIRS		26% SENS
		Sepsis-1 (severe)	92% SENS	
		NEWS > 6	41% SENS	36% SENS
			0.59 AUC	
Post-operative ICU patients [44] (*n* = 50)	Peritonitis + IAS requiring ICU		Multivariate Prediction of in-hospital death	
		APACHE II	HR 6.7 [95CI 2.7–17]	
		MPI	HR 9.8 095CI 1.3–73]	
		SAPS	NS	
		SSS	NS	
		MOF	NS	
		Ranson	NS	
		Imrie	NS	
			Predictions of death (day 1 SICU)	
Post-operative SICU patients (*n* = 145) Delibegovic 2011 [37]	Non-traumatic secondary peritonitis requiring laparotomy	TISS-28	AUC 0.87	
		APACHE II	AUC 0.86	
		MODS	AUC 0.83	
		SAPS	AUC 0.83	
		MPI	AUC 0.72	
		SSS	AUC 0.70	
Abdominal septic shock in ICU (*n* = 382) Hanisch 2011 [47]	Sepsis-1 criteria [61] for abdominal septic shock	SOFA	Death prediction first 3 ICU days	0.54 AUC
		APACHE II		0.52 AUC
		SAPS		0.52 AUC
		MODS		0.52 AUC
IAS pts requiring SCL (*n* = 211) Chan [48]	SCL and severe sepsis or septic shock as per Sepsis-1 (61)	APACHE-IV	Predicted mortality rate	0.67 AUC
IAS pts requiting re-laparotomy (*n* = 34) Das [32]	Secondary peritonitis	APACHE-II	Hospital mortality prediction	0.958 AUC
		SAPS-II		0.955 AUC
		P-POSSUM		0.931 AUC
IAS pts undergoing SCL (*n* = 221) Van Ruler [50]	APACHE > 10		Mortality	Need for Re-Laparotomy
		APACHE-II	0.74 AUC	0.49 AUC
		SAPS-II	0.80 AUC	0.56 AUC

Table 5 Previous assessments of predictive capabilities of sepsis scoring systems *(Continued)*

Population	Inclusion criteria	Scores tested	Outcome 1	Outcome 2 (if applicable)
		MPI	0.60 AUC	0.52 AUC
		SOFA	0.72 AUC	0.55 AUC
		MODS	0.76 AUC	0.55 AUC
		APS	0.68 AUC	.60 AUC

ED emergency department; *NEWS* National Early Warning Score; *Sepsis 1* use of the First Sepsis Consensus Definitions [61]; *SENS* sensitivity; *Sepsis-3* use of the Third Sepsis Consensus Definitions [2]; *qSOFA* quick SOFA score as per Sepsis-3 [2]; *SOFA* Sepsis-related Organ Failure Assessment [62]; *AUC* area under the curve of a receiver/operator curve; *SIRS* Systemic Inflammatory Response Syndrome Criteria as per Sepsis-1 consensus definitions [61]; *APACHE II* Acute Physiology and Chronic Health Evaluation II [31]; *MPI* Mannheim Peritonitis Index [41]; *SAPS* Simplified Acute Physiology Score [33]; *SSS* Sepsis Severity Score [33]; *MOF* multiple organ failure [35]; *TISS-28* Therapeutic Intervention Scoring System [38]; *IAS* intra-abdominal sepsis; *APACHE-IV* Acute Physiology and Chronic Health Evaluation IV [63]; *SCL* Source Control Laparotomy; *SAPS-II* Simplified Acute Physiology Score-II [64]; *P-POSSUM* Physiological and Operative Severity Score for the enumeration of Mortality and morbidity [36]; *APS* physiological part extracted from APACHE II [31]; *MODS* Multiple Organ Dysfunction Syndrome

The Predisposition, Infection, Response and Organ dysfunction (PIRO) staging system was designed as a stratification tool to deal with the inherent heterogeneity of septic patients [51]. The concept dates from recommendations made in the 2001 International Sepsis Definitions Conference to improve the traditional classification of sepsis [52, 53]. PIRO systems incorporate assessment of premorbid baseline susceptibility (predisposition), specific disorders responsible for illness (infection), responses of the host, and resulting degree of organ dysfunction. PIRO scores have been developed in patients with severe sepsis [54], community-acquired pneumonia (CAP) [55], and ventilator-associated pneumonia [56]. Evaluation in septic patients (25% intra-abdominal sepsis) in the emergency department suggested the PIRO score had a significantly improved AUC than both APACHE II and Mortality in the Emergency Department scores [51]. In Calgary, the CPIRO score showed consistent mortality discrimination outperforming both APACHE II and SOFA [57]. The mortality rate by CPIRO score was 37.6% for a CPIRO of 4 and 54.7% for a CPIRO of 5 during its development, and when tested with the Helsinki data, it had the highest AUC.

Another tool to potentially identify patients with intra-abdominal sepsis at a high risk of death is a World Society of Emergency Surgery Sepsis Severity Score of 8 points or more [7]. The World Society of Emergency Surgery (WSES) derived the WSESSSS from data and experience obtained from a global prospective observational study (CIAOW Study) that recruited patients in 132 medical institutions located in 54 countries [16, 17]. Seven hundred ninety-one patients (17.4%) were admitted in critical condition (septic shock or severe sepsis according to Sepsis-2 definitions [52]). The most significant variables, adjusted to clinical criteria, were used to create a severity score for patients with complicated intra-abdominal infections (cIAIs) including clinical conditions at admission (severe sepsis/septic shock), the origin of the cIAIs, the delay in source control, the setting of acquisition, and any risk factors such as age and immunosuppression. This predictive system carries the advantage of having been validated in a different worldwide population, giving great generalizability to the scoring system. In general, a score above 5.5 was the best predictor of mortality, but scores of 8 or more had a 41.7% mortality [7], very comparable to other groups of patients presenting with septic shock.

Combining the formal SOFA score with the WSESSSS had a marginally higher detection rate than combining the WSESSS, CPIRO, and septic shock (83.9 versus 82.8%). Practical considerations that both the CPIRO and WSESSS were designed to be used early in sepsis and include expanded patient-specific criteria that do not require periods of observation undergoing critical care were felt to mitigate the marginally improved detection of alternatively using the SOFA as an early marker. The qSOFA was developed as a simple clinical criterion to identify patients with suspected infection who were likely to have poor outcomes, but it was also suggested that this might constitute entry criteria for clinical trials, which the COOL investigators strongly considered. However, the qSOFA actually had the lowest AUC of the systems formally tested and one of the lowest prediction rates in this population. This finding in conjunction with a growing opinion that the qSOFA may not be sensitive enough tool for its intended purpose [39, 58–60] led the COOL advisory panel to remove this inclusion criteria from the study protocol. Nonetheless, a triggering of qSOFA criteria in any patient with complicated IAS who may require operative source control should alert the caregivers to assess further whether critical features of SCIAS are present (Fig. 3).

Conclusion

No one scoring system behaves perfectly, and all appear to be largely dominated by organ dysfunction. Utilizing both the CPIRO and WSESSSS scores in addition to the Sepsis-3 septic shock definition, combining the SOFA score with WSESSSS to detect seriously ill patients with

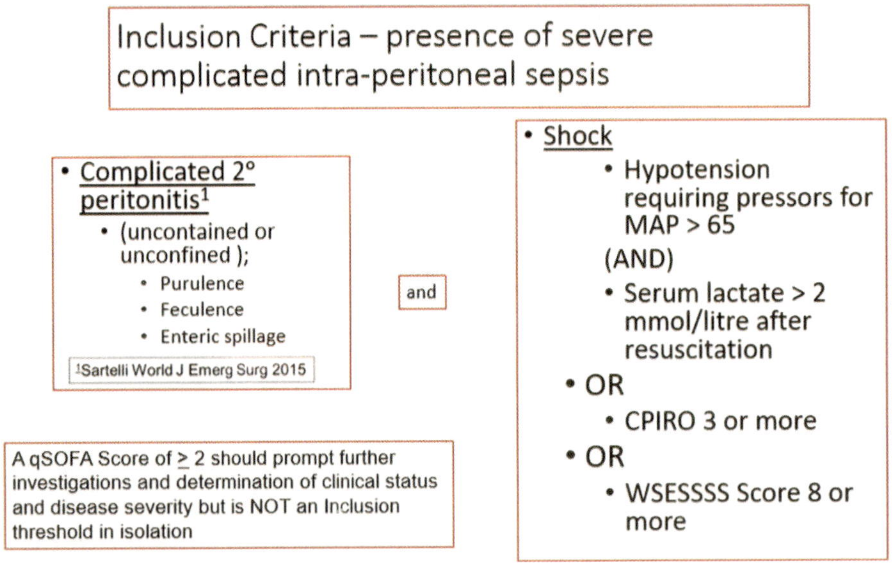

Fig. 3 Parma inclusion criteria for the COOL study as adopted at the Advisory Panel Meeting Parma, Italy

IAS, offered the widest "net" to recognize patients with a high chance of mortality and ICU admission. Given practical considerations, utilizing septic shock, CPIRO, and WSESSS will form the basis of patient recruitment into the COOL study in an additive fashion wherein patients meeting any of the severity score criterion will be eligible (Fig. 2). The qSOFA score was considered insufficiently sensitive to serve as an eligibility criterion but will nonetheless remain useful in a preoperative setting to identify patients who require further evaluation, investigation, and care and might be eligible with further information. Overall, efforts to refine predictive scoring will benefit investigators looking to optimize inception cohorts among other scientists attempting to understand and treat SCIAS.

Acknowledgements
Not applicable

Funding
No funding was received for the conduct of this analysis or the preparation of this manuscript. The COOL investigators as an entity were supported to conduct a protocol development meeting in Parma Italy on November 26, 2017 through an unrestricted grant from the Acelity Corporation in which Inclusion Criteria for Closed Or Open after Laparotomy (COOL) for Source Control in Severe Complicated Intra-Abdominal Sepsis (https://clinicaltrials.gov/ct2/show/NCT03163095) trial was discussed.

Authors' contributions
AWK, MT, and AR conceptualized the study. MT and AR performed the statistical analysis. MT, AWK, LA, MS, DJR, JLK, AL, CJD, FC, TF, CNJ, OC, PK, YK, GPF, BMP, JJD, MS, EEM, JR, CGB, RC, ED, WB, AM, PBM, JGPC, SDS, and JX discussed and critiqued the data and its interpretation. AWK drafted the initial manuscript. All authors read and approved the final manuscript.

Competing interests
Jessica L McKee declares that she has consulted for Innovative Trauma Care, Aceso, and the Acelity Corporations. Osvaldo Chiara reported having consulted for the Acelity Corporation. Jose J. Diaz reported having consulted for the Acelity Corporation. Michael Sugrue reported having consulted for the Smith and Nephew Corporation. Ernest E. Moore reported Research support and Intellectual property related to the Haemonetics, TEM Systems, Pryor Corporations, and being a Cofounder of Thrombo Therapeutics Inc. Andrew W Kirkpatrick serves in the Canadian Forces Medical Services and has consulted for the Innovative Trauma Care and Acelity Corporations. All other authors declared that they have no competing interests.

Author details
[1]Department of Abdominal Surgery, Abdominal Center, University of Helsinki and Helsinki University Central Hospital, Helsinki, Finland. [2]Emergency and Trauma Surgery Department, Bufalini Hospital, Cesena, Italy. [3]Unit of General and Emergency Surgery, Bufalini Hospital of Cesena, Cesna, Italy. [4]Department of Surgery, Macerata Hospital, Macerata, Italy. [5]Department of Surgery, University of Calgary, Calgary, Alberta, Canada. [6]Regional Trauma Services, Foothills Medical Centre, Calgary, Canada. [7]Departments of Critical Care Medicine and Community Health Sciences, Cumming School of Medicine, University of Calgary, Calgary, Canada. [8]Emergency Surgery Department, Parma University Hospital, Parma, Italy. [9]University of Tennessee Health Sciences Center, Memphis, TN, USA. [10]Department of Critical Care Medicine, University of Calgary, Calgary, Alberta, Canada. [11]General Surgery and Trauma Team Niguarda Hospital Milano, Milan, Italy. [12]Phoebe and Joan Snyder Institute for Chronic Diseases, University of Calgary, Calgary, Canada.

[13]Departments of Physiology and Pharmacology Cumming School of Medicine, University of Calgary, Calgary, Canada. [14]Rambam Health Care Campus, Haifa, Israel. [15]Division of Trauma Surgery, University of Campinas, Campinas, SP, Brazil. [16]Trauma/Acute Care Surgery and Surgical Critical Care, University of Campinas, Campinas, Brazil. [17]Department of Surgery, R Adams Cowley Shock Trauma Center, University of Maryland School on Medicine, Baltimore, MD, USA. [18]Letterkenny University Hospital, Donegal Clinical Research Academy, Donegal, Ireland. [19]Trauma and Critical Care Research, University of Colorado, Denver, CO, USA. [20]Department of Surgery, Jinling Hospital, Medical School of Nanjing University, Nanjing, China. [21]Acute Care, and Hepatobiliary Surgery, and Regional Trauma Services, University of Calgary, Calgary, Alberta, Canada. [22]Riverside University Health System Medical Center, Moreno Valley, USA. [23]Loma Linda University School of Medicine, Loma Linda, CA, USA. [24]Surgery, Oncology, and Community Health Sciences, City Wide Section of General Surgery, University of Calgary, Calgary, Alberta, Canada. [25]Trauma and Acute Care Surgery, Scripps Memorial Hospital La Jolla, La Jolla, California, USA. [26]Division of General Surgery Foothills Medical Centre, Department of Surgery, University of Calgary, Calgary, Canada. [27]The Trauma Program, University of Calgary, Calgary, Alberta, Canada. [28]Cambridge University Hospitals NHS Foundation Trust, Addenbrooke's Hospital, Cambridge, UK. [29]EG23 Foothills Medical Centre, Calgary, Alberta T2N 2T9, Canada.

References

1. Shankar-Hari M, Phillips GS, Levy ML, Seymour CW, Liu VX, Deutschman CS, et al. Developing a new definition and assessing new clinical criteria for septic shock: for the Third International Consensus Definitions for Sepsis and Septic Shock (Sepsis-3). JAMA. 2016;315(8):775–87.
2. Singer M, Deutschman CS, Seymour CW, Shankar-Hari M, Annane D, Bauer M, et al. The third international consensus definitions for Sepsis and septic shock (Sepsis-3). JAMA. 2016;315(8):801–10.
3. Marshall JC. Sepsis definitions: a work in progress. Crit Care Clin. 2018;34(1):1–14.
4. Angus DC, Linde Zwirble WT, Lidicker J, Clermont G, Carillo J, Pinsky MR. Epidemiology of severe sepsis in the United States: analysis of incidence, outcomes, and associated costs of care. Crit Care Med. 2001;29:1303–10.
5. Lagu T, Rothberg MB, Shieh MS, Pekow PS, Steingrub JS, Lindenauer PK. Hospitalizations, costs, and outcomes of severe sepsis in the United States 2003 to 2007. Crit Care Med. 2012;40(3):754–61.
6. Lagu T, Rothberg MB, Shieh MS, Pekow PS, Steingrub JS, Lindenauer PK. What is the best method for estimating the burden of severe sepsis in the United States? J Crit Care. 2012;27(4):414 e1–9.
7. Sartelli M, Abu-Zidan FM, Catena F, Griffiths EA, Di Saverio S, Coimbra R, et al. Global validation of the WSES Sepsis Severity Score for patients with complicated intra-abdominal infections: a prospective multicentre study (WISS Study). World J Emerg Surg. 2015;10:61.
8. Szakmany T, Lundin RM, Sharif B, Ellis G, Morgan P, Kopczynska M, et al. Sepsis prevalence and outcome on the general wards and emergency departments in Wales: results of a multi-centre, observational, point prevalence study. PLoS One. 2016;11(12):e0167230.
9. Jawad I, Luksic I, Rafnsson SB. Assessing available information on the burden of sepsis: global estimates of incidence, prevalence and mortality. J Glob Health. 2012;2(1):010404.
10. Roberts DJ, Ball CG, Kirkpatrick AW. Increased pressure within the abdominal compartment: intra-abdominal hypertension and the abdominal compartment syndrome. Curr Opin Crit Care. 2016;22(2):174–85.
11. Leligdowicz A, Dodek PM, Norena M, Wong H, Kumar A, Kumar A, et al. Association between source of infection and hospital mortality in patients who have septic shock. Am J Respir Crit Care Med. 2014;189(10):1204–13.
12. Sartelli M, Abu-Zidan FM, Ansaloni L, Bala M, Beltran MA, Biffl WL, et al. The role of the open abdomen procedure in managing severe abdominal sepsis: WSES position paper. World J Emerg Surg. 2015;10:35.
13. Sartelli M, Viale P, Catena F, Ansaloni L, Moore E, Malangoni M, et al. 2013 WSES guidelines for management of intra-abdominal infections. World J Emerg Surg. 2013;8(1):3.
14. Weber DG, Bendinelli C, Balogh ZJ. Damage control surgery for abdominal emergencies. Br J Surg. 2014;101(1):e109–18.
15. Stawicki SP, Brooks A, Bilski T, Scaff D, Gupta R, Schwab CW, et al. The concept of damage control: extending the paradigm to emergency general surgery. Injury. 2008;39(1):93–101.
16. Sartelli M, Catena F, Ansaloni L, Leppaniemi A, Taviloglu K, van Goor H, et al. Complicated intra-abdominal infections in Europe: a comprehensive review of the CIAO study. World J Emerg Surg. 2012;7(1):36.
17. Sartelli M, Catena F, Ansaloni L, Coccolini F, Corbella D, Moore EE, et al. Complicated intra-abdominal infections worldwide: the definitive data of the CIAOW Study. World J Emerg Surg. 2014;9:37.
18. Sartelli M, Catena F, Ansaloni L, Moore E, Malangoni M, Velmahos G, et al. Complicated intra-abdominal infections in a worldwide context: an observational prospective study (CIAOW Study). World J Emerg Surg. 2013;8(1):1.
19. Tellor B, Skrupky LP, Symons W, High E, Micek ST, Mazuski JE. Inadequate source control and inappropriate antibiotics are key determinants of mortality in patients with intra-abdominal sepsis and associated bacteremia. Surg Infect. 2015;16(6):785–93.
20. Rausei S, Pappalardo V, Ruspi L, Colella A, Giudici S, Ardita V, et al. Early versus delayed source control in open abdomen management for severe intra-abdominal infections: a retrospective analysis on 111 cases. World J Surg. 2017;42(3):707-712. https://doi.org/10.1007/s00268-017-4233-y.
21. Leppaniemi A, Kimball EJ, De Laet I, Malbrain ML, Balogh ZJ, De Waele JJ. Management of abdominal sepsis—a paradigm shift? Anaesthesiol Intensive Ther. 2015;47(4):400–8.
22. De Waele JJ. Abdominal sepsis. Curr Infect Dis Rep. 2016;18(8):23.
23. Vincent JL, Grimaldi D. Novel interventions: what's new and the future. Crit Care Clin. 2018;34(1):161–73.
24. Gentile LF, Moldawer LL. HMGB1 as a therapeutic target for sepsis: it's all in the timing! Expert Opin Ther Targets. 2014;18(3):243–5.
25. Opal SM, Dellinger RP, Vincent JL, Masur H, Angus DC. The next generation of sepsis clinical trial designs: what is next after the demise of recombinant human activated protein C? Crit Care Med. 2014;42(7):1714–21.
26. Khan A, Hsee L, Mathur S, Civil I. Damage-control laparotomy in nontrauma patients: review of indications and outcomes. J Trauma Acute Care Surg. 2013;75(3):365–8.
27. Bruns BR, Ahmad SA, O'Meara L, Tesoriero R, Lauerman M, Klyushnenkova E, et al. Nontrauma open abdomens: a prospective observational study. J Trauma Acute Care Surg. 2016;80(4):631–6.
28. Goussous N, Jenkins DH, Zielinski MD. Primary fascial closure after damage control laparotomy: sepsis vs haemorrhage. Injury. 2014;45(1):151–5.
29. Pommerening MJ, DuBose JJ, Zielinski MD, Phelan HA, Scalea TM, Inaba K, et al. Time to first take-back operation predicts successful primary fascial closure in patients undergoing damage control laparotomy. Surgery. 2014;156(2):431–8.
30. Chiara O, Cimbanassi S, Biffl W, Leppaniemi A, Henry S, Scalea TM, et al. International consensus conference on open abdomen in trauma. J Trauma Acute Care Surg. 2016;80(1):173–83.
31. Knaus WA, Draper EA, Wagner DP, Zimmerman JE. APACHE II: a severity of disease classification. Crit Care Med. 1985;13:818–29.
32. Das K, Ozdogan M, Karateke F, Uzun AS, Sozen S, Ozdas S. Comparison of APACHE II, P-POSSUM and SAPS II scoring systems in patients underwent planned laparotomies due to secondary peritonitis. Ann Ital Chir. 2014; 85(1):16–21.
33. Elebute EA, Stoner HB. The grading of sepsis. Br J Surg. 1983;70(1):29–31.
34. Gauzit R, Pean Y, Barth X, Mistretta F, Lalaude O, Top Study T. Epidemiology, management, and prognosis of secondary non-postoperative peritonitis: a French prospective observational multicenter study. Surg Infect. 2009;10(2):119–27.
35. Goris RJ, te Boekhorst TP, Nuytinck JK, Gimbrere JS. Multiple-organ failure. Generalized autodestructive inflammation? Arch Surg. 1985;120(10):1109–15.
36. Copeland GP, Jones D, Walters M. POSSUM: a scoring system for surgical audit. Br J Surg. 1991;78(3):355–60.
37. Delibegovic S, Markovic D, Hodzic S. APACHE II scoring system is superior in the prediction of the outcome in critically ill patients with perforative peritonitis. Med Arh. 2011;65(2):82–5.
38. Lefering R, Zart M, Neugebauer EA. Retrospective evaluation of the simplified Therapeutic Intervention Scoring System (TISS-28) in a surgical intensive care unit. Intensive Care Med. 2000;26(12):1794–802.
39. Szakmany T, Pugh R, Kopczynska M, Lundin RM, Sharif B, Morgan P, et al. Defining sepsis on the wards: results of a multi-centre point-prevalence study comparing two sepsis definitions. Anaesthesia. 2018;73(2):195-204. https://doi.org/10.1111/anae.14062. Epub 2017 Nov 17.
40. McGinley A, Pearse RM. A national early warning score for acutely ill patients. BMJ. 2012;345:e5310.

41. Linder MM, Wacha H, Feldmann U, Wesch G, Streifensand RA, Gundlach E. The Mannheim peritonitis index. An instrument for the intraoperative prognosis of peritonitis. Chirurg. 1987;58(2):84–92.
42. Ranson JH, Rifkind KM, Roses DF, Fink SD, Eng K, Localio SA. Objective early identification of severe acute pancreatitis. Am J Gastroenterol. 1974;61(6):443–51.
43. Imrie CW, Benjamin IS, Ferguson JC, McKay AJ, Mackenzie I, O'Neill J, et al. A single-centre double-blind trial of Trasylol therapy in primary acute pancreatitis. Br J Surg. 1978;65(5):337–41.
44. Bosscha K, Reijnders K, Hulstaert PF, Algra A, van der Werken C. Prognostic scoring systems to predict outcome in peritonitis and intra-abdominal sepsis. Br J Surg. 1997;84(11):1532–4.
45. Tolonen M, Sallinen V, Mentula P, Leppaniemi A. Preoperative prognostic factors for severe diffuse secondary peritonitis: a retrospective study. Langenbeck's Arch Surg. 2016;401(5):611–7.
46. Kirkpatrick AW. Closed or Open Abdomen for the Management of Abdominal Sepsis: NIH; 2017 [cited 2017 Sept 21 2017]. Available from: https://clinicaltrials.gov/ct2/show/NCT03163095.
47. Hanisch E, Brause R, Paetz J, Arlt B. Review of a large clinical series: predicting death for patients with abdominal septic shock. J Intensive Care Med. 2011;26(1):27–33.
48. Chan T, Bleszynski MS, Buczkowski AK. Evaluation of APACHE-IV predictive scoring in surgical abdominal sepsis: a retrospective cohort study. J Clin Diagn Res. 2016;10(3):PC16–8.
49. van Ruler O, Mahler CW, Boer KR, Reuland EA, Gooszen HG, Opmeer BC, et al. Comparison of on-demand vs planned relaparotomy strategy in patients with severe peritonitis: a randomized trial. JAMA. 2007;298(8):865–72.
50. van Ruler O, Kiewiet JJ, Boer KR, Lamme B, Gouma DJ, Boermeester MA, et al. Failure of available scoring systems to predict ongoing infection in patients with abdominal sepsis after their initial emergency laparotomy. BMC Surg. 2011;11:38.
51. Chen YX, Li CS. Risk stratification and prognostic performance of the predisposition, infection, response, and organ dysfunction (PIRO) scoring system in septic patients in the emergency department: a cohort study. Crit Care. 2014;18(2):R74.
52. Levy MM, Fink MP, Marshall JC, Abraham E, Angus D, Cook D, et al. 2001 SCCM/ESICM/ACCP/ATS/SIS international sepsis definitions conference. Crit Care Med. 2003;31(4):1250–6.
53. Levy MM, Fink MP, Marshall JC, Abraham E, Angus D, Cook D, et al. 2001 SCCM/ESICM/ACCP/ATS/SIS international sepsis definitions conference. Intensive Care Med. 2003;29(4):530–8.
54. Moreno RP, Metnitz B, Adler L, Hoechtl A, Bauer P, Metnitz PG. Sepsis mortality prediction based on predisposition, infection and response. Intensive Care Med. 2008;34(3):496–504.
55. Rello J, Rodriguez A, Lisboa T, Gallego M, Lujan M, Wunderink R. PIRO score for community-acquired pneumonia: a new prediction rule for assessment of severity in intensive care unit patients with community-acquired pneumonia. Crit Care Med. 2009;37(2):456–62.
56. Lisboa T, Diaz E, Sa-Borges M, Socias A, Sole-Violan J, Rodriguez A, et al. The ventilator-associated pneumonia PIRO score: a tool for predicting ICU mortality and health-care resources use in ventilator-associated pneumonia. Chest. 2008;134(6):1208–16.
57. Posadas-Calleja JG, Stelfox HT, Ferland A, Zuege DJ, Niven DJ, Berthiaume L, et al. Derivation of a PIRO score for prediction of mortality in surgical patients with intra-abdominal sepsis/severe sepsis/septic shock. Am J Crit Care. (in press)
58. Tusgul S, Carron PN, Yersin B, Calandra T, Dami F. Low sensitivity of qSOFA, SIRS criteria and sepsis definition to identify infected patients at risk of complication in the prehospital setting and at the emergency department triage. Scand J Trauma Resusc Emerg Med. 2017;25(1):108.
59. Askim A, Moser F, Gustad LT, Stene H, Gundersen M, Asvold BO, et al. Poor performance of quick-SOFA (qSOFA) score in predicting severe sepsis and mortality—a prospective study of patients admitted with infection to the emergency department. Scand J Trauma Resusc Emerg Med. 2017;25(1):56.
60. Raith EP, Udy AA, Bailey M, McGloughlin S, MacIsaac C, Bellomo R, et al. Prognostic accuracy of the SOFA score, SIRS criteria, and qSOFA score for in-hospital mortality among adults with suspected infection admitted to the intensive care unit. JAMA. 2017;317(3):290–300.
61. Bone RC, Balk RA, Cerra FB, Dellinger RP, Fein AM, Knaus WA, et al. Definitions for sepsis and organ failure and guidelines for the use of innovative therapies in sepsis. The ACCP/SCCM consensus conference committee. American College of Chest Physicians/Society of Critical Care Medicine. Chest. 1992;101(6):1644–55.
62. Vincent JL, Moreno R, Takala J, Willatts S, De Me A, Bruining H, et al. The SOFA (Sepsis-related Organ Failure Assessment) score to describe organ dysfunction/failure. Intensive Care Med. 1996;22:707–10.
63. Zimmerman JE, Kramer AA, McNair DS, Malila FM. Acute Physiology and Chronic Health Evaluation (APACHE) IV: hospital mortality assessment for today's critically ill patients. Crit Care Med. 2006;34(5):1297–310.
64. Le Gall JR, Lemeshow S, Saulnier F. A new simplified acute physiology score (SAPS II) based on a European/North American multicenter trial. JAMA. 1993;270:2957–63.

22

Acute care surgery: a means for providing cost-effective, quality care for gallstone pancreatitis

Patrick B. Murphy[1*], Dave Paskar[2], Richard Hilsden[1], Jennifer Koichopolos[1], Tina S. Mele[1,3]
and on behalf of Western Ontario Research Collaborative on Acute Care Surgery

Abstract

Background: Modern practice guidelines recommend index cholecystectomy (IC) for patients admitted with gallstone pancreatitis (GSP). However, this benchmark has been difficult to widely achieve. Previous work has demonstrated that dedicated acute care surgery (ACS) services can facilitate IC. However, the associated financial costs and economic effectiveness of this intervention are unknown and represent potential barriers to ACS adoption. We investigated the impact of an ACS service at two hospitals before and after implementation on cost effectiveness, patient quality-adjusted life years (QALY) and impact on rates of IC.

Methods: All patients admitted with non-severe GSP to two tertiary care teaching hospitals from January 2008–May 2015 were reviewed. The diagnosis of GSP was confirmed upon review of clinical, biochemical and radiographic criteria. Patients were divided into three time periods based on the presence of ACS (none, at one hospital, at both hospitals). Data were collected regarding demographics, cholecystectomy timing, resource utilization, and associated costs. QALY analyses were performed and incremental cost effectiveness ratios were calculated comparing pre-ACS to post-ACS periods.

Results: In 435 patients admitted for GSP, IC increased from 16 to 76% after implementing an ACS service at both hospitals. There was a significant reduction in admissions and emergency room visits for GSP after introduction of ACS services ($p < 0.001$). There was no difference in length of stay or conversion to an open operation. The implementation of the ACS service was associated with a decrease in cost of $1162 per patient undergoing cholecystectomy, representing a 12.6% savings.
The time period with both hospitals having established ACS services resulted in a highly favorable cost to quality-adjusted life year ratio (QALY gained and financial costs decreased).

Conclusions: ACS services facilitate cost-effective management of GSP. The result is improved and timelier patient care with decreased healthcare costs. Hospitals without a dedicated ACS service should strongly consider adopting this model of care.

Keywords: Acute care surgery, Quality, Cost effectiveness, Gallstone pancreatitis, Cholecystectomy

* Correspondence: pbatesmurphy@gmail.com;
patrick.murphy@londonhospitals.ca
Poster presentation of preliminary work at the 2015 Canadian Association of General Surgery Conference, Quebec City, Quebec, Canada on September 17-20, 2015.Work performed at the London Health Sciences Centre and Western University
[1]Division of General Surgery, Department of Surgery, Schulich School of Medicine and Dentistry, Western University, London, Canada
Full list of author information is available at the end of the article

Background

Dedicated ACS services continue to be implemented in North America and around the globe. Increasingly comparable to trauma systems, ACS is a growing field with developing fellowships [1], centralization of care, and on-going research particularly with respect to appendicitis [2] and acute biliary disease [3, 4]. The benefits of ACS services are many, and include the optimization of health care delivery from the perspectives of surgeons, patients, and hospitals; these positive changes have been summarized and reported in two systematic reviews to date [5, 6].

GSP is one of the most common gallstone-related emergency general surgery (EGS) conditions, the definitive management of which is index cholecystectomy (IC) [7–13]. IC is recommended as the burden of recurrence requiring additional emergency room visits and re-admissions to hospital is high if definitive management (cholecystectomy) is not provided on the index admission [14–21]. A recent randomized trial, the PONCHO trial, has confirmed the safety and efficacy of index cholecystectomy for non-severe gallstone pancreatitis [22]. A Cochrane meta-analysis further suggests that early IC (<72h) for GSP is safe [23]. However, the facilitation of IC remains a challenge in many centers [15–19]. Lack of emergency general surgical resources, specifically dedicated operating room (OR) time, is the most significant barrier to the provision of early definitive care (IC) [24]. Additional challenges include surgeon acceptance of index (vs. delayed) cholecystectomy and competition with elective practice demands. As such, significant variation persists with respect to the management of acute biliary disease, gallstone pancreatitis in particular [25].

Our previous work has demonstrated an ACS service that can facilitate IC for GSP, leading to decreased GSP recurrence and subsequently reduced emergency room (ER) visits and re-admissions [4]. The cost of ACS provision has been described for acute cholecystitis, and in general, results in cost savings [24–26]. However, no study, to our knowledge, has reported on the impact of patient quality of life, nor performed a formal health economic analysis, following the implementation of an ACS service.

It is well established that delay of definitive management confers an approximately 25% risk of re-admission for gallstone-related illness prior to elective cholecystectomy [14–23]. This potentially impacts patient quality of life with respect to pain, anxiety, and lost days of work and other forms of social functioning. A model-based cost-utility analysis using data from the recent Cochrane review has suggested IC, particularly within 72 h, is cost effective for mild acute gallstone pancreatitis [26].

In our first study, a notable increase in IC rate for GSP at a single center was noted following the initiation of an ACS service (with a non-ACS center serving as a time-control). This second institution has since added an ACS service, allowing us to examine whether the improved outcomes for GSP can be replicated. In addition, we sought to assess the sustainability of a high IC rate within a mature ACS service over time, by continuing to track performance at the first site. Moreover, we investigated the fiscal and quality of life impacts associated with implementing an ACS service by performing a formal health economic analysis from the perspective of the GSP population. We hypothesize a sustainable rate of IC in keeping with our previous results after implementing ACS as well as cost savings and improved quality of life for patients compared to non-index cholecystectomy.

Methods

Ethics approval was obtained from the Health Sciences Research Ethics Board at Western University (HSREB# 104525). The study was conducted at London Health Sciences Centre, a tertiary care, academic institution comprised of two hospital campuses (site A and site B for the purposes of this study) in London, Ontario, Canada. In July 2010, one campus (site A) implemented an ACS service and in July 2014, site B implemented a similar service. A complete description of our ACS model is available [4]. Briefly, in our model, a surgeon suspends his or her elective practice to cover emergency surgical consults, admissions, and surgeries, both through the emergency department and via other in-hospital services, for 1 week. Site A has dedicated daily emergency operative time while site B shares time with other surgical services.

We retrospectively reviewed the charts of all patients admitted to general surgery at both hospitals for the period of January 2008 to May 2015 with an initial diagnosis of pancreatitis. This group of patients was then further refined to include only those with GSP. Our inclusion criteria were as follows: age 18 years old or older, a lipase greater than 300 U/L, had not undergone ERCP within 7 days prior to presentation, and the presence of gallstones on imaging. In order to identify all potential candidates for IC, patients were excluded only if they were pregnant and/or had an intensive care unit (ICU) admission within 48 h of admission to a hospital. ICU admission was used to exclude patients with probable severe pancreatitis and/or had significant co-morbidities, and thus likely not suitable candidates for IC. All patient health records were complete for all parameters of interest, and thus, no patient had missing data. In addition, our network of partner community hospitals shares an electronic health record with our institution, so we were able to detect if patients sought surgical care at these sites.

We divided this population into three time periods. Period 1 (January 1, 2008, to June 30, 2010; 2.5 years) represents when neither hospital had an ACS service. During period 2 (July 1, 2010, to June 30, 2014; 4 years), an ACS service was only present at site A. Finally, period 3 (July 1, 2014, to May 15, 2015; 10.5 months) represents the era when both sites had an ACS service.

Descriptive statistics including demographics, use of ERCP (index or not), time to OR from ER presentation, OR duration, conversion to open cholecystectomy, and site of index admission were collected. Re-admission and repeat ER visits rates for GSP, gallstone-related complaints or postoperative concerns were also tracked.

Cost analysis

The cost effectiveness was evaluated from the perspective of a single government payer, which is consistent with the public healthcare systems employed in Canada. The time horizon for the cost effectiveness analysis was either 1 year or the actual duration of illness related to gallstone pancreatitis, for patients whose disease experience in the study extended beyond 1 year. No patients in this study were awaiting management beyond 2 years. A discount rate of 3.5% per year was applied to both health effects and costs, in line with the National Institute for Health and Care Excellence (NICE) guidelines for health economic analysis [27]. Patients who presented with GSP but did not ultimately receive surgical management were excluded from the cost analysis. These patients were excluded as it cannot be assumed that non-surgical management restored these patients to their pre morbid health state.

Costs for providing management to each individual patient were estimated using financial data available from the Ontario Case Costing Program which contains publicly available data, maintained by the Province of Ontario, Table 1 [28]. This database contains both direct and indirect costs of managing patients with particular diagnoses and of performing certain procedures, as reported by participating hospitals. Using the database, the cost of each component of care for a patient with GSP was estimated, and then was applied to each individual patient in this study, Table 1.

Quality analysis

Quality-adjusted life years (QALY) were used to evaluate health effects. All patients were assigned a QALY of 1 (full health) to represent their health condition prior to developing gallstone pancreatitis. The health multipliers for health states associated with GSP were as follows: no biliary disease—1.0, laparoscopic cholecystectomy—0.91 [29], recurrent biliary colic—0.80 [29], open cholecystectomy—0.77 [30], and acute pancreatitis—0.44 [29]. While admitted to hospital, patients were assigned the acute pancreatitis multiplier. Patients that were discharged from hospital, but who did not have IC, were assigned the recurrent biliary colic QALY multiplier to represent failure to return to normal health. Finally, patients treated surgically were assigned the QALY multiplier that represents the surgery they received for the remaining study time horizon. An incremental cost effectiveness ratio (ICER) comparing the study time periods was calculated. As per health economic analysis convention, it was predetermined that only positive ICERs would be reported in the final analysis. Outcomes that both save money and improve clinical outcomes are "dominant strategies" whose magnitude of effect cannot be described by the ICER, nor are the "dominated strategies" that result in greater economic expenditures and lead to worse outcomes. Both of these situations result in negative ICERs whose magnitude offers no practical relevance in terms of decision-aiding.

Table 1 Cost and QALY data

Cost	Value	Source
Outpatient laparoscopic cholecystectomy	$1389	Avg direct cost (OCCP)
Inpatient open cholecystectomy	$10,423	Avg direct cost (OCCP)
Inpatient laparoscopic cholecystectomy	$4349	Avg direct cost (OCCP)
ERCP	$839	Avg direct cost (OCCP)
Ultrasound abdomen	$356	Avg direct cost (OCCP)
CT abdomen	$491	Avg direct cost (OCCP)
ER visit acute cholecystitis	$286	Avg direct cost (OCCP)
Hospital admission cost per day[a]	$776	Derived from OCCP data
Surgeon fee	$478	2011 OMA SOB
Anesthesia unit fee	$15.01	2011 OMA SOB
Cholecystectomy units	7 + time units	2011 OMA SOB
QALY—health states	Value	Source
No biliary disease	1	
Laparoscopic cholecystectomy	0.91	Bass, et. al. 1993 [30]
Recurrent biliary colic	0.8	Cook, et. al. 1993 [29]
Open cholecystectomy	0.77	Bass, et. al. 1993 [30]
Acute pancreatitis	0.44	Cook, et. al. 1993 [29]
Death	0	

OCCP Ontario Case Costing Program 2011 values, *OMA SOB* Ontario Medical Association Schedule of Benefits
[a]Includes indirect costs related to hospital admission

Statistical analysis

Continuous parameters were expressed as mean with standard deviation and nonparametric data were expressed as median and interquartile range. Categorical data were expressed as proportions. We performed one-way ANOVA analysis of variance, Pearson Chi-squared or Mann-Whitney *U* tests to determine statistical significance, with an alpha of 0.05, depending on the nature of the variable. Multivariate logistic regression was used to determine factors influencing IC performance. The primary clinical outcome was IC rate, and the primary cost end-point was an incremental cost effectiveness ratio (ICER). The student's *t* test was used to compare each time period (periods 2 and 3) to the reference period of neither site having ACS (period 1). Secondary end-points included length of stay, OR duration, number of ER visits, and re-admissions for gallstone pancreatitis. SPSS Version 20 (IBM Inc., 2011) was used as a statistical platform.

Results

There were a total of 435 patients admitted to general surgery with GSP during the study periods, Table 2. There was no difference with respect to the sex and age of patients in any of the periods. The implementation of an ACS service drastically increased the rate of IC from 16% in period 1 to 76% in period 3 when both sites had an ACS service; Table 3, Fig. 1. When examining the sites separately, there was an increase in IC rate from 19 to 70% ($p < 0.001$) and 25 to 83% ($p < 0.001$) following ACS implementation at sites A and B, respectively. The median ER to OR time for IC was 3.3 days (2.4–4.6) and for elective operation was 53.6 days (18.6–101.4) ($p < 0.001$). In a multivariate model of predicting IC that included age, sex, site of admission, and presence of an ACS service, only age (OR 0.97; 95% CI 0.95–0.98) and the presence of an ACS service (OR 13.6; 95% CI 7.5–24.8) were statistically significant.

A total of 342 patients received definitive surgical management for GSP. The re-admission rate and the number of ER visits for GSP were significantly reduced with the addition of an ACS service, Table 3 and Fig. 1. When considering index, elective, and non-surgery groups, the rates of re-admission were 3, 30, and 29%, respectively ($p < 0.001$). OR duration, postoperative stay, and total length of stay were no different between time periods, Table 3. There was significant cost savings realized when both sites had an ACS service compared to when neither did, Table 3. When comparing influence on patient quality of life, all periods with an ACS service resulted in improved QALY over the fully non-ACS period. During period 2, the average per patient improved by 0.032 QALY ($p < 0.001$) vs period 1 and period 3 the average patient improved by 0.039 QALY ($p = 0.013$), Fig. 2. Regarding costs, implementation of ACS at site A during period 2 resulted in a non-significant average cost increase of $52 ($p = 0.954$). During period 3, when both sites had established ACS, there was a cost savings of $1162 ($p = 0.05$) per case compared to period 1. The primary outcome of ICER for period 2 compared to that for period 1 was $1626/QALY. The ICER for period 3 compared to that for period 1 was negative, and thus, the magnitude is not meaningful and therefore not reported (dominant strategy). Figure 2 displays a cost by QALY chart where the bottom right quadrant represents the ideal scenario of simultaneous cost saving with improved QALY outcomes. ACS at both sites (period 3) suggests both a significant cost saving and improved quality of life for patients.

There was an increase in Monday to Friday, daytime (7 a.m.–5 p.m.) operating room use, 46 to 62% when IC was performed, although this was not significant ($p = 0.32$). There were more ultrasounds performed on patients undergoing an elective operation compared to IC; >25% of patients undergoing an elective operation required more than one ultrasound compared to <10% of patients undergoing an IC ($p < 0.001$). ERCP rates were not statistically different between periods although less ERCPs were performed when both sites had ACS. Patients who did not undergo operative management were more likely to undergo ERCP compared to those undergoing operative management of GSP, 53% compared to 34% ($p < 0.001$).

Table 2 Patient demographics of the three periods, based on the presence of an ACS service

	Period 1	Period 2	Period 3	*p* value
Number, n	139	241	55	–
Site A, *n* (%)	73 (53)	127 (53)	32 (58)	0.74
Age, year, mean (SD)	55 (21)	58 (20)	57 (21)	0.45
Male, *n* (%)	50 (36)	97 (40)	23 (40)	0.65

Period 1: 2008–2010 (no ACS at either site)
Period 2: 2010–2014 (ACS at site A)
Period 3: 2014–2015 (ACS at both sites)

Discussion

The standard of care for uncomplicated GSP is IC, and our results confirm that the presence of ACS services can enable high rates of IC which are robust over time and replicable. Further, our results suggest that IC is exceptionally cost effective, resulting in both fiscal cost savings and improved patient quality of life outcomes. The most favorable ICER was the final period of study, where both sites had an ACS service, suggesting that ACS services deliver high quality and cost-effective care for GSP.

GSP management has shifted over the past decade from the previous preference for a "cooling off" period prior to outpatient cholecystectomy to the modern approach of performing early IC [23, 31–34]. The PONCHO trial, a randomized trial comparing IC to outpatient cholecystectomy confirms the safety and efficacy of definitive management for non-severe GSP on the index admission. Even with the short delay (25–30 days) for elective operation, 18% of patients in this study

Table 3 Comparison of clinical outcomes and total cost between three time periods, based on the presence of an ACS service

	Period 1	Period 2	Period 3	*p* value
Number, *n*	139	241	55	–
Index OR, *n* (%)	22 (16)	120 (50)	42 (76)	<0.001
Elective OR, *n* (%)	85 (61)	67 (28)	6 (11)	<0.001
Inpatient ERCP, *n* (%)	61 (44)	87 (36)	16 (29)	0.11
ER to OR, d, mean (SD)	95 (194)	32 (66)	23 (107)	<0.001
OR duration, minutes	65 (32)	68 (29)	63 (34)	0.44
Open, *n* (%)	6 (4)	9 (4)	0 (0)	–
Postoperative stay, d, mean (SD)	1.5 (1.8)	1.4 (5.7)	1.1 (1.9)	0.87
Total LOS on index admission, days, mean (SD)	5 (3)	6 (9)	5 (3)	0.10
More than one admission for GSP, *n* (%)	47 (34)	30 (12)	4 (7)	<0.001
More than one ER visit for GSP, *n* (%)	58 (42)	32 (13)	9 (16)	<0.001
Time of index OR				
Mon–Fri (7 a.m.–5 p.m.)	10 (46)	73 (61)	26 (62)	0.675
Mon–Fri (5 p.m.–Midnight)	2 (9)	9 (8)	2 (5)	
Mon–Fri (Midnight–7 a.m.)	0 (0)	0 (0)	0 (0)	
Weekend	10 (46)	38 (32)	14 (33)	
Total cost (2011 dollars), mean (SD)	$9255 (324)	$9307 (648)	$8093 (505)	<0.001

Period 1: 2008–2010 (no ACS at either site)
Period 2: 2010–2014 (ACS at site A)
Period 3: 2014–2015 (ACS at both sites)
LOS Length of stay, *ERCP* endoscopic retrograde cholangiopancreatography, *ER* emergency room, *OR* operating room

required re-admission for gallstone-related problems. Our re-admission rate for patients undergoing planned elective surgery was significantly higher, likely due to an even longer delay (194 days) to definitive management in this group. This was similar to the re-admission rate of ~30% seen in the group of patients who did not undergo surgical management. Our findings are consistent with other reports on mild non-severe gallstone pancreatitis [14, 15, 35]. Our previous work demonstrated that our institution had very low IC rates historically, and that the passage of time following the publication of mounting evidence and guidelines encouraging IC only

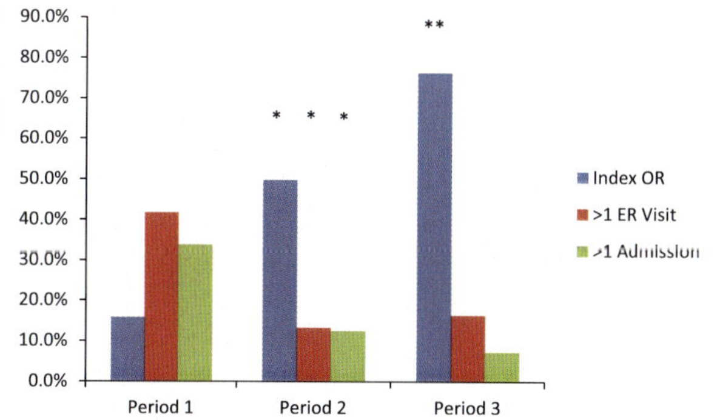

Fig. 1 Rate of index cholecystectomy, emergency room visits, and admissions across the three time periods. (*<0.05 compared to period 1, **<0.05 compared to period 2

marginally improved our IC rates [4]. It was clear, that at our institution, barriers to IC performance included a lack of operative resources accessible to emergency patients and competition with busy elective practices. Encountering intraoperative surgical difficulty with the "hot gallbladder" has been suggested as another potential additional barrier but has not been confirmed as a valid reason for delaying surgery. Numerous reports suggest cholecystectomy may be easier in the setting of GSP [36, 37]. Indeed, the PONCHO trial included a rating scale of intraoperative surgical difficulty and found no difference [4]. We also did not see an increase in operative time, length of stay, or rate of conversion associated with the increased rate of IC. Implementation of an ACS service with dedicated daytime emergency operative time allowed surgeons to suspend elective practice and facilitated IC achievement.

De Mestral et al. clearly demonstrate the variation in management of acute biliary disease. In this study, the authors found a fourfold difference in the likelihood of IC at various centers within the province of Ontario, Canada, even for young, healthy male patients with acute cholecystitis [25]. While our study represents some of the first work to demonstrate the increase of IC for uncomplicated GSP resulting from ACS adoption, others have demonstrated similar findings in acute cholecystitis. Pepingco et al. found an increase from 55 to 90% in the rate of IC for acute cholecystitis after the

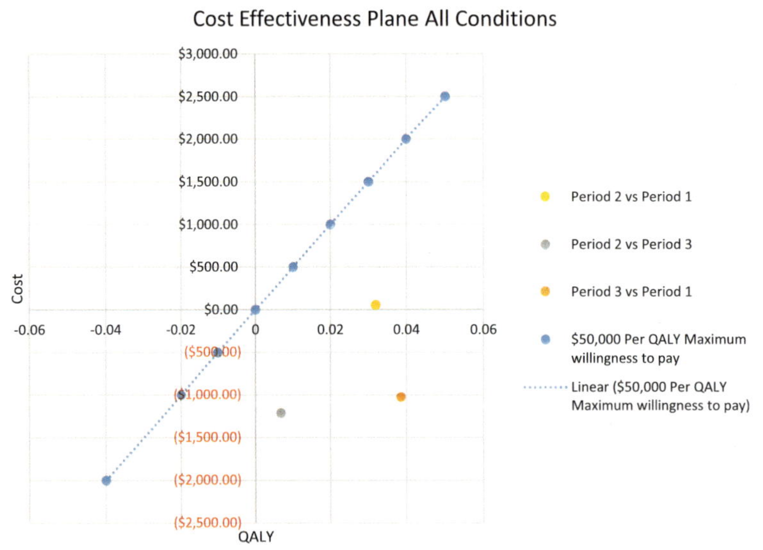

Fig. 2 Cost effectiveness plane for each time period; period 3 (ACS at both sites favored)

addition of an ACS service [5]. Our ACS service has dedicated daytime operating time at one site which we believe facilitates our improved IC rate. We obtained a rate of 76% without a subsequent increase in after-hours or weekend operations. Reports of operative timing for acute cholecystitis vary with some centers reporting an increase in after-hours/weekend operations [38], and others reporting a decrease [5, 9, 11]. Unfortunately, the role of a dedicated operating room is challenging to discern as the reporting on the design of the ACS services in the collective literature is generally poor.

Waiting for an elective operation, including cholecystectomy, significantly impacts quality of life from both potential physical and emotional aspects [39]. Further, quality of life can be impacted by the financial implications of missing work due to emergency room visits, outpatient clinic visits, and hospital re-admissions [40, 41]. For example, the number of patients reporting pain while waiting for surgery in the interval cholecystectomy group in the PONCHO trial was >50%. While other studies have demonstrated the cost savings associated with an ACS service for acute cholecystitis, none have done so for gallstone pancreatitis. We demonstrate significant cost savings of over $1000 per patient when both sites had an ACS service (period 3). This has significant health care resource utilization implications on a national scale given: (1) the number of cholecystectomies are performed on an annual basis and (2) gallstone-related disease is the leading cause of gastrointestinal admission to hospital [42]. Coupled with improved quality of life following cholecystectomy, the resulting negative incremental cost effectiveness ratio suggests both improvement of quality of life and a net cost benefit. Using the results of a Cochrane review on the management of GSP, Morris et al. demonstrated divergent results. In the analysis performed by Morris et al., early laparoscopic cholecystectomy (<72 h) demonstrated a cost reduction which was attributed to decreased length of stay [26]. In contrast, our cost savings results were largely driven by decreased re-admission rates, imaging utilization, and ER visits (while length of stay remained largely unchanged).

Our study is retrospective and is limited by the inherent biases associated with this study design, including identification of GSP patients. Further, we cannot be completely certain that the care of the study patients was contained to our institution and that they did not present elsewhere. Our electronic record does include most neighboring community hospitals and as such, we believe that the potential to miss re-presentations to nearby hospitals is very low but not impossible. Therefore, our results represent a minimum re-admission rate for GSP. In addition, we cannot adequately discern the reason for not undergoing IC and certainly mitigating factors such as patient preference may influence the timing of an operation. Finally, there are numerous other patient and societal factors that we cannot measure directly such as missed work and social welfare costs.

Conclusions

A dedicated ACS service significantly improves rates of IC for GSP in a cost-effective manner that improves quality of life for patients. The increased rate of IC is associated with a similar magnitude in decreased re-admissions, ER visits, and ancillary testing. We believe that our results provide an important quality benchmark (rate of IC) and moreover, suggests that financial costs may no longer be (or at least less of) a barrier to the creation of ACS services than some may have previously thought. In fact, ACS adoption may allow surgical hospitals to achieve the "ultimate outcome", generation of cost savings while providing better quality of care. General surgeons seeking to improve their care of emergency surgery patients via the adoption of an ACS service should consider our results when advocating and negotiating for resources with hospital administration and other stakeholders.

Abbreviations

ACS: Acute care surgery; EGS: Emergency general surgery; ER: Emergency room; ERCP: Endoscopic retrograde cholangiopancreatography; GSP: Gallstone pancreatitis; IC: Index cholecystectomy; ICER: Incremental cost effectiveness ratio; LOS: Length of stay; OR: Operating room; QALY: Quality-adjusted life years

Acknowledgements

Not applicable.

Funding

There was no funding source.

Authors' contributions

All authors contributed to the study design. PM and JK performed data collection and data analysis. RH performed the cost analysis. All authors critically interpreted all data analysis. PM and JK composed the manuscript, and all the remaining authors provided critical edits to the final draft. All authors read and approved the final manuscript.

Competing interests

The authors declare that they have no competing interests.

Author details

[1]Division of General Surgery, Department of Surgery, Schulich School of Medicine and Dentistry, Western University, London, Canada. [2]Divisions of General Surgery Trauma & Critical Care Medicine, University of Toronto, Toronto, Canada. [3]Divisions of Critical Care, Department of Surgery, Schulich School of Medicine and Dentistry, Western University, London, Canada.

References

1. Dinan KA, Davis JW, Wolfe MM, Sue LP, Cagle KM. An acute care surgery fellowship benefits a general surgical residency. J Trauma Acute Care Surg. 2014;77:209–12.
2. Earley AS, Pryor JP, Kim PK, et al. An acute care surgery model improves outcomes in patients with appendicitis. Ann Surg. 2006;244:498–504.
3. Murphy PB, Vogt KN, Mele TS, Hameed SM, Ball CG, Parry NG. Timely Surgical Care for Acute Biliary Disease: An Indication of Quality. Ann Surg. 2016;264(6):913–4.
4. Murphy PB, Paskar D, Parry NG, et al. Implementation of an acute care surgery service facilitates modern clinical practice guidelines for gallstone pancreatitis. J Am Coll Surg. 2015;222:975–81.
5. Pepingco L, Eslick GD, Cox MR. The acute surgical unit as a novel model of care for patients presenting with acute cholecystitis. Med J Aust. 2012;196:509–10.
6. Chana P, Burns EM, Arora S, Darzi AW, Faiz OD. A systematic review of the impact of dedicated emergency surgical services on patient outcomes. Ann Surg. 2015;261:1.
7. Britt RC, Bouchard C, Weireter LJ, Britt LD. Impact of acute care surgery on biliary disease. J Am Coll Surg. 2010;210:595–9. 599–601.
8. Kulvatunyou N, Joseph B, Gries L, et al. A prospective cohort study of 200 acute care gallbladder surgeries: the same disease but a different approach. J Trauma Acute Care Surg. 2012;73:1039–45.
9. Lau B, Difronzo LA. An acute care surgery model improves timeliness of care and reduces hospital stay for patients with acute cholecystitis. Am Surg. 2011;77:1318–21.
10. Lehane CW, Jootun RN, Bennett M, Wong S, Truskett P. Does an acute care surgical model improve the management and outcome of acute cholecystitis? ANZ J Surg. 2010;80:438–42.
11. Lim DW, Ozegovic D, Khadaroo RG, Widder S. Impact of an acute care surgery model with a dedicated daytime operating room on outcomes and timeliness of care in patients with biliary tract disease. World J Surg. 2013; 37:2266–72.
12. Burch JM, Feliciano DV, Mattox KL, Jordan GL. Gallstone pancreatitis. The question of time. Arch Surg. 1990;125:853–9. discussion 859–60.
13. Yadav D, Lowenfels AB. Trends in the epidemiology of the first attack of acute pancreatitis: a systematic review. Pancreas. 2006;33:323–30.
14. Mustafa A, Begaj I, Deakin M, et al. Long-term effectiveness of cholecystectomy and endoscopic sphincterotomy in the management of gallstone pancreatitis. Surg Endosc. 2014;28:127–33.
15. van Baal MC, Besselink MG, Bakker OJ, et al. Timing of cholecystectomy after mild biliary pancreatitis: a systematic review. Ann Surg. 2012;255:860–6.
16. Ito K, Ito H, Whang E. Timing of cholecystectomy for biliary pancreatitis: do the data support current guidelines? J Gastrointest Surg. 2008;12:2164–70.
17. Sanjay P, Yeeting S, Whigham C, et al. Management guidelines for gallstone pancreatitis. Are the targets achievable? JOP. 2009;10:43–7.
18. Sakowska M, McKay J, Lake S, Deacon A. Index cholecystectomy: a continuing challenge for a provincial hospital. N Z Med J. 2013;126:53–9.
19. Creedon L, Neophytou C, PC L, Awan A. Are we meeting the British Society of Gastroenterology guidelines for cholecystectomy post-gallstone pancreatitis? ANZ J Surg. 2016;86(12):1021–7.
20. Tucker JJ, Grim R, Bell T, Martin J, Mueller M, Ahuja V. Changing demographics in laparoscopic cholecystectomy performed in the United States hospitalizations from 1998–2010. J Surg Res. 2014;186:611–2.
21. de Mestral C, Rotstein OD, Laupacis A, Hoch JS, Zagorski B, Nathens AB. A population-based analysis of the clinical course of 10,304 patients with acute cholecystitis, discharged without cholecystectomy. J Trauma Acute Care Surg. 2013;74:26–30. discussion 30–1.
22. da Costa DW, Bouwense S a, Schepers NJ, et al. Same-admission versus interval cholecystectomy for mild gallstone pancreatitis (PONCHO): a multicentre randomised controlled trial. Lancet. 2015;386:1261–8.
23. Gurusamy KS, Nagendran M, Davidson BR. Early versus delayed laparoscopic cholecystectomy for acute gallstone pancreatitis. Cochrane Database Syst Rev. 2013;9:CD010326.
24. Lankisch PG, Weber-Dany B, Lerch MM. Clinical perspectives in pancreatology: compliance with acute pancreatitis guidelines in Germany. Pancreatology. 2005;5:591–3.
25. de Mestral C, Laupacis A, Rotstein OD, et al. Early cholecystectomy for acute cholecystitis: a population-based retrospective cohort study of variation in practice. CMAJ. 2013;1:E62–7.
26. Morris S, Gurusamy KS, Patel N, Davidson BR. Cost-effectiveness of early laparoscopic cholecystectomy for mild acute gallstone pancreatitis. Br J Surg. 2014;101:828–35.
27. National Institute for Health and Clinical Excellence. Methods for the development of NICE public health guidance. London: National Institute for Health and Clinical Excellence; 2012.
28. Ministry of Health and Long Term Care. Ontario Case Costing Program. Available at: https://hsimi.on.ca/hdbportal/. Accessed 15 Oct 2015.
29. Cook J, Richardson JRJ, National Centre for Health Program Evaluation. Quality of life measurement of patients receiving treatments for gallstone disease: options, issues and results. Fairfield: National Centre for Health Program Evaluation; 1993.
30. Bass EB, Pitt HA, Lillemoe KD. Cost-effectiveness of laparoscopic cholecystectomy versus open cholecystectomy. Am J Surg. 1993;165:466–71.

31. Tenner S, Baillie J, DeWitt J, Vege S. American College of Gastroenterology guideline: management of acute pancreatitis. Am J Gastroenterol. 2013;108:1400–15.
32. Forsmark CE, Baillie J. AGA Institute technical review on acute pancreatitis. Gastroenterology. 2007;132:2022–44.
33. UK Working Party on Acute Pancreatitis. UK guidelines for the management of acute pancreatitis. Gut. 2005;54:iii1–9.
34. Uhl W, Warshaw A, Imrie C, et al. IAP guidelines for the surgical management of acute pancreatitis. Pancreatology. 2002;2:585–73.
35. Hwang S, Bonnie H, Philip I. Gallstone pancreatitis without cholecystectomy. JAMA Surg. 2013;148:867–72.
36. Sinha R. Early laparoscopic cholecystectomy in acute biliary pancreatitis: the optimal choice? HPB (Oxford). 2008;10:332–5.
37. Monkhouse SJW, Court EL, Dash I, Coombs NJ. Two-week target for laparoscopic cholecystectomy following gallstone pancreatitis is achievable and cost neutral. Br J Surg. 2009;96:751–5.
38. Michailidou M, Kulvatunyou N, Friese RS, et al. Time and cost analysis of gallbladder surgery under the acute care surgery model. J Trauma Acute Care Surg. 2014;76:710–4.
39. Gurusamy KS, Koti R, Fusai G, Davidson BR. Early versus delayed laparoscopic cholecystectomy for uncomplicated biliary colic. Cochrane Database Syst Rev. 2013;6:CD007196.
40. Garner JP, Sood SK, Robinson J, Barber W, Ravi K. The cost of ignoring acute cholecystectomy. Ann R Coll Surg Engl. 2009;91:39–42.
41. Oudhoff JP, Timmermans DRM, Knol DL, Bijnen AB, van der Wal G. Waiting for elective general surgery: impact on health related quality of life and psychosocial consequences. BMC Public Health. 2007;7:164.
42. Shaheen NJ, Hansen RA, Morgan DR, et al. The burden of gastrointestinal and liver diseases, 2006. Am J Gastroenterol. 2006;101:2128–38.

Should ambulatory appendectomy become the standard treatment for acute appendicitis?

Benoit Gignoux[1], Marie-Cecile Blanchet[1], Thomas Lanz[2], Alexandre Vulliez[2], Mo Saffarini[3*], Hugo Bothorel[3], Maud Robert[4] and Vincent Frering[1]

Abstract

Background: Appendectomy is increasingly performed as a 'short stay' or 'ambulatory' procedure, yet there is no consensus for selection of patients with acute appendicitis for ambulatory surgery (AS). We aimed to compare characteristics and outcomes of complicated and uncomplicated appendectomies performed in ambulatory vs. conventional settings, and to determine factors associated with unexpected re-consultations and re-hospitalizations.

Methods: The authors reviewed a consecutive series of 185 laparoscopic appendectomies. Whenever possible, patients were offered AS, defined as 'discharge on the same working day.' Multivariable regressions were performed to determine associations of unexpected re-consultations and re-hospitalizations with surgery type (ambulatory or conventional) and patient characteristics (age, gender, obesity, symptoms, appendicolith, perforations, appendix diameter, serologic results, American Society of Anesthesiologists score, and Saint-Antoine score).

Results: From the initial cohort, 117 patients (63.2%) were eligible for AS, of which 8 had peri- or post-operative contraindications. Therefore, 109 patients (58.9%) were operated by AS, with median length of stay 8.5 h (range, 3.3–20.5). Ambulatory cases had a lower incidence of complications (11.9%) than conventional cases (25.0%) ($p = 0.029$). Uni- and multi-variable regressions revealed that unexpected re-consultations were not significantly associated with any of the pre- or peri-operative variables but that unexpected re-hospitalizations were 4 times more likely for patients with appendicolith (OR, 4.32; $p = 0.04$).

Conclusions: Ambulatory surgery could be considered as a standard procedure for both complicated and uncomplicated acute appendicitis. Appendicolith was found to be an independent risk factor for unexpected re-hospitalization and should therefore trigger closer monitoring.

Keywords: Laparoscopic appendectomy, Complicated appendicitis, Ambulatory surgery, Conventional hospitalization, Appendicolith

Background

Acute appendicitis is the most common indication for emergency surgery worldwide, with a lifetime risk of 8.6% for men and 6.7% for women [1, 2]. Despite the promotion of antibiotic therapy as a non-invasive alternative, laparoscopic appendectomy remains the standard treatment for acute appendicitis [3–5]. It is a common surgery, performed mostly in young healthy patients, with standardized management, operating time under 1 h, low morbidity, and low average length of hospital stay, all of which render it safe to perform in ambulatory settings [6]. Over the past decades, appendectomy has been increasingly performed as 'short stay' (< 24 h hospital stay) [7–10] or 'ambulatory' (no overnight hospital stay) [6, 11, 12] procedures, with satisfactory outcomes and low complication rates [13–16]. Yet, conventional hospitalization (with overnight stay) remains the routine procedure for acute appendicitis [6, 16].

There is no present consensus on the selection of patients with acute appendicitis for ambulatory surgery

* Correspondence: journals@resurg.eu
[3]Medical Technology, ReSurg SA, ch. de la Vuarpilliere 35, 1260 Nyon, Switzerland
Full list of author information is available at the end of the article

(AS). Recently, Lefrançois et al. [6] proposed a new score, which classifies patients into 6 risk levels, to select patients for ambulatory appendectomy without compromising outcomes. In their series, only 20% were discharged on the same day of surgery. The percentage of appendectomy procedures performed in ambulatory settings reported in the literature varies greatly (20–88%) [6, 8, 11–13, 15–18], likely due to inconsistent definitions of AS and to different criteria for enrollment of ambulatory patients.

For over 5 years, the authors have been performing ambulatory surgery for increasingly complex procedures, including colectomy [19], and have implemented a standardized care protocol for appendectomy following the guidelines of AS for common elective procedures [20]. The primary goal of the present study was to evaluate a consecutive series of appendectomies, complicated and uncomplicated, performed at our center and compare characteristics and outcomes of patients operated in ambulatory vs. conventional settings. The secondary goal was to investigate factors associated with unexpected re-consultations and re-hospitalizations, and thereby improve patient selection for ambulatory appendectomy.

Methods

The authors retrospectively reviewed a consecutive series of 185 patients who underwent emergency laparoscopic appendectomy for acute appendicitis by 5 surgeons, between January 2015 and June 2016. The series comprised 104 men and 81 women aged 34.1 ± 18.2 (median, 28; range 8–87) at the index operation. Acute appendicitis was suspected on the basis of clinical signs (pain, abdominal tenderness, and muscle guarding in the right lower quadrant), laboratory test results (abnormal white blood cell (WBC) count and serum C-reactive protein (CRP) level), and systematically confirmed by ultrasound (53%) and/or Computed Tomography (CT) (47%).

Following the definition of the International Association for Ambulatory Surgery (IAAS), we defined true AS as 'a procedure where the patient is discharged on the same working day,' that is, a procedure with no overnight stay. Ambulatory appendectomy was offered to all patients diagnosed with uncomplicated or complicated acute appendicitis, who presented none of the following *pre-operative* contraindications: (i) cases that could not be operated before 5 pm and could not be postponed to the next day (ii) home-hospital journey over 1 h, (iii) patient living alone, and (iv) severe comorbidities which required monitoring. Furthermore, based on the experience of the emergency team, surgeons reverted to conventional appendectomy in the event of one or more of the following *peri-* and *post-operative* contraindications: (v) generalized peritonitis or abscess requiring administration of intravenous antibiotics (vi) anaphylaxis, (vii) enduring pain that could not be treated by oral analgesic, (viii) fever, or (ix) vomiting.

Surgical technique

A standard laparoscopic technique was used for all patients. A 10-mm optic trocar was first introduced at the umbilicus and used for a 12-mmHg pneumoperitoneum inflation followed by the introduction of two 5-mm suprapubic and left iliac fossa ports. After a thorough exploration of the abdominal cavity, the appendix was excised and extracted in a bag through the optic tract. Abdominal drainage was restrictively placed in cases with severe infections. Ropivacaine (40 mL, 200 mg) was applied at each trocar site by infiltration as well as at the level of the diaphragmatic cupolas. General anesthesia was performed according to the recommendations of the Enhanced Recovery After Surgery Society [21]. Upon induction of general anesthesia, a single intravenous dose of amoxicillin plus clavulanic acid (2 g) was injected. We followed the guidelines of the French Society of Anesthesia and Resuscitation Medicine regarding the administration of antibiotics. In addition, for an improved rehabilitation and for preventing post-operative nausea and vomiting, intravenous injections of droperidol (1.25 mg) and dexamethasone (8 mg) were administered [22]. Multimodal analgesics were anticipated from the start of surgery using an anti-hyperalgesic agent (ketamine 20 mg) [23], step 1 analgesics (Nefopam + paracetamol + NSAID unless contra-indicated) and completing local and peritoneal infiltrations by local long-acting analgesics [24]. In case of complicated acute appendicitis, patients were given antibiotics postoperatively for at least 48 h.

Patient management

Hospital facilities included two theaters dedicated to planned and emergency digestive surgery with wide and flexible admission times. Patients diagnosed late afternoon with uncomplicated appendicitis returned home and were operated on the next day. Patients eligible for AS signed a consent form, which included complete information about appendicitis, surgical procedure, and their commitment to inform the clinic about any post-operative complications. AS patients operated on weekdays and discharged from the theater before 5 pm were admitted to the *ambulatory* recovery unit and discharged on the same day. AS patients operated on weekends, and those operated on weekdays but discharged from the theater after 5 pm, were admitted to the *conventional* recovery unit and discharged on the same day. All AS patients were monitored until full awakening and retained until they fulfilled the clinical discharge criteria for ambulatory procedures [25]. Each patient was contacted 1 day following discharge to verify their status and was invited for a follow-up consultation at 1 month. Out of 185 patients operated, 33 (17.8%) patients could not be re-contacted and did not inform the clinic of any complications. They were therefore assumed to have no unexpected re-consultation, re-hospitalization, or re-operation at any other clinic.

The following information was collected for each patient: age, gender, length of hospital stay, operating time, complications within 30 days from discharge, in addition to any unexpected re-consultation, unexpected re-hospitalization, and unexpected re-operation (Table 1). Complications were classified according to the modified Clavien system [26]. Data was collected as part of routine post-operative follow-up and all patients provided informed consent for the use of their data for research purposes. The institutional review board approval was therefore not required for this study.

Statistical analysis

Descriptive statistics were used to summarize the data. Shapiro-Wilk tests were used to assess the normality of distributions. For non-Gaussian quantitative data, differences between groups were evaluated using Wilcoxon rank sum tests (Mann Whitney *U* test). For non-Gaussian categorical data, differences between groups were evaluated using Fisher's exact tests. Multivariable logistic regression analyses were performed to determine associations between two outcomes (unexpected re-consultations and re-hospitalization) and 12 independent variables (gender, BMI > 28, symptoms > 48 h, appendicolith, perforation signs, ambulatory care, age, appendix diameter, CRP, WBC, American Society of Anesthesiologists (ASA) score, Saint-Antoine score. p values < 0.05 were considered statistically significant. Statistical analyses were performed using R version 3.3.2 (R Foundation for Statistical Computing, Vienna, Austria). p values < 0.05 were considered statistically significant.

Results

From the initial cohort of 185 patients, 117 (63.2%) were eligible for AS, of which 8 had peri-operative or post-operative contraindications (3 severe infections, 1 anaphylaxis, 2 generalized peritonitis, 2 excessive pain), which left a total of 109 (58.9%) patients operated in ambulatory settings. Their median length of stay, starting from hospital admission, was 8.5 h (range, 3.3–20.5). Compared to conventional cases, ambulatory cases were significantly younger (27.8 ± 13 vs 43.2 ± 20; $p < 0.001$), with lower preoperative CRP blood levels (27.8 ± 37 vs 63.7 ± 102; $p = 0.016$), smaller appendix diameters (10.0 ± 3.2 vs 11.7 ± 4.2, $p < 0.001$), fewer appendix perforations (10.1 vs 25%; $p = 0.008$), better Saint-Antoine scores (3.8 ± 1.1 vs 3.3 ± 1.2; $p = 0.009$), and shorter operation times (30.8 ± 12 min vs 37.7 ± 16.5 min; $p = 0.004$)

Table 1 Descriptives of the categoric and continuous variables for ambulatory and conventional cases

	Ambulatory cases (n = 109)			Conventional cases (n = 76)			p value
	Mean ± SD	Median	Range	Mean ± SD	Median	Range	
Pre-operative variables							
Age (years)	27.8 ± 13.8	23.0	(8.0–82.0)	43.2 ± 19.9	42.0	(15.0–87.0)	< 0.001
Appendix diameter (mm)	10.0 ± 3.2	9.0	(5.8–26.0)	11.7 ± 4.2	11.0	(5.0–30.0)	< 0.001
CRP level	27.8 ± 37.3	12.0	(1.0–233.0)	63.7 ± 101.7	21.0	(1.0–485.0)	0.016
WBC	12.8 ± 4.9	13.0	(4.1–23.0)	14.1 ± 5.2	13.4	(6.0–28.0)	0.136
ASA score	1.2 ± 0.5	1.0	(1.0–3.0)	1.3 ± 0.6	1.0	(1.0–3.0)	0.393
SA score	3.8 ± 1.1	4.0	(1.0–5.0)	3.3 ± 1.2	3.0	(0.0–5.0)	0.009
Male gender	57.8%			53.9%			0.653
BMI > 28	7.3%			7.9%			1.000
Symptoms > 48 h	38.5%			54.1%			0.049
Appendix diameter > 10 mm	27.8%			52.0%			0.001
Appendicolith	26.6%			27.6%			1.000
Perforation signs	10.1%			25.0%			0.008
Per-operative variables							
Operation-time (mn)	30.8 ± 12.0	30.0	(14.0–88.0)	37.7 ± 16.5	34.0	(15.0–102.0)	0.004
Post-operative variables							
Unexpected re-consultation	11.9%			22.4%			0.069
Unexpected re-hospitalization	4.6%			9.2%			0.236
Unexpected re-operation	0.9%			4.0%			0.306

(Table 1). Moreover, there were no statistical differences between ambulatory and conventional cases in terms of rates of unexpected re-consultations (11.9 vs 22.4%, $p = 0.069$), re-hospitalizations (4.6 vs 9.2%, $p = 0.236$), and re-operations (0.9 vs 4.0%, $p = 0.306$).

Of the 185 patients operated, postoperative complications were noted in 32 (17.3%), and included excessive pain or fever in 13 (7.0%), wound infections in 8 (4.3%), abdominal abscess in 5 (2.7%), liver abscess in 1 (0.5%), ileus in 2 (1.1%), phlegmon in 1 (0.5%), hematoma in 1 (0.5%), and acute urine retention in 1 (0.5%). The 109 ambulatory cases had a lower incidence of complications (11.9%) than the 76 conventional cases (25.0%) ($p = 0.029$). According to the modified Clavien system, the postoperative complications for ambulatory cases were of grade I in 7 (6.4%) patients and grade II in 6 (5.5%) patients, while for conventional cases, they were of grade I in 11 (14.5%) patients, grade II in 6 (7.9%) patients, and grade IIIb in 2 (2.6%) patients. Among the 32 patients with complications, 12 were re-hospitalized for the following reasons: pain or fever without abscess ($n = 6$), abdominal abscess ($n = 3$), liver abscess ($n = 1$), ileus ($n = 1$), and phlegmon ($n = 1$).

Uni- and multi-variable regressions for the entire cohort ($n = 185$) revealed that unexpected re-consultations were not significantly associated with any of the pre- or peri-operative variables (Table 2) but that unexpected re-hospitalizations were 4 times more likely for patients with appendicolith (OR, 4.32; $p = 0.04$) (Table 3). It is worth noting that among the 12 patients who were re-hospitalized, 7 (58%) had appendicolith, with a median time to rehospitalization of 3 days (range, 2–8).

Discussion

Studies on appendectomy refer to various labels, definitions, and criteria for 'ambulatory' surgery, making it difficult to compare the proportions of procedures performed in true ambulatory settings. Some defined 'ambulatory' surgery as 'outpatient procedures' with a length of hospital stay < 24 h (with or without overnight stay). Although it seems logical to calculate length of stay from the time of hospital admission [8, 13, 15, 18], many authors calculate it from the end of surgery [6, 12, 13, 15, 17, 18]. Over the last decade, definitions of AS changed from day-case surgery with possible overnight stay [17] to a procedure with no overnight stay [6, 11, 12, 16]. We followed the current guidelines of the IAAS and defined ambulatory surgery as 'a procedure where the patient is discharged on the same working day.'

In this series, 59% of all appendectomies were performed as ambulatory procedures, which is higher than the rates reported in studies with a similar definition of AS (Table 4), whose IIT population comprised complicated appendicitis [6, 11, 12]. Sabbagh et al. [12], Lefrançois et al. [6], and Grelpois et al. [11] reported ambulatory surgery in 18, 20, and 32% of cases, respectively. Cash et al. [13] and Frazee et al. [15, 18], who discharged patients within 24 h, and whose cohorts with intention to treat (ITT) comprised *only* uncomplicated acute appendicitis, claimed remarkable outpatient rates ranging from 65 to 88%. Our rate of AS is all the more remarkable that 27% of patients presented appendicolith and 16% had perforation signs. In our series, 18% of appendectomies could not be performed in ambulatory settings because they were diagnosed or operated outside standard working hours. This was also observed by Scott

Table 2 Logistic regression analysis of re-consultation incidence associated with patient characteristics

Variable	Univariable			Multivariable		
	Odds ratio	95% CI	*p* value	Odds ratio	95% CI	*p* value
Categoric						
Male gender	1.02	(0.47–2.29)	0.957	1.04	(0.41–2.73)	0.931
BMI > 28	0.38	(0.02–2.01)	0.356	0.43	(0.02–3.18)	0.474
Symptoms > 48 h	1.09	(0.49–2.40)	0.823	0.85	(0.31–2.25)	0.746
Appendix diameter > 10 mm	1.12	(0.49–2.48)	0.777			
Appendicolith	1.44	(0.60–3.27)	0.397	1.66	(0.63–4.21)	0.290
Perforation signs	2.20	(0.83–5.42)	0.096	1.84	(0.46–6.55)	0.360
Ambulatory surgery	0.47	(0.21–1.03)	0.062	0.57	(0.21–1.55)	0.267
Continuous						
Age (years)	1.00	(0.97–1.02)	0.812	1.00	(0.97–1.03)	0.814
Appendix diameter	0.98	(0.87–1.08)	0.720	0.95	(0.81–1.10)	0.540
CRP level	1.00	(0.99–1.01)	0.882	1.00	(0.99–1.01)	0.705
WBC	1.06	(0.98–1.16)	0.126	1.05	(0.96–1.15)	0.295
ASA score	0.82	(0.33–1.69)	0.617	0.90	(0.27–2.66)	0.860
SA score	0.88	(0.62–1.27)	0.491			

Table 3 Logistic regression analysis of re-hospitalization incidence associated with patient characteristics

Variable	Univariable			Multivariable		
	Odds ratio	95% CI	*p* value	Odds ratio	95% CI	*p* value
Categoric						
Male gender	1.60	(0.49–6.19)	0.454	0.71	(0.15–3.47)	0.659
BMI > 28	1.12	(0.06–6.48)	0.917	1.44	(0.05–17.10)	0.788
Symptoms > 48 h	1.25	(0.38–4.15)	0.709	1.46	(0.32–6.56)	0.618
Appendix diameter > 10 mm	1.19	(0.34–3.90)	0.770			
Appendicolith	4.23	(1.29–14.96)	0.018	4.32	(1.09–19.08)	0.040
Perforation signs	2.83	(0.71–9.69)	0.109	3.23	(0.52–17.78)	0.184
Ambulatory surgery	0.47	(0.14–1.54)	0.218	0.85	(0.17–4.58)	0.842
Continuous						
Age (years)	1.01	(0.98–1.04)	0.559	1.03	(0.98–1.07)	0.174
Appendix diameter	1.01	(0.85–1.15)	0.873	0.95	(0.73–1.17)	0.698
CRP level	1.00	(1.00–1.01)	0.329	1.00	(0.98–1.01)	0.438
WBC	1.08	(0.96–1.22)	0.200	1.08	(0.93–1.24)	0.307
ASA score	0.38	(0.02–1.52)	0.306	0.21	(0.01–1.36)	0.180
SA score	0.81	(0.50–1.37)	0.422			

et al. [16] who demonstrated that surgeries completed after 8pm had 70% greater odds of retaining the patient overnight.

While there are guidelines for deciding on surgical or non-surgical treatment of acute appendicitis [27], there is no present consensus on medical indications to prefer conventional over ambulatory procedures for acute appendicitis [15], although ambulatory procedures have been shown to decrease post-operative morbidities [20]. In France, only 1.3% of appendectomy procedures in 2015 were performed in ambulatory settings [20]. Most surgeons see conventional hospitalization as the standard and look for patients eligible for AS. By contrast, we consider all patients eligible for AS by default, unless they (i) have severe comorbidities which require monitoring, (ii) cannot

Table 4 'Ambulatory' series for acute appendicitis reported in the literature

Author	Year	Indications (ITT)	N1	Contraindications[b] for AS	Treated by AS N2	(N2/N1%)	Re-consult	Re-hosp
Studies on patients with UAA and CAA								
This study	2017	AA	185	Severe[a] AA	109	59%	11.9%[d]	4.6%[d]
Aubry et al.	2017	AA	194	CAA, ASA ≥ 3, age < 15	89	46%		2%[c]
Grelpois et al.	2016	AA age < 18 ASA < 3	240	CAA	76	32%	13%[d]	4%[d]
LeFrancois et al.	2014	AA	184	CAA	37	20%	5%[d]	3%[d]
Sabbagh et al.	2012	AA	123	CAA, age < 18	22	18%	3.1%[d]	3.1%[d]
Dubois et al.	2010	AA	161	CAA, diabetes or immune disorder, age < 16 or > 65	72	45%	11.1%[d]	
Studies on patient with UAA only								
Scott et al.	2016	UAA age < 18	12,703	CAA	6710	53%		2.2%[d]
Frazee et al.	2016	UAA	563	CAA, age < 17	484	86%		1.2%[d]
Frazee et al.	2014	UAA	345	CAA, age < 17	305	88%		1%[d]
Cash et al.	2012	UAA	153	CAA, age < 18	99	65%		0%[c]

Abbreviations: *AA* acute appendicitis, *UAA* uncomplicated acute appendicitis, *CAA* complicated acute appendicitis [including perforated/gangrenous appendicitis or abscess], *ITT* intention to treat population, *ASA* American Society of Anesthesiologists score, *SA* Saint-Antoine score, *AS* ambulatory surgery, *IAAS* International Association for Ambulatory Surgery, *LOS* length of stay [from admission]

[a]Severe infections, anaphylaxis, generalized peritonitis, and excessive pain

[b]All studies considered the following characteristics as contraindications: history of abdominal surgery, patient's refusal, home > 1 h away, living alone, severe pre-op comorbidities

[c]Of patients admitted for AS

[d]Of patients treated by AS

be operated before 5 pm and cannot be postponed to the next day, (iii) do not meet ambulatory discharge criteria [25], and/or (iv) have severe infections or complications.

Lefrançois et al. [6] created a score to select patients for AS based on 5 preoperative criteria (BMI < 28 kg/m^2, preoperative CRP levels < 30 mg/dL, preoperative WBC counts < 15,000/mm^3, diameters of the appendix ≤ 10 mm, and no radiological signs of perforation). In our series, we found that patients with greater CRP levels, greater appendix diameters, perforation signs as well as older patients were less likely to have AS, but found no differences regarding BMI or WBC counts. Frazee et al. [15] and Cash et al. [13] also demonstrated that, in patients eligible for same-day discharge, pre-existing comorbidities as well as older age were factors that prompted conventional surgery. Scott et al. [16] underlined that the decision to discharge younger, healthier patients from the recovery room is often based on the subjective appreciation of operating surgeons rather than objective medical criteria. If so, then the practice of routine conventional hospitalization after appendectomy should be questioned.

In our series, complications were reported in 25% of conventional cases (Clavien grades I to IIIb) and in 12% of ambulatory cases (Clavien grades I and II). The higher rate of complications among conventional cases could be biased because they included patients with severe comorbidities. Among recent studies that used the definition of the IAAS, only Lefrançois et al. [6] reported the complication rate of 8% in their cohort of uncomplicated acute appendicitis treated by AS. In our series, the higher complication rate of 12% could be because we performed AS in a much larger proportion of patients, of whom 27% had appendicolith and 10% had perforation signs. Importantly, AS did not increase the rate of unexpected re-consultation, re-hospitalization, or re-operation. Our re-consultation, re-hospitalization, and re-operation rates amounted to 12, 4.5, and 1%, respectively, which is analogous to rates reported in recent studies [6, 11, 12, 16], even if our series included a larger proportion of ambulatory cases. Overall, the low rate of complications and re-hospitalizations of AS should challenge the current standard of routine conventional hospitalization for uncomplicated appendicitis. If AS is increasingly recognized as safe for uncomplicated cases, our findings suggest it could also be considered in some complicated cases without severe comorbidities.

Our uni- and multi-variable regressions revealed that no variable, including AS, were significantly associated with unexpected re-consultation. The only variable significantly associated with unexpected re-hospitalization was appendicolith, also known as fecalith, corpolith, or stercolith. Appendicolith, which is composed of firm feces and some mineral deposits, is a well-established risk factor for perforation [28–30], inflammation [31], and failure of antibiotics treatment [32] or post-operative adverse events [31, 33, 34]. In our series, BMI was not associated with unexpected re-consultations or re-hospitalizations. In our experience, the Saint-Antoine score is a good predictor of complicated appendicitis, but is too restrictive for selecting patients for AS, notably because of the criterion of BMI > 28. Our uni- and multi-variable regressions revealed that patients with appendicolith were 4 times more likely to be re-hospitalized. It is worth noting that Lefrançois et al. [6] did not include appendicolith in their multivariable analysis on which they based their Saint-Antoine score. Furthermore, as highlighted by Di Saverio et al. [35], each variable selected in the calculation of the total score was given an equal weight of 1 point instead of adjusting the propensity of each variable to its odds ratio. Interestingly, our series presented comparable proportions of appendicolith in ambulatory and conventional cases, which enabled detection of its associated risks, independently from AS or conventional hospitalization. Given the association of appendicolith with re-hospitalization, the authors recommend that appendicolith should therefore trigger closer monitoring.

Appendicolith is a known risk-factor for non-operative treatment of appendicitis [20, 36, 37], and its surgical treatment is recommended [38]. Before conducting this study, the authors did not expect that appendicolith was also a risk-factor in surgical treatment of appendicitis; therefore, they did not manage patients with appendicolith specifically. Recent studies have identified that retained appendicolith after appendectomy is associated with abscess formation and infection [39–42] and suggest that risk of spillage of appendicolith may be reduced by ensuring that the distal end of the appendix is intact after division [41] and by performing a double ligature of appendicular base [43]. Our findings suggest that appendicitis with appendicolith should be considered as "complicated," and therefore be treated with antibiotics post-operatively. Patients with appendicolith must be informed of increased risks of rehospitalization and be monitored regularly after appendectomy whether performed in conventional or ambulatory setting.

The limitations of this study are typical of retrospective investigation. Out of 185 patients operated, we could not re-contact 33 (17.8%) patients, which may have led us to underestimate the number of minor complications. The strengths of the study include a strict definition of AS rendering comparisons with the literature rigorous, a consecutive series, a multi-operators database, and a large inclusion of patients.

Conclusion

In the present consecutive series of complicated and uncomplicated appendectomies, 59% were performed as true ambulatory procedures, with patients discharged on the same working day. There were no significant differences in rates of unexpected re-consultations, re-hospitalizations, or re-operations between cases performed in ambulatory versus conventional settings. Therefore, ambulatory surgery seems safe and feasible for selected patients with both uncomplicated and complicated acute appendicitis. To better inform patients and manage their expectations, surgeons should be aware that appendicolith is an independent risk factor of unexpected re-hospitalization for appendectomy and should therefore trigger closer monitoring.

Acknowledgements
The authors are grateful to Mr. Vincent Petit for his assistance with data collection and to Mrs. Aude Michelet for her help in manuscript redaction.

Authors' contributions
BG, MB, TL, AV, MR, and VF made substantial contributions to study conception and design, or data acquisition. BG, MS, and HB made substantial contributions to data analysis and interpretation. BG, MB, MS, HB, and VF drafted the manuscript. All authors read and approved the manuscript.

Competing interests
The authors declare that they have no competing interests.

Author details
[1]Department of General, Visceral and Endocrine Surgery, Clinique de la Sauvegarde, Lyon, France. [2]Department of Anesthesiology, Clinique de la Sauvegarde, Lyon, France. [3]Medical Technology, ReSurg SA, ch. de la Vuarpilliere 35, 1260 Nyon, Switzerland. [4]Department of Digestive Surgery, University Hospital Edouard Herriot, Lyon, France.

References

1. Sammalkorpi HE, Mentula P, Leppaniemi A. A new adult appendicitis score improves diagnostic accuracy of acute appendicitis–a prospective study. BMC Gastroenterol. 2014;14:114.
2. Sabbagh C, Cosse C, Dupont H, Ntouba A, Lion T, Regimbeau JM. Ambulatory management of gastrointestinal emergencies: what are the current literature data? J Visc Surg. 2014;151:23–7.
3. Hansson J, Korner U, Khorram-Manesh A, Solberg A, Lundholm K. Randomized clinical trial of antibiotic therapy versus appendicectomy as primary treatment of acute appendicitis in unselected patients. Br J Surg. 2009;96:473–81.
4. Harnoss JC, Zelienka I, Probst P, Grummich K, Muller-Lantzsch C, Harnoss JM, Ulrich A, Buchler MW, Diener MK. Antibiotics versus surgical therapy for uncomplicated appendicitis: systematic review and meta-analysis of controlled trials (PROSPERO 2015: CRD42015016882). Ann Surg. 2017;265: 889–900.
5. Sartelli M, Viale P, Catena F, Ansaloni L, Moore E, Malangoni M, Moore FA, Velmahos G, Coimbra R, Ivatury R, Peitzman A, Koike K, Leppaniemi A, Biffl W, Burlew CC, Balogh ZJ, Boffard K, Bendinelli C, Gupta S, Kluger Y, Agresta F, Di Saverio S, Wani I, Escalona A, Ordonez C, Fraga GP, Junior GA, Bala M, Cui Y, Marwah S, Sakakushev B, Kong V, Naidoo N, Ahmed A, Abbas A, Guercioni G, Vettoretto N, Diaz-Nieto R, Gerych I, Trana C, Faro MP, Yuan KC, Kok KY, Mefire AC, Lee JG, Hong SK, Ghnnam W, Siribumrungwong B, Sato N, Murata K, Irahara T, Coccolini F, Segovia Lohse HA, Verni A, Shoko T. 2013 WSES guidelines for management of intra-abdominal infections. World J Emerg Surg. 2013;8:3.
6. Lefrancois M, Lefevre JH, Chafai N, Pitel S, Kerger L, Agostini J, Canard G, Tiret E. Management of acute appendicitis in ambulatory surgery: is it possible? How to select patients? Ann Surg. 2015;261:1167–72.
7. Alvarez C, Voitk AJ. The road to ambulatory laparoscopic management of perforated appendicitis. Am J Surg. 2000;179:63–6.
8. Aubry A, Saget A, Manceau G, Faron M, Wagner M, Tresallet C, Riou B, Lucidarme O, le Saché F, Karoui M. Outpatient appendectomy in an emergency outpatient surgery unit 24 h a day: an intention-to-treat analysis of 194 patients. World J Surg. 2017;41(10):2471–9.
9. Gilliam AD, Anand R, Horgan LF, Attwood SE. Day case emergency laparoscopic appendectomy. Surg Endosc. 2008;22:483–6.
10. Ramesh S, Galland RB. Early discharge from hospital after open appendicectomy. Br J Surg. 1993;80:1192–3.
11. Grelpois G, Sabbagh C, Cosse C, Robert B, Chapuis-Roux E, Ntouba A, Lion T, Regimbeau JM. Management of uncomplicated acute appendicitis as day case surgery: feasibility and a critical analysis of exclusion criteria and treatment failure. J Am Coll Surg. 2016;223:694–703.
12. Sabbagh C, Brehant O, Dupont H, Browet F, Pequignot A, Regimbeau JM. The feasibility of short-stay laparoscopic appendectomy for acute appendicitis: a prospective cohort study. Surg Endosc. 2012;26:2630–8.
13. Cash CL, Frazee RC, Abernathy SW, Childs EW, Davis ML, Hendricks JC, Smith RW. A prospective treatment protocol for outpatient laparoscopic appendectomy for acute appendicitis. J Am Coll Surg. 2012;215:101–5 discussion 105-106
14. Cash CL, Frazee RC, Smith RW, Davis ML, Hendricks JC, Childs EW, Abernathy SW. Outpatient laparoscopic appendectomy for acute appendicitis. Am Surg. 2012;78:213–5.
15. Frazee RC, Abernathy SW, Davis M, Hendricks JC, Isbell TV, Regner JL, Smith RW. Outpatient laparoscopic appendectomy should be the standard of care for uncomplicated appendicitis. J Trauma Acute Care Surg. 2014;76:79–82. discussion 82-73
16. Scott A, Shekherdimian S, Rouch JD, Sacks GD, Dawes AJ, Lui WY, Bridges L, Heisler T, Crain SR, Cheung MW, Aboulian A. Same-day discharge in laparoscopic acute non-perforated appendectomy. J Am Coll Surg. 2017; 224:43–8.
17. Dubois L, Vogt KN, Davies W, Schlachta CM. Impact of an outpatient appendectomy protocol on clinical outcomes and cost: a case-control study. J Am Coll Surg. 2010;211:731–7.
18. Frazee RC, Abernathy SW, Isbell CL, Isbell T, Regner JL, Smith RD. Outpatient laparoscopic appendectomy: is it time to end the discussion? J Am Coll Surg. 2016;222:473–7.
19. Gignoux B, Gosgnach M, Lanz T, Vulliez A, Blanchet M-C, Frering V, Faucheron J-L, Chasserant P. Short-term outcomes of ambulatory colectomy for 157 consecutive patients. Ann Surg. 2018;In Press.
20. Vons C, Johanet H, Beaussier M. Chirurgie ambulatoire générale et digestive [In French]; In: Rapport au 119eme congrès français de chirurgie. Monographie de l'association française de chirurgie. ISBN: 978-2-7184-1459-1. Paris: John Libbey Eurotext; 2017. https://www.decitre.fr/livres/chirurgie-ambulatoire-generale-et-digestive-9782718414591.html.
21. Nygren J, Thacker J, Carli F, Fearon KC, Norderval S, Lobo DN, Ljungqvist O, Soop M, Ramirez J, Enhanced Recovery After Surgery Society fPC, European Society for Clinical N, Metabolism, International Association for Surgical M, Nutrition. Guidelines for perioperative care in elective rectal/pelvic surgery: enhanced recovery after surgery (ERAS((R))) society recommendations. World J Surg. 2013;37:285–305.
22. Kranke P, Eberhart LH. Possibilities and limitations in the pharmacological management of postoperative nausea and vomiting. Eur J Anaesthesiol. 2011;28:758–65.
23. Aubrun F, Gaulain KN, Fletcher D, Belbachir A, Beloeil H, Carles M, Cuvillon P, Dadure C, Lebuffe G, Marret E, Martinez V, Olivier M, Sabourdin N, Zetlaoui P, Réanimation Sfdaed. Réactualisation de la recommandation sur la douleur postopératoire. Anesth Reanim. 2016;2:421–30. www.em-consulte.com/revue/anrea.

24. Kahokehr A, Sammour T, Srinivasa S, Hill AG. Systematic review and meta-analysis of intraperitoneal local anaesthetic for pain reduction after laparoscopic gastric procedures. Br J Surg. 2011;98:29–36.
25. Chung F, Chan VW, Ong D. A post-anesthetic discharge scoring system for home readiness after ambulatory surgery. J Clin Anesth. 1995;7:500–6.
26. Dindo D, Demartines N, Clavien PA. Classification of surgical complications: a new proposal with evaluation in a cohort of 6336 patients and results of a survey. Ann Surg. 2004;240:205–13.
27. Di Saverio S, Birindelli A, Kelly MD, Catena F, Weber DG, Sartelli M, Sugrue M, De Moya M, Gomes CA, Bhangu A, Agresta F, Moore EE, Soreide K, Griffiths E, De Castro S, Kashuk J, Kluger Y, Leppaniemi A, Ansaloni L, Andersson M, Coccolini F, Coimbra R, Gurusamy KS, Campanile FC, Biffl W, Chiara O, Moore F, Peitzman AB, Fraga GP, Costa D, Maier RV, Rizoli S, Balogh ZJ, Bendinelli C, Cirocchi R, Tonini V, Piccinini A, Tugnoli G, Jovine E, Persiani R, Biondi A, Scalea T, Stahel P, Ivatury R, Velmahos G, Andersson R. WSES Jerusalem guidelines for diagnosis and treatment of acute appendicitis. World J Emerg Surg. 2016;11:34.
28. Imran JB, Madni TD, Minshall CT, Mokdad AA, Subramanian M, Clark AT, Phelan HA, Cripps MW. Predictors of a histopathologic diagnosis of complicated appendicitis. J Surg Res. 2017;214:197–202.
29. Singh JP, Mariadason JG. Role of the faecolith in modern-day appendicitis. Ann R Coll Surg Engl. 2013;95:48–51.
30. Singh M, Kadian YS, Rattan KN, Jangra B. Complicated appendicitis: analysis of risk factors in children. Afr J Paediatr Surg. 2014;11:109–13.
31. Kim MS, Kim MS, Kim DH, Park HW, Park HJ, Hong HP, Kwon HJ. Pre-operative CT predictors associated with 30-day adverse events in patients with appendiceal inflammatory masses who underwent immediate appendectomies. Abdom Imaging. 2015;40:2263–71.
32. Vons C, Barry C, Maitre S, Pautrat K, Leconte M, Costaglioli B, Karoui M, Alves A, Dousset B, Valleur P, Falissard B, Franco D. Amoxicillin plus clavulanic acid versus appendicectomy for treatment of acute uncomplicated appendicitis: an open-label, non-inferiority, randomised controlled trial. Lancet. 2011;377:1573–9.
33. Fike FB, Mortellaro VE, Juang D, Sharp SW, Ostlie DJ, St Peter SD. The impact of postoperative abscess formation in perforated appendicitis. J Surg Res. 2011;170:24–6.
34. Henry MC, Walker A, Silverman BL, Gollin G, Islam S, Sylvester K, Moss RL. Risk factors for the development of abdominal abscess following operation for perforated appendicitis in children: a multicenter case-control study. Arch Surg. 2007;142:236–41. discussion 241
35. Di Saverio S, Catena F, Tarasconi A, Tugnoli G, Jovine E. How to select patients with acute appendicitis for appendectomy in ambulatory surgery? Ann Surg. 2016;263:e64.
36. Mahida JB, Lodwick DL, Nacion KM, Sulkowski JP, Leonhart KL, Cooper JN, Ambeba EJ, Deans KJ, Minneci PC. High failure rate of nonoperative management of acute appendicitis with an appendicolith in children. J Pediatr Surg. 2016;51:908–11.
37. Yoon HM, Kim JH, Lee JS, Ryu JM, Kim DY, Lee JY. Pediatric appendicitis with appendicolith often presents with prolonged abdominal pain and a high risk of perforation. World J Pediatr. 2018;14(2):184–90.
38. Steiner Z, Buklan G, Stackievicz R, Gutermacher M, Litmanovitz I, Golani G, Arnon S. Conservative treatment in uncomplicated acute appendicitis: reassessment of practice safety. Eur J Pediatr. 2017;176:521–7.
39. Ajitha M, Ramya Y, Sharath Kumar K. Dropped appendicolith: complications and management. Int J Biomed Res. 2015;6:65–70.
40. Muyldermans K, Brussaard C, Willekens I, de Mey J. Liver abscess due to dropped appendicolith after laparoscopic appendectomy. J Belgian Soc Radiol. 2015;99:47–9.
41. Maatouk M, Bunni J, Schuijtvlot M. Perihepatic abscess secondary to retained appendicolith: a rare complication managed laparoscopically. J Surg Case Rep. 2011;2011:6.
42. Singh AK, Hahn PF, Gervais D, Vijayraghavan G, Mueller PR. Dropped appendicolith: CT findings and implications for management. AJR Am J Roentgenol. 2008;190:707–11.
43. Guillem P, Mulliez E, Proye C, Pattou F. Retained appendicolith after laparoscopic appendectomy: the need for systematic double ligature of the appendiceal base. Surg Endosc. 2004;18:717–8.

24

Advanced gallbladder inflammation is a risk factor for gallbladder perforation in patients with acute cholecystitis

Stefan Jansen[1], Maciej Stodolski[1], Hubert Zirngibl[1], Daniel Gödde[2] and Peter C. Ambe[1,3*]

Abstract

Background: Acute perforated cholecystitis (APC) is probably the most severe benign gallbladder pathology with high rates of morbidity and mortality. The cause of APC has not been fully understood. We postulated that APC is a complication of advanced gallbladder inflammation. The aim of this study was to investigate the extent of gallbladder inflammation in patients with APC.

Methods: Patients with intraoperative and histopathologic diagnosis of APC were compared with cases with acute cholecystitis without perforation with respect to the extent of inflammation on histopathology as well as surgical outcomes.

Results: Fifty patients with APC were compared to 150 cases without perforation. Advanced age > 65 years and elevated CRP were confirmed on multivariate analysis as independent risk factors for APC. Advanced gallbladder inflammation was seen significantly more often in patients with APC (84.0 vs. 18.7%). Surgery lasted significantly longer 131.3 ± 55.2 min vs. 100.4 ± 47.9 min; the rates of conversion (22 vs. 4%), morbidity (24 vs. 7%), and mortality (8 vs. 1%) were significantly higher in patients with APC. ICU management following surgery was needed significantly more often in the APC group (56 vs. 15%), and the overall length of stay (11.2 ± 12.0 days vs. 5.8 ± 6.5 days) was significantly longer compared to the group without perforation.

Conclusion: Acute gallbladder perforation in patients with acute cholecystitis represents the most severe complication of cholecystitis. Acute perforated cholecystitis is a sequela of advanced gallbladder inflammation like empyematous and gangrenous cholecystitis and is associated with poor outcome compared to non-perforated cases.

Keywords: Acute perforated cholecystitis, Gallbladder perforation, Laparoscopic cholecystectomy, Bile duct injury, Morbidity and mortality

Background

Acute perforated cholecystitis (APC) defines gallbladder perforation in the setting of acute cholecystitis. This condition is probably one of the most severe benign gallbladder pathology with an associated high risk of morbidity and mortality [1]. Patients with APC generally present with elevated inflammatory markers like white blood count (WBC) and C-reactive protein (CRP) [2, 3]. Besides, advanced age, relevant concomitant medical conditions, and the male sex have been identified as possible patient-dependent risk factors for APC [4–8]. These features, however, have been described in connection with other severe forms of cholecystitis and therefore are not directly indicative of APC [9, 10]. It is therefore non-conclusive whether these clinical factors are secondary to APC per se or herald de facto the presence of advanced gallbladder inflammation. We postulate that APC must be a sequela of severe gallbladder inflammation. The aim of this study, therefore, was to investigate the extent of gallbladder inflammation in patients undergoing emergency or urgent gallbladder surgery and APC.

* Correspondence: peter.ambe@uni-wh.de
[1]Department of Surgery, Helios University Hospital Wuppertal, Witten-Herdecke University, Heusnerstr. 40, 42283 Wuppertal, Germany
[3]Department of Visceral, Minimally Invasive and Oncologic Surgery, Marien Hospital Düsseldor, Rochusstr. 2, 40479 Düsseldorf, Germany
Full list of author information is available at the end of the article

Methods

The study protocol was reviewed and approved by the institutional board of review at the Witten/Herdecke, Germany University. A prospectively maintained database of patients undergoing gallbladder surgery in the department of surgery of a university hospital in Germany was reviewed to identify patients undergoing emergency or urgent cholecystectomy for APC between 2013 and 2016. A written consent was received from all patients. The operative notes of identified cases were reviewed to confirm the intraoperative diagnosis of APC and determine the type of perforation. Gallbladder perforation was graded using a modification of Niemeier's classification [11]. According to this classification, free perforation into the peritoneal cavity is graded as type I, perforation with pericholecystic abscess walled off by adhesions as type II, while a chronic perforation with cholecystoenteric fistula is graded as type III. The surgical specimens of identified cases were re-examined to confirm the diagnosis of APC and determine the extent of inflammation. Patients undergoing emergency or urgent from 2013 to 2016 were randomly chosen from the database to create a control group. The size of the control group was calculated with a 90% power and a 5% alpha assuming that 30% of cases with APC had advanced cholecystitis on histopathology compared to 10% in cases without perforation. The surgical specimens of all patients included in the control group were re-examined by a blinded experienced pathologist, and the extent of inflammation was determined.

Acute cholecystitis in our department is an indication for emergency or urgent surgery. Generally, laparoscopic cholecystectomy (LC) represents the standard of care for acute cholecystitis (AC) in our institution. All emergency or urgent procedures are performed either by an attending surgeon or by a surgical fellow with profound experience in minimal invasive surgery. We perform a four-port LC as described elsewhere [12]. The decision to convert is reached by the attending surgeon. Primary open cholecystectomy is seldom performed in our department. Drains were used as needed. All patients with APC were put on broadband antibiotics following surgery.

Demographic information including age, sex, and body mass index (BMI) were recorded for each patient. Relevant preoperative findings including WBC, CRP, and gallbladder wall thickness measured by abdominal ultrasound as well as the American Society of Anesthesiologists (ASA) score at the time of surgery were documented. Intraoperative data including the duration of surgery defined as time from incision to suture, the type of surgery (LC, conversion from LC to open surgery and primary open surgery), and rate of conversion after attempted LC was noted. The preoperative severity of AC was classified using the previously published severity scoring system by Ambe et al. [13]. Postoperative findings including the need for intensive care unit (ICU) management, the rate of relevant morbidity, and death as well as the length of stay (LOS) defined as the time interval from surgery to discharge were documented.

Blinded hematoxylin and eosin (HE)-stained sections of gallbladder specimens of all patients included in the study were re-examined by an experienced pathologist. Edematous cholecystitis was classified as uncomplicated while gangrenous and empyematous cholecystitis were classified as complicated as described elsewhere [14–16]. To achieve our goal, the extent of gallbladder inflammation following histopathology was compared in both groups.

The data generated was analyzed using the Statistics Package for Social Sciences version 24 (SPSS, IMB Corp, Armonk, NY, USA). The variables were described using absolute number and percentages, while central tendencies were reported using means with the corresponding standard deviations where necessary. Analytic statistics was performed using the chi-square test, Mann-Withney U test, or t test where necessary. Univariate and multivariate analyses were performed as needed. A 95% confidence interval was used for all calculations. Results were reported as statistically significant whenever $p < 0.05$.

The primary outcome was the extent of gallbladder inflammation defined as complicated vs. uncomplicated. Secondary outcomes included duration of surgery, rate of conversion following attempted LC, rate of relevant morbidity defined as Clavien–Dindo ≥ 3 [17], need for ICU management, rate of mortality, and LOS.

Results

Seventy-five cases of APC were identified based on operative records. Histopathology confirmed APC in 50 cases, which were included in the study group. Type I perforation was seen in one case (2%). Type II perforation was present in 48 cases (96%) including 30 cases (60.0%) with perforation into the large omentum and 18 cases (36%) with perforation towards the liver, while one case (2%) with a cholecysto-duodenal fistula (type III perforation) was recorded. Following sample size analysis as stated above, 150 cases of AC without perforation were included in the control group. Figure 1 shows the distribution of the study population. The demographic characteristics of the study population are presented in Table 1.

The mean WBC was 14.2 ± 6.6/μl in the study group and 12.4 ± 6.3/μl in the control. This difference was not statistically significant, $p = 0.112$. Equally, the mean gallbladder wall thickness did not differ amongst both groups, 6.1 ± 2.6 mm vs. 5.5 ± 2.7 mm, $p = 0.332$. However, the mean CRP was significantly higher in the study group compared to the control group, 19.9 ± 13.5 mg/dl vs. 8.9 ± 10.3 mg/dl, $p = 0.001$.

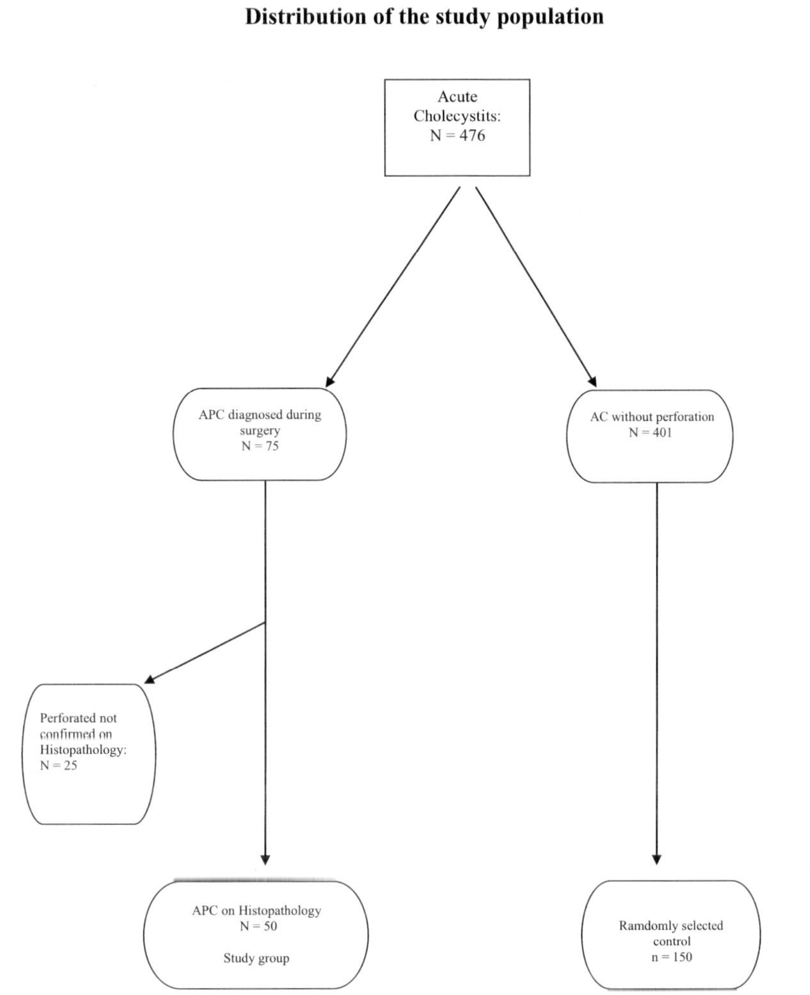

Fig. 1 Distribution of the study population. APC: Acute Perforated Cholecystitis

Table 1 Demographic characteristics of the study population

Features	Study group	Control group	*p* value
Sex			
Female	17 (34.0%)	61 (40.7%)	0.403
Male	33 (66.0%)	9 (59.5%)	
Mean age (years)	73.4 ± 10.0	63.4 ± 16.7	0.001
Mean BMI (kg/m^2)	28.6 ± 7.2	28.9 ± 13.3	0.870
ASA scores			
1	6 (12.0%)	41 (27.3%)	
2	18 (36.0%)	66 (44.0%)	0.003
3	19 (38.0%)	39 (26.0%)	
> 3	7 (14.0%)	4 (2.7%)	

ASA American Society of Anesthesiology score, *BMI* body mass index

Attempted LC was performed in all cases in the control group, while primary open surgery was performed in four (8%) cases in the study group. Conversion from laparoscopic to open surgery was performed in six cases in the control group (4.0%) compared to 11 cases in the study group (22.0%). This difference was statistically significant, $p = 0.001$. The duration of surgery in both groups is presented in Fig. 2. Surgery lasted significantly longer in the study group.

Postoperative ICU management was needed significantly more often in the study group, 28 (56.0%) cases vs. 23 (15.3%) cases, $p = 0.001$. Grade ≥ 3 complications were recorded in 12 cases (24.0%) in the study group including four (8%) deaths (1× myocardial infarction and 3× sepsis with multi-organ failure), four (8%) cases with bile duct injury, three cases (6%) with intra-abdominal abscess, and one case with surgical site infection. Eleven (7.3%) grade ≥ 3 complications were recorded in the control group including four cases with bile leak (3.0%), two with intra-abdominal abscess, two relevant wound

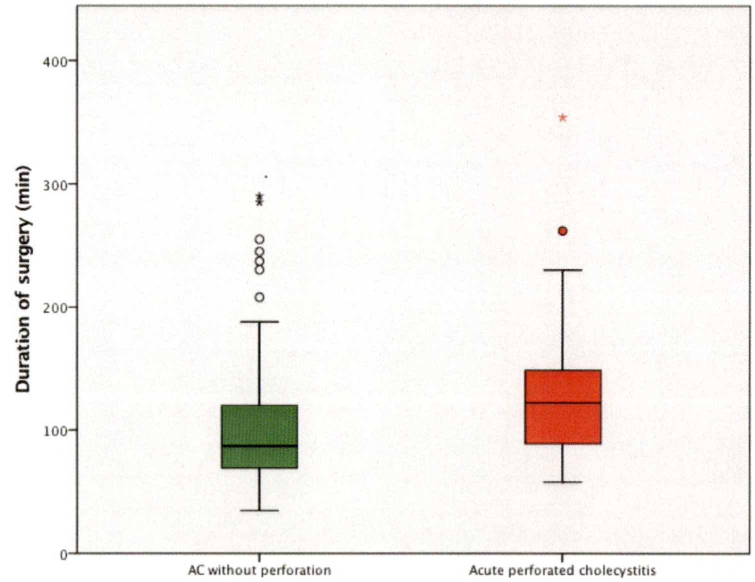

Fig. 2 Duration of surgery. Surgery lasted significantly longer in the APC group: 131. 3 ± 55.2 min vs. 100.4 ± 47.9 min, $p = 0.001$

complications, and one case of bleeding, pneumonia, and death (0.7%) following respiratory failure. The rates of morbidity ($p = 0.003$) and mortality ($p = 0.001$) were significantly higher in the APC group. The mean length of hospital stay was significantly longer in the APC group 11.2 ± 12.0 days vs. 5.8 ± 6.5 days, $p = 0.001$.

Histopathology confirmed an advanced form of gallbladder inflammation in the form of empyematous or gangrenous cholecystitis in significantly more cases in the APC group compared to the control group, (84.0 vs. 18.7%, $p = 0.001$), Fig. 3.

Discussion

This study investigated the extent of gallbladder inflammation in patients undergoing emergency or urgent surgery for APC. Fifty patients with confirmed APC following intraoperative and histological diagnosis were compared to 150 randomly chosen cases undergoing LC for AC without perforation. Advanced gallbladder inflammation with empyematous and gangrenous cholecystitis was recorded significantly more often in the APC group compared to the control. Patients with APC were significantly older and had significantly higher CRP

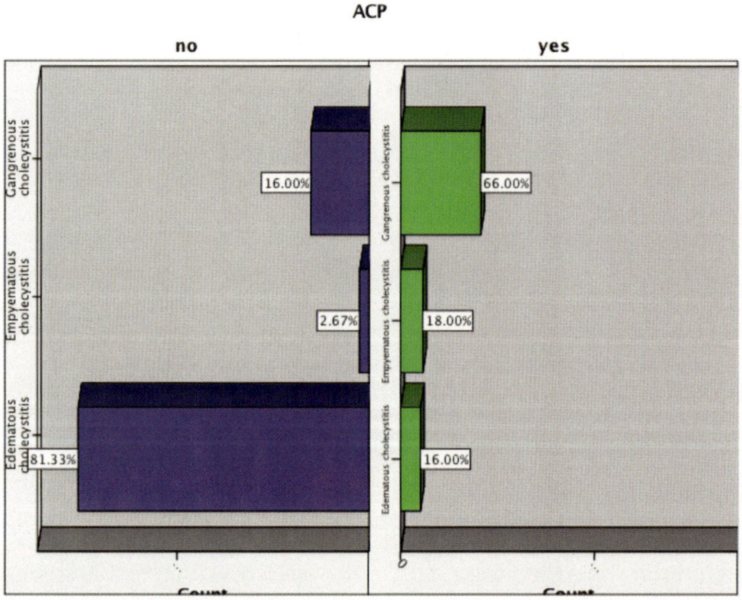

Fig. 3 Extent of gallbladder inflammation on histopathology

in comparison to the controls. Surgery lasted significantly longer; the rates of conversation, morbidity, and mortality were significantly higher in the APC group. ICU management was needed significantly more often in the APC group, and the overall LOS was significantly longer in the APC group compared to the group without perforation.

Gallbladder perforation in the setting of acute cholecystitis has been suggested in our recently published register study to be a risk factor for poor outcome in patients undergoing cholecystectomy for AC [1]. The outcomes of 5704 cases with APC undergoing emergency or urgent cholecystectomy were compared to those of 39,661 patients without perforation. The duration of surgery, the rates of conversation, morbidity, and mortality were significantly higher in patients with APC compared to those without APC. The results of the present study are in accordance with the results reported in the above study.

A great drawback to the register study by Jansen et al. which was clearly stated by the authors in the limitation section was the inability to characterize the extent of gallbladder inflammation because the register data used in their study did not contain histology findings. This shortcoming was investigated in the present study. Complicated cholecystitis defined as advanced gallbladder inflammation in the form of empyematous or gangrenous cholecystitis was confirmed in a significant portion of the APC group compared to the control group.

Advanced age > 65 years and elevated CRP were identified as risk factors for APC. These factors were further confirmed on multivariate analysis as independent risk factors for APC. These same factors have been previously described in connection with other forms of severe cholecystitis and therefore are not specific for APC [18, 19].

The significantly longer duration of surgery and higher rate of conversion to open surgery following attempted LC in the APC group in comparison to the group without perforation are de facto arguments for the surgical challenge associated with the management of patients with APC. Besides, the 8% rate of bile duct injury and 6% rate of postoperative intra-abdominal abscess formation in the APC group herald the severity of this entity. The mortality rate in this study was 8%. This rate is almost twice the reported rate by Jansen et al. [1] but comparable with the 9.5% rate of death reported in a retrospective analysis of 137 patients with APC by Ausania et al. in 2015 [20]. The heterogeneity in the reported risk of mortality in this and as well as in previous publications must be interpreted in context with the study population. Furthermore, the significantly higher rates of ICU management, as well as the significantly longer LOS, must be interpreted as indicators of the astringent nature of APC.

Another interesting finding in this study was the fact that four patients (8%) in the APC group underwent primary open cholecystectomy compared to none in the control group. These patients underwent explorative laparotomy for acute abdomen with peritonitis, and the diagnosis of APC was reached during surgery. Type I perforation with bilious peritonitis was evident during laparotomy in these patients. This finding should be interpreted as a further demonstration of the severe clinical nature of APC.

The retrospective study design and the small size of the study population must be stated as possible limitations to this study. Thus, further investigations with larger populations would be needed to further investigate the trends shown here. Besides, the results reported in this study might be secondary to the profound expertise in laparoscopic surgery in our department. Therefore, the results of this study might not be readily projected on other institutions. All cases included in this study were managed surgically. Interventional treatment like percutaneous cholecystostomy is not routinely performed in our center. Although the current literature on the role of percutaneous cholecystostomy is not conclusive [21–25], it remains speculative if the outcomes recorded in this study might have been altered by such an interventional management.

Surgeons and clinicians must be aware of the severe nature of APC with associated high risks of morbidity and mortality. The surgical management of such patients warrants profound expertise, and conversion from laparoscopic to open surgery should never be considered a failure. A vigilant postoperative care including the use of broadband antibiotics and close monitoring, e.g., in the ICU, should be considered in such cases.

Taken together, the results of this study confirm APC as a severe complication of AC with significantly higher rates of morbidity and mortality. Advanced gallbladder inflammation including empyematous and gangrenous cholecystitis was seen significantly more often in patients with APC compared to those without perforation. Thus, gallbladder perforation in APC must be secondary to advanced gallbladder inflammation.

Conclusion

Acute gallbladder perforation in patients with acute cholecystitis represents the most severe complication of cholecystitis. Acute perforated cholecystitis is a sequela of advanced gallbladder inflammation like empyematous and gangrenous cholecystitis and is associated with poor outcome compared to non-perforated cases.

Abbreviations

AC: Acute cholecystitis; APC: Acute perforated cholecystitis; ASA: American Society of Anesthesiologists; BMI: Body mass index; CRP: C-reactive protein; HE: Hematoxylin and eosin; ICU: Intensive care unit; LC: Laparoscopic cholecystectomy; LOS: Length of stay; WBC: White blood count

Acknowledgements

Not applicable

Funding

None

Authors' contributions

PA contributed to the study concept. PA, SJ, DG, and HZ contributed to the study design. MS, PA, SJ, and DG contributed to the data collection. DG performed the histopathology. PA and SH contributed to the statistical analysis. PA, SJ, DG, HZ, and MS interpreted the results. SH and PA drafted the manuscript. PA, SJ, HZ, DG, and MS critically reviewed and approved the manuscript.

Competing interests

The authors declare that they have no competing interests.

Author details

[1]Department of Surgery, Helios University Hospital Wuppertal, Witten-Herdecke University, Heusnerstr. 40, 42283 Wuppertal, Germany. [2]Department of Pathology and Molecular Pathology, Helios University Hospital Wuppertal, Witten-Herdecke University, Heusnerstr. 40, 42283 Wuppertal, Germany. [3]Department of Visceral, Minimally Invasive and Oncologic Surgery, Marien Hospital Düsseldor, Rochusstr. 2, 40479 Düsseldorf, Germany.

References

1. Jansen S, Doerner J, Macher-Heidrich S, Zirngibl H, Ambe PC. Outcome of acute perforated cholecystitis: a register study of over 5000 cases from a quality control database in Germany. Surg Endosc. 2017;31(4):1896–900.
2. Ambe PC, Jansen S, Macher-Heidrich S, Zirngibl H. Surgical management of empyematous cholecystitis: a register study of over 12,000 cases from a regional quality control database in Germany. Surg Endosc. 2016;30(12): 5319–24.
3. Aydin C, Altaca G, Berber I, Tekin K, Kara M, Titiz I. Prognostic parameters for the prediction of acute gangrenous cholecystitis. J Hepato-Biliary-Pancreat Surg. 2006;13(2):155–9.
4. Ambe PC, Kohler L. Is the male gender an independent risk factor for complication in patients undergoing laparoscopic cholecystectomy for acute cholecystitis? Int Surg. 2015;100(5):854–9.
5. Botaitis S, Polychronidis A, Pitiakoudis M, Perente S, Simopoulos C. Does gender affect laparoscopic cholecystectomy? Surg Laparosc Endosc Percutan Tech. 2008;18(2):157–61.
6. Kanakala V, Borowski DW, Pellen MG, Dronamraju SS, Woodcock SA, Seymour K, Attwood SE, Horgan LF. Risk factors in laparoscopic cholecystectomy: a multivariate analysis. Int J Surg. 2011;9(4):318–23.
7. Kortram K, van Ramshorst B, Bollen TL, Besselink MGH, Gouma DJ, Karsten T, Kruyt PM, Nieuwenhuijzen GAP, Kelder JC, Tromp E, et al. Acute cholecystitis in high risk surgical patients: percutaneous cholecystostomy versus laparoscopic cholecystectomy (CHOCOLATE trial): study protocol for a randomized controlled trial. Trials. 2012;13
8. Laurila J, Syrjala H, Laurila PA, Saarnio J, Ala-Kokko TI. Acute acalculous cholecystitis in critically ill patients. Acta Anaesthesiol Scand. 2004;48(8):986–91.
9. Cho JY, Han HS, Yoon YS, Ahn KS. Risk factors for acute cholecystitis and a complicated clinical course in patients with symptomatic cholelithiasis. Archives of surgery (Chicago, Ill : 1960). 2010;145(4):329–33. discussion 333
10. Fagan SP, Awad SS, Rahwan K, Hira K, Aoki N, Itani KM, Berger DH. Prognostic factors for the development of gangrenous cholecystitis. Am J Surg. 2003;186(5):481–5.
11. Niemeier OW. Acute free perforation of the gall-bladder. Ann Surg. 1934; 99(6):922–4.
12. Papadakis M, Ambe PC, Zirngibl H. Critically ill patients with acute cholecystitis are at increased risk for extensive gallbladder inflammation. World J Emerg Surg. 2015;10:59.
13. Ambe PC, Papadakis M, Zirngibl H. A proposal for a preoperative clinical scoring system for acute cholecystitis. J Surg Res. 2016;200(2):473–9.
14. Ambe PC, Christ H, Wassenberg D. Does the Tokyo guidelines predict the extent of gallbladder inflammation in patients with acute cholecystitis? A single center retrospective analysis. BMC Gastroenterol. 2015;15(1):142.
15. Kimura Y, Takada T, Kawarada Y, Nimura Y, Hirata K, Sekimoto M, Yoshida M, Mayumi T, Wada K, Miura F, et al. Definitions, pathophysiology, and epidemiology of acute cholangitis and cholecystitis: Tokyo guidelines. J Hepato-Biliary-Pancreat Surg. 2007;14(1):15–26.
16. Kimura Y, Takada T, Strasberg SM, Pitt HA, Gouma DJ, Garden OJ, Buchler MW, Windsor JA, Mayumi T, Yoshida M, et al. TG13 current terminology, etiology, and epidemiology of acute cholangitis and cholecystitis. J Hepatobiliary Pancreat Sci. 2013;20(1):8–23.
17. Dindo D, Demartines N, Clavien PA. Classification of surgical complications: a new proposal with evaluation in a cohort of 6336 patients and results of a survey. Ann Surg. 2004;240(2):205–13.
18. Nazeer MA, Ali M, Ahmed K, Saleem R, Ali M, Suleman B. Outcomes of laparoscopic cholecystectomy in the elderly versus young patients. Pak J Med Health Sci. 2012;6(3):544–6.
19. Indar AA, Beckingham IJ. Acute cholecystitis. BMJ. 2002;325(7365):639–43.
20. Ausania F, Guzman Suarez S, Alvarez Garcia H, Senra del Rio P, Casal Nunez E. Gallbladder perforation: morbidity, mortality and preoperative risk prediction. Surg Endosc. 2015;29(4):955–60.
21. Ambe PC, Kaptanis S, Papadakis M, Weber SA, Jansen S, Zirngibl H. The treatment of critically ill patients with acute cholecystitis. Dtsch Arzteblatt Int. 2016;113(33–34):545–51.
22. Ambe PC, Zirngibl H. The fate of patients managed with percutaneous cholecystostomy for acute cholecystitis. Surgery. 2016;159(5):1479–80.
23. Anderson JE, Inui T, Talamini MA, Chang DC. Cholecystostomy offers no survival benefit in patients with acute acalculous cholecystitis and severe sepsis and shock. J Surg Res. 2014;190(2):517–21.
24. Gurusamy KS, Rossi M, Davidson BR. Percutaneous cholecystostomy for high-risk surgical patients with acute calculous cholecystitis. Cochrane Database Syst Rev. 2013;8:CD007088.
25. Winbladh A, Gullstrand P, Svanvik J, Sandstrom P. Systematic review of cholecystostomy as a treatment option in acute cholecystitis. HPB (Oxford). 2009;11(3):183–93.

25

Implementation and adoption of advanced care planning in the elderly trauma patient

K. Verhoeff[1], P. Glen[2], A. Taheri[2], B. Min[1], B. Tsang[2], V. Fawcett[2] and S. Widder[2*]

Abstract

Background: Geriatric trauma has high morbidity and mortality, often requiring extensive hospital stays and interventions. The number of geriatric trauma patients is also increasing significantly and accounts for a large proportion of trauma care. Specific geriatric trauma protocols exist to improve care for this complex patient population, who often have various comorbidities, pre-existing medications, and extensive injury within a trauma perspective. These guidelines for geriatric trauma care often suggest early advanced care planning (ACP) discussions and documentation to guide patient and family-centered care.

Methods: A provincial ACP program was implemented in April of 2012, which has since been used by our level 1 trauma center. We applied a before and after study design to assess the documentation of goals of care in elderly trauma patients following implementation of the standardized provincial ACP tool on April 1, 2012.

Results: Documentation of ACP in elderly major trauma patients following the implementation of this tool increased significantly from 16 to 35%. Additionally, secondary outcomes demonstrated that many more patients received goals of care documentation within 24 h of admission, and 93% of patients had goals of care documented prior to intensive care unit (ICU) admission. The number of trauma patients that were admitted to the ICU also decreased from 17 to 5%.

Conclusion: Early advanced care planning is crucial for geriatric trauma patients to improve patient and family-centered care. Here, we have outlined our approach with modest improvements in goals of care documentation for our geriatric population at a level 1 trauma center. We also outline the benefits and drawbacks of this approach and identify the areas for improvement to support improved patient-centered care for the injured geriatric patient. Here, we have provided a framework for others to implement and further develop.

Keywords: Quality improvement, Geriatric trauma, Advanced care planning, Patient and family-centered care

Background

The number of Canadian seniors is increasing significantly, with people over the age of 65 expected to compose 25% of the country's population by 2036 [1]. A proportional increase in geriatric trauma is expected [2, 3]. Geriatric trauma is associated with longer intensive care unit (ICU) admissions, more life-threatening complications while in hospital, and significantly higher mortality despite similar injury severity when compared to younger patients [2–6].

The American College of Surgeons Committee on Trauma (ACS COT) has defined specific protocols for geriatric trauma in order to improve management of comorbid conditions, polypharmacy, poor physiologic reserve, and elderly specific complications (i.e., delirium) [2]. ACS COT suggests involving the patient, surrogate decision-makers, family, and the health care team in a discussion about the patient's treatment priorities. This conversation aims to establish and document the commonly termed "goals of care" (GOC) within the first 72 h after admission and is meant to weigh the benefits of escalating treatments against the risks of complications [2].

Despite trauma being a leading cause of death in Canada, there is a relative dearth of studies focusing on GOC discussions in trauma patients [7]. Advanced care planning (ACP) facilitates discussions around patient's health care goals (i.e., cardiopulmonary resuscitation) along with a realistic presentation of what intensive,

* Correspondence: Sandy.Widder2@albertahealthservices.ca
[2]Department of Surgery, 2D4.27 Mackenzie Health Sciences Centre, University of Alberta, 8440-112 St. Edmonton, Edmonton, Alberta T6G 2B7, Canada
Full list of author information is available at the end of the article

invasive treatments can provide. ACP processes can guide complex treatment decision-making (including end-of-life discussions between allied health professionals, patients, and their families) to promote patient and family-centered care (PFCC) and eliminate uncertainty regarding the patient's wishes [8, 9].

The province of Alberta implemented an ACP tool in April of 2012, including within our level 1 trauma center. The program involved providing every patient and family with information sheets regarding ACP, prompting a discussion about future care between the patient and care providers regarding the patient's care goals, and ultimately documenting these goals of care in the chart (see Additional file 1). A specific GOC order sheet was also provided to practitioners for process standardization (see Additional file 1). We sought to determine the effect of this ACP tool on establishing documented GOC for geriatric trauma patients. We also aimed to outline the benefits and drawbacks of this approach and identify the areas for improvement to assist others who wish to implement an ACP system within their trauma systems.

Methods

We applied a before and after study design to assess the documentation of GOC in elderly trauma patients following implementation of the standardized provincial ACP tool on April 1, 2012 (see Additional file 1). The Alberta Trauma Registry is a prospective database that collects information on all major trauma patients (Injury Severity Score ≥ 12). This database was retrospectively queried for a cohort of patients over the age of 65 who were admitted from April 1, 2010, to September 30, 2014, representing a period of 24 months before and 30 months after ACP implementation. Charts for this cohort were individually reviewed to determine patient demographics, whether GOC were documented, whether it was done within 24 h of admission and prior to ICU admission, the source of the GOC information, and the patient's post-hospitalization disposition.

Data was separated into a pre-intervention group ($n = 177$) that included patients 24 months prior to April 2012 and a post-intervention group ($n = 294$) that included patients 30 months after ACP program implementation. A 2-year before and after time frame was chosen to adequately assess for change following the project implementation. As the ACP tool was implemented provincially, an additional 6 months was included within the analysis for the after group to allow for a period of institutional uptake of these processes. The groups were compared based on Injury Severity Score (ISS), sex, age, length of stay, and mechanism of injury, using chi-squared tests of independence. The primary outcome measure of this study was whether the ACP intervention was associated with a change in the documentation of GOC in the chart overall; a comparison between both time periods was made using Fisher's exact test. Secondary measures assessed documentation of GOC within 24 h and upon admission to ICU. These were also assessed with Fisher's exact test.

Results

The two groups of geriatric trauma patients in this study were similar with regard to age, sex, mechanism of injury, length of stay, ISS, and disposition after discharge (Table 1). Patients were approximately 77 years old in both groups with 35% of patients before 2012 and 40% after 2012 being female (Table 1). Importantly, the mean ISS for patients in both groups was statistically similar, being 23 before the ACS program and 22 after. Patients primarily suffered blunt traumatic injuries from either falls or motor vehicle accidents, a distribution that did not change between study periods (Table 1).

Analysis of the primary outcome demonstrated a statistically significant change ($p < 0.01$) in GOC documentation following the ACP program implementation. Twenty-four months prior to the ACP program implementation, only 16% of major geriatric trauma

Table 1 Patient demographics

	Before ($n = 177$)	After ($n = 294$)	p value
Mean age (years)	76.50	77.02	0.51
Mean ISS	22.65	22.13	0.50
Median LOS (days)	9	7	N/A
Number female (proportion)	60 (0.34)	117 (0.40)	0.92
Number male (proportion)	117 (0.66)	177 (0.60)	0.94
Injury	*n* (%)	*n* (%)	
Blunt	174 (98)	289 (98)	0.99
Fall	118 (68)	207 (72)	0.96
Motor vehicle	35 (20)	57 (20)	0.99
Pedestrian	8 (5)	9 (3)	0.94
Other	13 (7)	16 (6)	0.94
Penetrating	0 (0)	1 (0)	0.94
Burn	3 (2)	4 (1)	0.98
Other	0 (0)	1 (0)	0.94
Disposition			
Home	73 (41)	127 (43)	0.97
Home support	13 (7)	10 (3)	0.84
Other hospital	35 (20)	49 (17)	0.94
Rehabilitation	13 (7)	30 (10)	0.92
Chronic care	20 (11)	27 (9)	0.95
Nursing home	7 (4)	4 (1)	0.83
Died	16 (9)	47 (16)	0.84

Characteristics of geriatric trauma population before and after the implementation of the advanced care planning project at our hospital

patients had documented GOC by the end of their hospital stay (Table 2). This improved to 35% in the study period following ACP project implementation.

Secondary outcomes demonstrated that GOC documentation within 24 h was significantly higher after the intervention (Table 2). For the 30 months following April 2012, 21% of geriatric major trauma patients had this documentation done within 24 h as compared to 11% in the 24 months prior to ACP implementation.

The rate of admission to the ICU was significantly lower after the ACP program implementation when compared to before (Table 3). There was also a significant increase in the documentation of GOC for patients admitted to the ICU with 93% of admitted ICU patients having this documented after the ACP implementation, as compared to 20% prior to this project.

Discussion

Despite the importance of ACP, a 2008 report from the US Congress demonstrated the widespread failure of implementation [10]. Some publications have advocated to abandon advanced care directives, citing reasons such as patient uncertainty about their use, inadequate prognostication to guide discussions, and poor compliance by health care practitioners with patient wishes [11–13]. However, when achieved ACP has been shown to significantly reduce anxiety, depression, and post-traumatic stress disorder in the relatives of patients who die [8, 14, 15]. Even when ACP was done but not enacted, patient and family satisfaction with their care was significantly improved [14]. This correlation addresses the vital importance of patient autonomy and PFCC to guide treatment decisions. It is also vitally important to separate the notion of ACP and end of life care decision-making. The two are independent, with the ACP discussion establishing patient care priorities.

Table 2 Successful goals of care documentation

Goals of care	Before ($n = 177$)	After ($n = 294$)	p value
	n (%)	n (%)	
Documented			
Yes	28 (16)	103 (35)	
No	149 (84)	191 (65)	< 0.01
Within 24 h			
Yes	20 (11)	61 (21)	
No	157 (89)	233 (79)	< 0.01
Source			
Patient	1 (4)	2 (2)	
Substitute decision-maker	26 (93)	87 (84)	
Advance directive	1 (4)	14 (14)	ns

Documentation of goals of care before and after the implementation of the advanced care planning project at our hospital

Table 3 Admission to ICU and rate of GOC documentation

	Before ($n = 177$)	After ($n = 294$)	p value
	n (%)	n (%)	
Admitted to ICU	30 (17)	14 (5)	< 0.01
Goals documented			
Yes	6 (20)	13 (93)	
No	24 (80)	1 (7)	< 0.01

Documentation of goals of care before and after the implementation of the advanced care planning project for patients admitted to the intensive care unit (ICU)

If the patient's priorities do not fit with achievable improvements in their condition, then end of life care discussions may be required. However, the initial discussion should focus on establishing priorities in care. We outline our institution's improvements for geriatric trauma patients following the implementation of a provincial ACP tool and discuss the areas for potential improvement.

As the management of traumatic injuries improves and patient expectations of autonomy are reinforced, the practice of ACP will become increasingly important [3–6]. Prior to the implementation of Alberta's provincial ACP program, only 16% of our level one trauma center's major trauma patients over 65 years old had documented GOC by the end of their hospital stay (Table 2). Following the implementation of a provincial ACP program, GOC documentation changed significantly, with an increase to 34% (Table 2). Although we achieved improvement, this result shows that many patients did not have their goals documented—indicating that barriers continue to exist that limit ACP discussions. The source of the GOC decision was documented in our study and shows that in both the before and after groups, most decisions regarding GOC were provided by a substitute decision-maker or an advanced care directive (Table 2). This is likely because geriatric trauma patients have injuries, co-morbidities, and complications (i.e., delirium) that would prevent them from making GOC decisions. This also highlights the importance of care conferences that focus on PFCC early during geriatric trauma admission to support GOC decisions.

Due to the high risk of intervention, prolonged ICU admission, life-threatening complications, and mortality in geriatric trauma, early ACP discussion is key [2, 4–6]. Following implementation of our ACP tool, new ACS COT guidelines suggested ACP and documentation of GOC within 72 h of admission for geriatric trauma patients [2]. Secondary outcomes to evaluate GOC documentation in the first 24 h and prior to ICU admission were chosen as two identifiable time points when geriatric patients were likely to undergo interventions. However, if ACS COT guidelines were released prior to study implementation, a 72-h period may have been chosen to assess our compliance with these guidelines. Despite that, our ACP program implementation was associated with increased early GOC documentation within the first 24 h (Table 2).

A substantial increase in GOC prior to ICU admission is also noted from 20 to 93% with an associated decrease in ICU admission from 17 to 5% (Table 3). There was an obvious culture shift within the ICU to initiate GOC documentation on transfer to their unit, which may have even prevented undesired transfers to the ICU, whereby risks of intensive invasive care would have outweighed benefits to the patient. We suggest that ICU providers are likely accustomed to undergoing ACP discussion due to their highly acute patient population and specialized training around PFCC and communication, lending to the ease of transition for their unit. It may be beneficial to involve these types of practitioners in GOC discussion early in a geriatric trauma patient's hospital admission. Having these practitioners involved with medical education to provide tools and approaches for these discussions may also be beneficial.

Of note, there was a statistically insignificant mortality increase after ACP project implementation (Table 1). This may relate to fewer patients desiring ICU care and heroic lifesaving measures. There was also an accompanying statistically insignificant trend towards fewer patients sent to chronic care or a nursing home following their trauma admission. However, these results should be evaluated cautiously, as our study lacked the power to isolate the significance of these trends.

Successful programs such as "Respecting Choices," "Physician Orders for Life-Sustaining Treatment," and others outlined important tools for ACP implementation that our provincial program modeled [14, 16]. These included a need for leaders to enact change, implementation in a medical culture receptive to change, and complex ACP that focused on discussions rather than specific interventions [14, 16]. Ensuring ACP and documentation of GOC prior to deterioration in condition is vitally important to ensure escalated care can be accessed expediently, when appropriate [10, 16]. The ACP program also increased GOC documentation in the first 24 h (Table 2), which is important for geriatric trauma patients who often require rapid interventions soon after admission. A final important aspect of successful ACP project implementation that we modeled is an openness to department-specific quality improvement, as ACP is diverse and can take many forms even within a single hospital [14–16]. This will allow our project to continue building on its success in the future within our own institution as we seek opportunities to educate our physicians on the importance of having ACP discussions.

Despite ACP program implementation and a significant change in GOC documentation, we are seeking ways to increase the documentation beyond the 35% level we have achieved in our current study. Achievable, identifiable, and clinically significant pathways to implementing effective ACP have been demonstrated, and we continue to follow these models to further improve our ACP practices [8, 14–16]. The barriers to ACP in these studies include staff availability and time, their ability to confidently and accurately discuss ACP, and organizational commitment and support for ACP programs [14, 17–19]. Similarly, focusing on specific advanced directives, rather than a complex and complete understanding of the patient's GOC, leads to non-documented and ineffective ACP [13, 14, 19, 20].

Lessons and limitations

Future initiatives that may assist our trauma services division to improve ACP for geriatric trauma patients exist. Ensuring ACP prior to emergency care, such as by primary care providers in family practice—so-called advance directives—has been used by other programs to improve ACP and reduce time constraints for acute care providers in the emergency setting [10, 16]. It is important to recognize that while ACP was increased through this project, 93% of GOC decisions in the before group and 84% in the after group were made via a substitute decision maker; this highlights the importance of discussing ACP while patients are healthy to maintain their autonomy in acute scenarios. Initiating these family discussions and decisions should be standard of care for all patients that are admitted to hospital and should be encouraged in the outpatient population as well. Emphasizing the importance of ACP during trauma educational initiatives and outreach programs within the community may improve pre-trauma GOC documentation or discussion; as mentioned, involving experienced intensivists to assist education may provide insight into tools and approaches for these difficult discussions.

Time constraint concerns both in the primary care and emergency care settings were identified by practitioners early in the development of model ACP programs and may be an area for future examination [16]. While the resources do not exist to employ individuals solely for the purposes of ACP discussion, the provincial program suggested that all health care practitioners (including nurses, social workers, respiratory therapists, spiritual health practitioners, and all allied health professionals) play a role in ACP by following five "Core Elements of ACP" (Fig. 1) [16]. Involving specialists, such as intensivists, geriatricians, and palliative care specialists, early in the care of geriatric trauma patients is likely beneficial, especially if a shared mental model between the care team and patient and family cannot be achieved. In order to implement these elements in our program and limit time constraint issues, the culture and approach to ACP will likely require champions for change

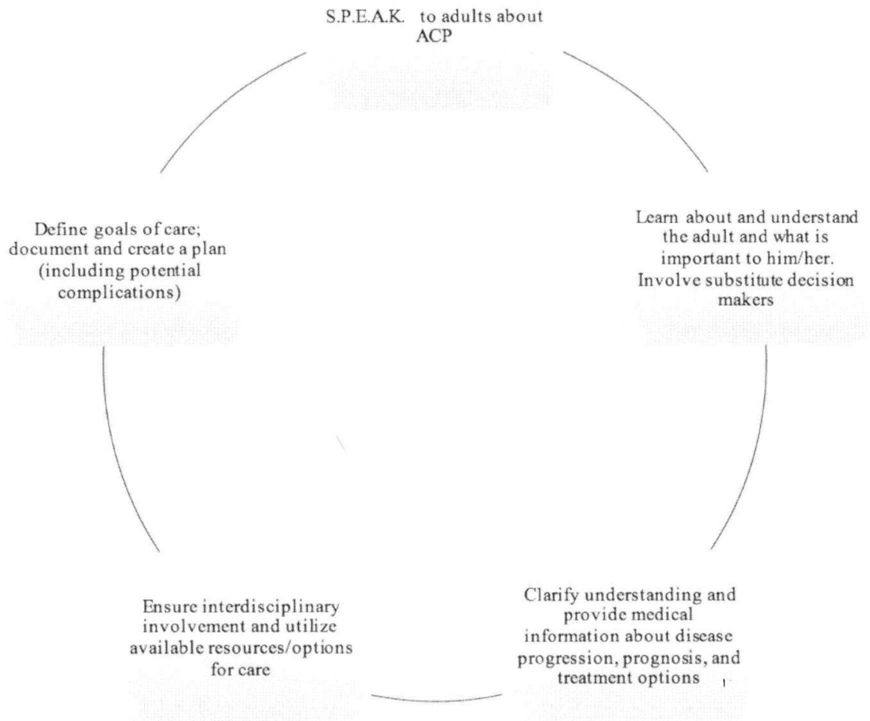

Fig. 1 The five "Core Elements of ACP." Five elements of advanced care planning identified by our provincial advanced care planning program to help involve allied health professionals in goals of care discussions [16]

to lead the way, as other successful programs have demonstrated [14, 16].

Despite demonstrating improved GOC documentation, the authors recognize certain shortcomings of this method for evaluating ACP program implementation. A before and after study design cannot exclude that other changes or that baseline improvement led to the results we discovered. An interrupted time series analysis to describe the baseline increase in GOC documentation could help attribute the results of our study more directly to the intervention. Also, our comparison groups would ideally be similar in size; however, this is likely accounted for by increasing geriatric trauma volume at our center and the 6-month transition period in our post-intervention group. Our study also associated GOC documentation with ACP discussions; however, we did not evaluate the comprehensiveness of the ACP discussions, or whether they led to a change in intervention and procedures for geriatric trauma patients. Additional studies would be needed to evaluate if the change in GOC documentation and ACP over the study period altered or improved care. Our study attempted to assess mortality and disposition but did not possess sufficient power to determine any change. Future studies may endeavor to include these changes and assess other clinical outcomes to better evaluate the implementation of their ACP programs.

Conclusion

The provincial advanced care planning program applied to major geriatric trauma patients at our hospital successfully increased GOC documentation from 16 to 35%. Additionally, 21% of patients received had documentation within the first 24 h of their admission versus 11% prior to the project. This demonstrates that ACP programs can improve GOC documentation within the geriatric trauma environment. Additional quality improvement is required to further increase ACP use at our hospital; however, many other programs have shown successful ACP implementation in similar patients and provide various areas for improvement [14–16]. We posit that the most significant factors for ACP improvement using our program will involve additional educational support on the importance of these discussions, the involvement of specialists' adept at these discussions, and leaders to promote effective culture change about ACP at our hospital. While this process can be slow, as demonstrated by others, effective ACP is required for proper patient-centered care for the growing geriatric trauma patient population.

Abbreviations

ACP: Advanced care planning; ACS COT: American College of Surgeons Committee on Trauma; GOC: Goals of care; ICU: Intensive care unit; ISS: Injury Severity Score; PFCC: Patient and family-centered care

Acknowledgements

The authors wish to thank the staff from the Health Records at the University of Alberta Hospital for their assistance and effort towards the collection of patient charts for this project.

Funding

This work was not supported by any funding, and no funding body was involved with the design of the study; collection, analysis, and interpretation of data; or with any writing for this manuscript.

Authors' contributions

KV collected the patient data, drafted the manuscript, and assisted with the editing. PG assessed the data, drafted the manuscript, and assisted with the editing. AT assisted with the data assessment and editing. BM collected the patient data and assisted with the drafting of the manuscript. BT and VF assisted with the project strategy and edited the manuscript. SW initiated the project implementation and strategy and edited the manuscript. All authors have read and approved the final manuscript.

Competing interests

The authors declare that they have no competing interests.

Author details

[1]Faculty of Medicine and Dentistry, University of Alberta, 8440-112 St. Edmonton, Edmonton, Alberta T6G 2B7, Canada. [2]Department of Surgery, 2D4.27 Mackenzie Health Sciences Centre, University of Alberta, 8440-112 St. Edmonton, Edmonton, Alberta T6G 2B7, Canada.

References

1. Canadian Institute for Health Information. Health Care in Canada. A focus on seniors and aging. Ottawa. Ontario: CIHI; 2011. p. 2011.
2. American College of Surgeons Committee on Trauma. ACS TQIP Geriatric Trauma Management Guidelines. https://www.facs.org/~/media/files/.../trauma/tqip/geriatric%20guide%20tqip.ashx. Accessed 1 Jan 2015.
3. Chu I, Vaca F, Stratton S, Chakravarthy B, Hoonpongsimanont W, Lotfipour S. Geriatric trauma care: challenges facing emergency medical services. Cal J Emerg Med. 2007;8:51–5.
4. Perdue PW, Watts DD, Kaufmann CR, Trask AL. Differences in mortality between elderly and younger adult trauma patients: geriatric status increases risk of delayed death. J Trauma-Injury Infec Crit Care. 1998;45:805–10.
5. Gowing R, Jain MK. Injury patterns and outcomes associated with elderly trauma victims in Kingston. Ontario Can J Surg. 2007;50:437–44.
6. Champion HR, Copes WS, Buyer D, Flanagan ME, Bain L, Sacco WJ. Major trauma in geriatric patients. Am J Public Health. 1989;79:1278–82.
7. Leading causes of death, Canada, 2008, males and females combined, counts (age-specific death rate per 100,000) [https://www.canada.ca/en/public-health/services/reports-publications/leading-causes-death-hospitalization-canada/2008-males-females-combined-counts-specific-death-rate.html]. Oct 12th 2017.
8. Brinkman-Stoppelenburg A, Rietjens JA, van der Heide A. The effects of advance care planning on end-of-life care: a systematic review. Palliat Med. 2014;28:1000–25.
9. Gordy S, Klein E. Advance directives in the trauma intensive care unit: do they really matter? Int J Crit Illn Sci. 2011;1:132–7.
10. U.S. Department of Health and Human Services, U.S. Department of Health and Human Services Assistant Secretary for Planning and Evaluation Office of Disability Aging and Long-Term Care Policy, Advance Directive and Advance Care Planning. Washington, D.C: Report to Congress. https://aspe.hhs.gov/system/files/pdf/75811/ADCongRpt.pdf. Accessed 10 Oct 2017.
11. Fagerlin A, Schneider CE. Enough. The failure of the living will. Hast Cent Rep. 2004;34:30–42.
12. Perkins HS. Controlling death: the false promise of advance directives. Ann Intern Med. 2007;147:51–7.
13. Danis M, Southerland LI, Garrett JM, Smith JL, Hielema F, Pickard CG, Egner DM, Patrick DL. A prospective study of advance directives for life-sustaining care. N Engl J Med. 1991;324:882–8.
14. Detering KM, Hancock AD, Reade MC, Silvester W. The impact of advance care planning on end of life care in elderly patients: randomised controlled trial. BMJ. 2010;23:c1345.
15. Hammes BJ, Rooney BL, Gundrum JD. A comparative, retrospective, observational study of the prevalence, availability, and specificity of advance care plans in a county that implemented an advance care planning microsystem. J Am Geriatr Soc. 2010;58:1249–55.
16. Hoffman CB. Passion, persistence, and pennies. In: Rogne LM, Lauraine S, editors. Advance care planning: communicating about matters of life and death. New York: Springer Publishing Company, LLC; 2014.
17. Morrison RS, Morrison EW, Glickman DF. Physician reluctance to discuss advance directives. An empiric investigation of potential barriers. Arch Intern Med. 1994;154:2311–8.
18. Winzelberg GS, Hanson LC, Tulsky JA. Beyond autonomy: diversifying end-of-life decision-making approaches to serve patients and families. J Am Geriatr Soc. 2005;53:1046–50.
19. Prendergast TJ. Advance care planning: pitfalls, progress promise. Crit Care Med. 2001;29:N34–9.
20. Teno J, Lynn J, Wenger N, Phillips RS, Murphy DP, Connors AF, Desbiens N, Fulkerson W, Bellamy P, Knaus WA. Advance directives for seriously ill hospitalized patients: effectiveness with the patient self-determination act and the SUPPORT intervention. SUPPORT investigators. Study to understand prognoses and preferences for outcomes and risks of treatment. J Am Geriatr Soc. 1997;45:500–7.

Outcomes following repair of incarcerated and strangulated ventral hernias with or without synthetic mesh

Sameh Hany Emile*, Hesham Elgendy, Ahmad Sakr, Waleed Ahmed Gado, Ahmed Aly Abdelmawla, Mahmoud Abdelnaby and Alaa Magdy

Abstract

Background: The use of synthetic mesh for ventral hernia repair under contaminated conditions is a controversial issue due to the considerable risk of surgical site infection (SSI). This study aimed to review the outcomes of repair of incarcerated and strangulated ventral hernias with or without synthetic mesh in compliance with established clinical guidelines regarding the incidence of SSI and hernia recurrence.

Methods: The records of patients with complicated ventral hernias who were treated with or without synthetic mesh repair were reviewed. Variables collected included the characteristics of patients and of ventral hernias, type of repair, and incidence of SSI and recurrence.

Results: One hundred twenty-two patients (56 males) of a mean age of 56 years were included. Fifty-two (42.6%) and 70 (57.4%) patients presented with incarcerated and strangulated ventral hernias, respectively. Sixty-six (54%) patients were treated with on-lay mesh repair, and 56 (46%) were managed with suture repair. Twenty-one patients required bowel resection. SSI was detected in eight (6.5%) patients. There was no significant difference between both groups regarding the incidence of SSI (7.5% for mesh group vs 5.3% for suture group). Recurrence occurred in seven patients. Median follow-up period was 24 months. The suture repair group had a significantly higher incidence of recurrence than the mesh group. Diabetes mellitus, previous recurrence, and intestinal resection were significant predictors for SSI.

Conclusion: Following established guidelines, synthetic mesh repair of incarcerated and strangulated ventral hernias attained lower recurrence rate, comparable incidence of SSI, and higher rate of seroma formation than suture repair.

Keywords: Mesh, synthetic, Ventral hernia, Incarcerated, Strangulated, Outcome, infection

Background

Ventral hernias include all hernias arising from a defect in the anterior abdominal wall as epigastric, umbilical, and incisional hernias. Ventral hernias are susceptible for various complications, particularly incarceration and strangulation, that warrant urgent operative intervention which is usually associated with high rates of postoperative recurrence and complications [1].

The diagnosis of incarceration/strangulation on the verdict of clinical examination alone is not an easy task. Strangulation should be recognized in a timely manner as it warrants immediate surgical intervention. Early operative intervention for strangulated hernia is crucial since any delay in the diagnosis can lead to further compromise of the bowel viability and eventually bowel resection. In addition to the risk of anastomotic leak after bowel resection and anastomosis, strangulation increases the contamination of the operative field which subsequently increases the incidence of postoperative surgical site infection (SSI) and hernia recurrence [2].

The World Society for Emergency Surgery (WSES) [2] has issued a grade 1A recommendation for the use of synthetic mesh repair in the cases of incarcerated ventral

* Correspondence: Sameh200@hotmail.com
General surgery department, faculty of Medicine, Mansoura University Hospitals, Elgomhuoria Street, Mansoura city, Egypt

hernia without signs of bowel strangulation or concurrent intestinal resection [3, 4]. On the other hand, owing to the increased likelihood of SSI in the cases of strangulated hernias with concomitant bowel resection [5, 6], synthetic mesh repair should be used with caution in these circumstances (grade 2C recommendation).

The use of prosthetic mesh in potentially-contaminated and contaminated settings is not frequently described in the literature. Despite the wide variations of data and the conflicting reports, prosthetic materials are not generally recommended for the repair of ventral hernias in contaminated settings. Choi and colleagues [7] used the records of the National Surgical Quality Improvement Program of the United States and evaluated the prosthetic repair of strangulated ventral hernia for more than 33,000 patients in clean-contaminated and contaminated settings. The authors reported that clean-contaminated cases had a significantly higher incidence of wound disruption, and superficial, and deep SSIs along with significantly increased odds for complications overall.

Xourafas et al. [8] evaluated the feasibility of using a synthetic mesh in ventral hernia repair with simultaneous bowel resection. The authors found a significantly higher incidence of postoperative SSI in patients treated with prosthetic mesh compared to those treated without mesh (22 vs 5%).

The present study aimed to review the outcomes following the repair of incarcerated and strangulated ventral hernias with or without synthetic mesh in compliance with the established clinical guidelines of WSES in terms of the incidence of SSI and recurrence of hernia postoperatively.

Methods

Study design and setting

Prospectively collected data of consecutive patients with incarcerated or strangulated ventral hernia who were treated with or without synthetic mesh were reviewed. The study took place at the general surgery departments of Mansoura University principal hospital and Emergency hospital. Data collection involved patients treated between January 2014 and June 2016.

Ethical approval for the study was obtained from the institutional review board of Mansoura Faculty of medicine. The study was registered on www.researchregistry.com under the unique identifying number (UIN): *researchregistry1891.*

Eligibility criteria

Adult patients of both genders who presented with incarcerated or strangulated ventral hernia were included. Ventral hernias comprised all hernias arising from a defect in the anterior abdominal wall including umbilical, epigastric, incisional, and Spigelian hernias. Patients who underwent resection of gangrenous bowel and anastomosis were also included.

We excluded patients with other types of hernia other than ventral hernias, patients who underwent elective hernia repair after manual reduction of irreducible hernia, patients who underwent bowel resection with stoma formation, patients with incarcerated or strangulated omentum only without bowel involvement, and patients with associated necrotizing fasciitis of the anterior abdominal wall. Patients with incomplete records were also excluded.

Definition of procedures and outcomes

Incarcerated ventral hernia was defined as irreducible hernia associated with symptoms of bowel obstruction, yet with no compromise of the blood supply of the bowel. Strangulated hernia presented with partial or complete interruption of the blood supply of the intestine. After application of hot fomentation to the doubtful bowel loop, it was considered either viable and returned to the peritoneal cavity or non-viable and resection with anastomosis of the bowel ends was conducted.

Incisional hernias were defined as hernias occurring at the site of abdominal incision performed for procedures other than hernia repair. Recurrent hernias are the hernias occurring at the site of incision made for previous hernia repair. According to the Center for Disease Control and Prevention (CDC) surgical wound classification [9], incarcerated hernias were considered as class I (clean), strangulated hernias without bowel resection as class II (clean contaminated), and strangulated hernias with simultaneous bowel resection as class III (contaminated).

Anesthetic fitness of patients, especially those with associated comorbidities (diabetes mellitus, hepatic disease, hypertension, etc.), was classified according to the American Society of Anesthesiologists (ASA) score into class I to class V. Perioperative antibiotics (2 g of third generation cephalosporines) were administered to patients in both groups in accordance with Surgical Care Improvement Project protocol. The bio-burden reduction technique was followed by careful debridement of all non-viable tissues and removal of mesh in the cases of complicated recurrent hernias after prior mesh repair. The surgical field was thoroughly irrigated with gentamycin-saline solution. Upon completion of repair, subcutaneous drains were routinely placed above the mesh in all patients per hospital protocol and were removed when their drainage was less than 30 cc per day.

Prosthetic mesh repair was performed by approximation of the edges of the abdominal wall defect using continuous running polyprolene 0 sutures then the abdominal wall was reinforced by using a synthetic polyprolene 15 × 15 cm or 30 × 30 cm mesh (Prolene® mesh, Ethicon, Johnson-Johnson Inc. Langhorne, PA, USA) according to the size of the defect. The on-lay technique of mesh repair was used in all patients. Non-mesh suture repair was performed either by direct approximation of the edges of the abdominal wall defect (simple primary repair) or by overlapping the abdominal wall fascia (Mayo's repair).

The decision on the technique of repair was made by the attending staff surgeon in accordance with the WSES guidelines [2] and depending on the degree of contamination of the surgical field and the general condition of the patients. Patients were primarily offered mesh repair unless they were hemodynamically unstable or had significant comorbidities (i.e., ASA III or higher) warranting a quick intervention such as suture repair. In addition, if patients had significant gross contamination of the surgical field (i.e., spillage of intestinal content, CDC class III) rendering the application of synthetic mesh risky, then suture repair was performed.

Follow-up was conducted at the outpatient clinic by a surgical resident to eliminate risk of investigator bias, and then by one of the operating consultants at 1 week, two weeks, one, six, and 12 months postoperatively then every six months after the first year. Surgical site occurrence (SSO) was defined as SSI, cellulitis, necrosis, chronic and/or non-healing wound, serous or purulent drainage, seroma, hematoma, wound dehiscence, or fistula at the surgical site [10]. SSI was defined according to the standard criteria devised by CDC [9]. Recurrence was defined as the re-appearance of the ventral hernia at the site of previous repair as detected by clinical examination during follow-up.

Data collection

The records of the patients were searched for the following data: patients' characteristics as age, sex, ASA grade, and associated comorbidities, type of ventral hernia and type of emergent presentation (incarceration or strangulation), operation performed and whether intestinal resection was done or not, operation time, incidence of SSO, SSI, and recurrence of hernia. The primary outcome of the study was the incidence of postoperative SSI. Secondary end points included the incidence of hernia recurrence after the procedure, SSO, and other postoperative complications.

Statistical analysis

Excel program and SPSS (Statistical Package for Social Science) version 21 under Microsoft Windows were used to analyze the data. The data was described in the form of mean ± standard deviation (SD) for quantitative data, while frequency and proportion were used to describe qualitative data. Student *t* test was used to compare the quantitative data of the two groups. Fisher's exact test and Chi square test were used for the analysis of qualitative variables. Multivariate analysis of the risk factors for SSI was performed using the binary logistic regression test. *P* value less than 0.05 was considered significant. Post-hoc analysis of the incidence of recurrence of ventral hernia in both groups (0 vs 12.5%) revealed a study power of 83% with alpha set at 0.05.

Results

Patients' characteristics

Among 145 patients with complicated ventral hernias who were treated within the study period, 122 patients fit the eligibility criteria and were included. Patients were 56 (46%) males and 66 (54%) females. The mean age of patients was 56 ± 10.3 (range, 21–82) years. Ninety-seven (79.5%) patients had associated comorbid conditions: 30 (24.6%) had diabetes mellitus (D.M), 33 (27%) had chronic liver disease (CLD), and 34 (27.8%) had cardiac problems. Eleven (9%) patients had more than one comorbidity. Ninety-nine (81.1%) patients had ASA grade of I-II, whereas 23 (18.9%) patients had ASA grade III-IV. Both groups had comparable demographic data (Table 1).

Characteristics of ventral hernia

One hundred and three (84.4%) hernias were umbilical, six (5%) were epigastric, ten (8.1%) were incisional, and

Table 1 Characteristics of patients in both groups

Variable	Mesh repair	Suture repair	Total	*P* value
Number	66	56	122	–
Mean age ± SD (range)	54.6 ± 10.2 (33–82)	57.6 ± 10.4 (21–80)	–	0.11
Male/female	34/32	22/34	56/66	0.24
ASA grade I–II (%)	54 (81.8)	45 (80.3)	99 (81.1)	0.83
ASA grade III–IV (%)	12 (18.1)	11 (19.6)	23 (18.9)	0.83
Diabetes mellitus (%)	16 (24.2)	14 (25)	30 (24.6)	0.92
Hepatic disease (%)	19 (28.7)	14 (25)	33 (27)	0.68
Cardiac disease (%)	19 (28.7)	15 (26.7)	34 (27.8)	0.96
More than 1 comorbidity (%)	7 (10.6)	4 (7.1)	11 (9)	0.54

three (2.4%) were Spigelian. Thirteen patients (10.6%) had a recurrent umbilical hernia after previous operations (four previous mesh repairs and nine suture repairs). The median size of hernia defect was 7 (range, 5–14) cm.

Fifty-two (42.6%) and 70 (57.4%) patients presented with incarcerated and strangulated ventral hernias, respectively. No significant differences were noted between the two groups regarding the characteristics of ventral hernias as illustrated in Table 2.

Treatment and outcomes

Sixty-six (54%) patients were treated with prosthetic mesh repair, and 56 (46%) were managed with suture repair (simple primary repair in 39 and Mayo's repair in 17 patients). Mesh repair was done in 31 (60.7%) of 52 incarcerated hernias and 35 (50%) of 70 strangulated hernias (Table 3, Fig. 1).

Twenty-one (17.2%) patients underwent resection of gangrenous bowel with anastomosis of the bowel ends. Two (9.5%) of those 21 patients were treated with mesh hernioplasty and 19 (90.5%) were treated with suture repair.

The suture group had a significantly higher rate of contaminated (CDC class III) wounds. Overall, there were 52 (42.6%) class I wounds, 49 (40.1%) class II wounds, and 21 (17.2%) class III wounds. Contents of the incarcerated and strangulated hernia comprised small bowel alone ($n = 88$), small bowel and omentum ($n = 12$), large bowel alone ($n = 8$), large bowel and omentum ($n = 14$).

SSO was detected in 34 (27.8%) patients including SSI ($n = 8$), seroma ($n = 19$), hematoma ($n = 4$), and wound dehiscence ($n = 3$). The mesh hernioplasty group had significantly ($p = 0.038$) higher rate of SSO overall, particularly seroma formation, than the suture group.

SSI in the form of superficial incisional infection was detected in eight (6.55%) patients, seven of them presented with strangulated ventral hernia and one with incarcerated hernia, three (5.3%) of which were in the non-mesh group and five (7.5%) were in the mesh group. Patients who developed SSI were treated conservatively on outpatient basis with antibiotics for 7–14 days according to the culture results and drainage if necessary. Only one patient in the mesh group was re-admitted for 3 days to have his mesh surgically removed owing to resistant SSI unresponsive to conservative treatment. All cases of SSI were detected within 30 days after surgical repair; there were no cases of latent mesh infection on further follow-up for at least 12 months.

There was no significant difference ($p = 0.72$) between both groups regarding the overall incidence of SSI (7.5% [95%CI: 2.9–16.9%] for the mesh group vs 5.3% [95%CI: 1.2–15.1%] for the suture group). Similarly, on subgroup analysis, no significant differences in the rates of SSI were observed between mesh and suture repairs in the cases of incarcerated hernias ($p = 1$) and strangulated hernias ($p = 1$).

Seven (5.7%) patients developed recurrence of ventral hernia within a period ranging from 6–18 months after repair, all recurrences were in the suture repair group. The suture repair group had a significantly ($p = 0.003$) higher incidence of recurrence than the mesh group (Table 3).

The median duration of follow-up was 24 months (range, 6–32 months). Ninety-two (75.4%) patients were followed for more than 18 months, 21 (17.3%) were followed for 12-18 months, and nine (7.3%) were followed for less than 12 months.

Risk factors for SSI

Univariate analysis (Table 4) of the risk factors for SSI after surgical repair revealed that D.M ($p = 0.02$),

Table 2 Characteristics of ventral hernia in both groups

Variable		Mesh repair ($n = 66$)	Suture repair ($n = 56$)	Total ($n = 122$)	*P* value
Primary/recurrent hernia		58/8	51/5	109/13	0.78
Anatomic location	Umbilical (%)	57 (86.3)	46 (82.1)	103 (84.4)	0.69
	Epigastric (%)	4 (6)	2 (3.57)	6 (5)	0.68
	Spigelian (%)	1 (1.5)	2 (3.57)	3 (2.4)	0.59
	Incisional (%)	4 (6)	6 (10.7)	10 (8.1)	0.51
Incarcerated hernia (%)		31 (47)	21 (37.5)	52 (42.6)	0.38
Strangulated hernia (%)		35 (53)	35 (62.5)	70 (57.4)	0.38
CDC wound classification	Class I	31 (47)	21 (37.5)	52 (42.6)	*0.00003*
	Class II	33 (50)	16 (28.5)	49 (40.1)	
	Class III	2 (3)	19 (34)	21 (17.2)	

CDC center for disease control
The italicized figures indicate a signficant *p*-value less than 0.05

Table 3 Outcome of surgical treatment in both groups

Variable		Mesh repair ($n = 66$)	Suture repair ($n = 56$)	Total ($n = 122$)	P value
Median operation time in minutes (range)		88 (70–120)	68 (46–128)	77 (46–128)	–
Resection anastomosis (%)		2 (3)	19 (34)	21 (17.2)	*<0.0001*
SSO (%)	SSI (%)	5 (7.5)	3 (5.3)	8 (6.5)	0.72
	Seroma (%)	15 (22.7)	4 (7.1)	19 (15.5)	*0.02*
	Hematoma (%)	3 (4.5)	1 (1.7)	4 (3.2)	0.62
	Wound dehiscence (%)	1 (1.5)	2 (3.5)	3 (2.4)	0.59
	Total (%)	24 (36.3)	10 (17.8)	34 (27.8)	*0.038*
SSI (%)	In incarcerated hernia	1/31 (3.2)	0/21 (0)	1/52 (1.9)	1
	In strangulated hernia	4/35 (11.5)	3/35 (8.5)	7/70 (10)	1
Recurrence (%)		0	7 (12.5)	7 (5.7)	*0.003*
Median follow-up in months (range)		24 (6–32)	22 (6–30)	–	–

SSI surgical site infection, *SSO* surgical site occurrence
The italicized figures indicate a signficant *p*-value less than 0.05

previous recurrence ($p = 0.04$), and intestinal resection ($p = 0.03$) were the significant predictors for SSI. All previously recurrent hernias that developed SSI had prior mesh repair. Four of 21 patients who had resection of gangrenous bowel with re-anastomosis developed SSI, two of which had mesh repair and another two had suture repair.

Binary logistic regression analysis revealed the most significant risk factors for SSI included D.M (OR = 11.2, $p = 0.004$), previous recurrence (OR = 6.2, $p = 0.02$), and intestinal resection with CDC class III wound (OR = 5.7, $p = 0.02$).

Patients' age, gender, and ASA grade; type of ventral hernia; type of emergent presentation; and type of repair

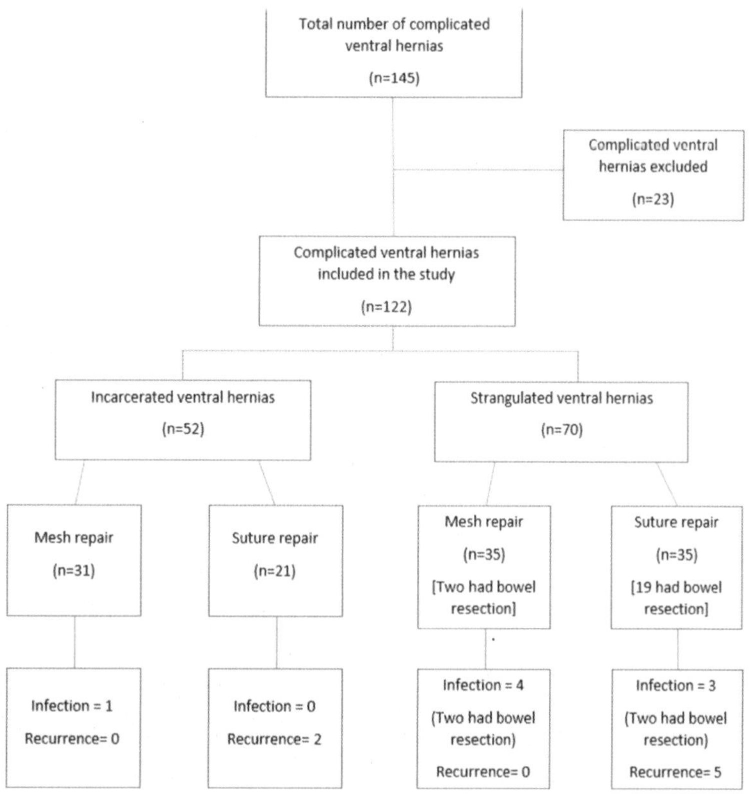

Fig. 1 Flow diagram illustarting the treatment and outcomes of patients with complicated ventral hernias

Table 4 Univariate and multivariate analysis of the risk factors for SSI

Variable	Infection ($n = 8$)	No infection ($n = 114$)	Univariate analysis	Multivariate analysis		
			P value	Odds ratio	95% CI	*P* value
Mean age ± SD	56.2 ± 5.8	56 ± 10.6	0.96	–	–	–
Male patient (%)	3 (37.5)	53 (46.5)	0.72	–	–	–
Female patient (%)	5 (62.5)	61 (53.5)	0.72	–	–	–
Diabetes mellitus (%)	6 (75)	24 (21)	*0.002*	11.2	2.13–59.31	*0.004*
Hepatic disease (%)	3 (37.5)	30 (26.3)	0.44	–	–	–
More than 1 comorbidity (%)	2 (25)	9 (7.9)	0.15	–	–	–
ASA grade III–IV (%)	1 (12.5)	22 (19.3)	1	–	–	–
Previous recurrence (%)	3 (37.5)	10 (8.8)	*0.04*	6.24	1.29–30	*0.02*
Umbilical hernia (%)	7 (87.5)	96 (84.2)	1	–	–	–
Incisional hernia (%)	1 (12.5)	9 (7.9)	0.5	–	–	–
Strangulation (%)	7 (87.5)	63 (55.2)	0.13	–	–	–
CDC class III wound	4 (50)	17 (14.9)	*0.03*	5.7	1.3–25.03	*0.02*
Resection anastomosis (%)	4 (50)	17 (14.9)	*0.03*	5.7	1.3–25.03	*0.02*
Mesh repair	5 (62.5)	61 (53.5)	0.72	–	–	–
Suture repair	3 (37.5)	53 (46.5)	0.72	–	–	–

The italicized figures indicate a signficant *p*-value less than 0.05

were not significant risk factors for the development of SSI postoperatively.

Discussion

The debate on the optimal management of complicated ventral hernias continues. The use of prosthetic mesh has been considered the standard treatment for elective ventral hernia repair since simple repair with sutures is associated with significantly higher rates of recurrence of hernia that can reach up to 67% on long term follow-up [11, 12]. On another hand, the emergency management of complicated ventral hernias can be more cumbersome owing to the potential contamination of the operative field which can preclude the use of synthetic mesh. Alternatives to synthetic mesh, as bioprosthesis and biosynthetic mesh, appeared to solve the problem; nevertheless, these alternatives are not readily available everywhere because of their cost. This leaves the surgeon on the horns of a dilemma that entails higher risk for SSI when synthetic mesh is used and higher incidence of recurrence when the mesh is abandoned.

The WSES [2] has issued a useful set of recommendations for the emergency repair of complicated ventral hernias including a grade A1 recommendation for the use of synthetic mesh for incarcerated hernias, grade 2C recommendation for the use of synthetic mesh with caution in strangulated hernias with or without concurrent bowel resection, and grade 2C recommendation for using biologic mesh instead of synthetic mesh in the cases of acute strangulation with bowel perforation.

We employed the WSES clinical guidelines for emergency ventral hernia repair on 122 patients and examined the outcome of synthetic mesh repair versus suture repair performed in accordance with the guidelines. Patients included were adults of a mean age of 56 years close to the mean age of paraumbilical hernia reported by Bedewi et al. [13]. The majority of the patients had at least one associated comorbidity, yet less than 20% of them had high ASA grade. Umbilical hernias represented around 85% of the ventral hernias included in the study, in accord with Aguirre and colleagues [14] defined this type as the most common type of ventral hernia.

Both groups (suture and mesh repair) had comparable patients' demographics and hernia characteristics which can minimize the inherent risk of selection bias associated with retrospective studies. Although according to WSES guidelines, incarcerated hernias are recommended to be managed with synthetic mesh repair invariably, only 60% of these patients were treated with mesh repair in our study. The reason for this can be the overall general condition and associated comorbidities of the patients that called for a rapid maneuver such as simple suture repair. On the other hand, only half of the patients with strangulation and around 10% of the patients with concomitant bowel resection underwent mesh repair which is in line with the WSES recommendations to use synthetic mesh cautiously in these potentially contaminated conditions.

Although mesh hernioplasty had higher incidence of SSO overall, there was no significant difference in the incidence of SSI between mesh repair and suture repair. The overall 30-day SSI after mesh repair in our series was 7.5% ranging between 3% for incarcerated hernias and 11.5% for strangulated hernias. The rates of SSI after prosthetic repair of strangulated hernias are generally higher than those of incarcerated hernia which can be attributed to the ischemia of the bowel wall that predisposes to bacterial translocation, as well as the risk of bowel resection that can further increase the contamination of the surgical field. That is why the operative field in the cases of strangulated hernias was classified as clean-contaminated or contaminated [2].

A randomized controlled trial [15] found prosthetic repair of incarcerated umbilical hernias a safe option with lower recurrence rates than suture repair. Similarly, other retrospective studies [16–18] concluded that synthetic mesh repair was not associated with higher risk of SSI in the treatment of complicated ventral and groin hernias. Unlike the present study, the study by Bessa and Abdel-Razek [17] lacked the presence of a control group (suture repair) to compare the outcomes with.

The incidence of SSI in the present series was comparable to that disclosed by Nieuwenhuizen et al. [18], slightly higher than the incidence (6%) reported by Abd Ellatif and colleagues [19], yet much lower than the rate of SSI (14%) Carbonell and colleagues [20] reported after the application of synthetic mesh in contaminated ventral hernia repair. Nonetheless, since causes of contamination in Carbonell's series were quite variable including infected previous mesh, violation of the gastrointestinal tract, and ostomy creation or reversal along other causes whereas contamination in our series was caused by bowel strangulation only; the higher rate of SSI in their study can be explained. We excluded patients with stoma from the present report since the management of stoma in conjunction with ventral hernia is likely to be coupled with serious morbidities as Carbonell et al. have acknowledged.

The relatively low incidence of SSI after synthetic mesh repair in the current study can be attributed to the combined application of clinical guidelines along with the use of good clinical judgment. As a general rule, following guidelines and applying evidence-based medicine can serve to achieve better outcomes in the surgical practice. The incidence of SSI after prosthetic mesh repair of complicated ventral hernias can be further reduced by employing different techniques of mesh placement (i.e., retrorectus mesh) and negative pressure wound therapy.

Despite the low rates of SSI in our report, chronic infection after the use of synthetic mesh under contaminated conditions remains one of the most concerning consequences. Chronic infection can compromise the wound healing resulting in chronic draining sinuses. Additionally, involvement of the underlying abdominal viscera can sometimes result in enterocutaneous fistulas. Furthermore, re-admission and reoperation for the management of mesh-related infection, including mesh extraction, are linked with added morbidities to the patient and higher treatment-related costs.

Another controversial issue is the feasibility of synthetic mesh repair when bowel resection is being conducted in the same setting. Less than 10% of patients with bowel resection in our study were treated with a synthetic mesh. We found bowel resection and anastomosis to be a significant independent risk factor for SSI whether a mesh was used or not. Four of 21 patients with bowel resection developed SSI, attaining a rate of 19% close to the incidence (22%) reported by Xourafas and colleagues [8] when simultaneous intestinal resection took place with synthetic mesh repair of ventral hernia. Bowel resection with possibility of spillage of intestinal content into the operative field renders the field a class III, contaminated surgical wound. The use of synthetic mesh in such a contaminated setting should be employed with caution as per the WSES guidelines.

Conversely, other investigators found the use of synthetic mesh to be acceptable with bowel resection. Geisler and affiliates [21] examined the safety of non-absorbable mesh repair in the presence of open bowel and reported a wound-related morbidity rate of 7%. Campanelli et al [22] recommended prosthetic repair to be used in all cases of abdominal wall hernia even in potentially contaminated fields; nevertheless, since the authors operated on only ten patients, the outcome of their study should be interpreted with caution. Other studies [17, 19] came to a conclusion that intestinal resection should not be considered a contraindication to the use of synthetic mesh.

In addition to bowel resection, D.M and previous hernia surgery were recognized as significant predictors for SSI. D.M has been known to be associated with higher rates of infection after mesh repair of hernia [23] since it reduces the T cell response and neutrophil function and causes disorders of humoral immunity [24]. Previous surgeries for ventral hernias, especially when involving the use of prosthetic mesh, may render the repeat procedure technically demanding with difficult dissection, longer operation time, and increased risk of inadvertent bowel injury during dissection of the adhesions. Moreover, if the recurrence of hernia was associated with surgical site infection, further procedures for the treatment of recurrent hernia can have higher likelihood of SSI.

Although on-lay mesh hernioplasty was reported to have higher rates of recurrence and SSI than the sub-lay technique [25], we found the on-lay repair confers satisfactory results with no recorded cases of hernia recurrence and a rate of SSI comparable to those recorded after the sub-lay technique which ranged from 0–14.4%. We opt for employing the on-lay technique of repair as it appeared technically easier and faster to perform in the setting of emergency treatment of complicated ventral hernia, unlike the sub-lay technique that can be more technically demanding, time consuming, and requires better experience. Moreover, we thought that if SSI occurred, the removal of on-lay mesh would be technically easier and safer than the removal of a deeply-placed retromuscular mesh. Nevertheless, we think if the mesh was placed in retro-rectus position, better results could have been obtained with lower rates of SSO and SSI.

Reviewing the current literature, two opposite perspectives can be noted; the first discourages the use of mesh repair for ventral hernias at any level of contamination [7], and the second recommends using mesh repair even with evident contamination as in the cases of concomitant bowel resection [17, 19]. Based on the outcomes of the present study, we would choose a compromise between the two extremes. Since prosthetic mesh repair attained significantly lower incidence of recurrence of hernia than suture repair without significantly increasing the rates of SSI, we recommend the use of synthetic mesh hernioplasty for complicated ventral hernias, with exception of diabetic patients, previously recurrent hernias, and when bowel resection is to be simultaneously conducted.

Even with bowel resection, patients should not be denied the option of reinforcing the abdominal wall with mesh to minimize the likelihood of recurrence. Some options were devised in this context as the retro-rectus positioning of the polyprolene mesh. Proper preparation, washing, and accurate drainage of the preperitoneal space in addition to perfect hemostasis and local antibiotic treatment are crucial to guarantee the success of this method [22].

The use of bioprosthesis has been proposed as a safe and efficient approach for abdominal wall reconstruction under contaminated conditions, yet the long term durability of biologic mesh has not been verified [26]. Other alternatives include the use of long-term absorbable synthetic materials or the biosynthetic meshes. The use of biosynthetic (GORE BIO-A) has been evaluated in The Complex Open Bioabsorbable Reconstruction of the Abdominal Wall (COBRA) study [27] which concluded the efficacy of biosynthetic prosthesis in terms of long-term recurrence and life quality with a SSI of around 18%.

Limitations to the present study include being a single-institution, retrospective study, the small number of patients who had bowel resection, and the lack of some essential parameters as the body mass index, cigarette smoking, and steroid use that may have an impact on the incidence of SSI after the treatment of complicated ventral hernias. Furthermore, the technique of prosthetic repair used (on-lay mesh) is not widely used which may limit the generalizability of the study. Finally, the non-randomized nature of the study and the selection of patients for each treatment group according to the established guidelines and clinical judgment may have been the cause of the better outcomes reported, rather than the type of repair per se.

Conclusion

Following the WSES clinical guidelines in conjunction with good clinical judgment, synthetic mesh repair of incarcerated and strangulated ventral hernias achieved lower recurrence rate than suture repair. Although mesh hernioplasty was followed by a higher incidence of SSO and seroma formation, the incidence of SSI was comparable in both groups.

Bowel resection, D.M, and previously recurrent ventral hernias were the significant independent risk factors for SSI after repair of complicated ventral hernias. Well-powered randomized trials are needed to reach a strong conclusion about the safety of synthetic mesh when simultaneous bowel resection is conducted; until then, synthetic mesh should be used with caution in these conditions.

Abbreviations

CDC: Center of disease control; CLD: Chronic liver disease; D.M: Diabetes mellitus; OR: Odds ratio; SSI: Surgical site infection; SSO: Surgical site occurrence

Acknowledgements

Not applicable.

Funding

No funding sources to disclose.

Authors' contributions

SE and HE designed the study and contributed to data collection and analysis and writing of the manuscript. AS, WG, AA, MA participated in data analysis and acquisition, drafting, and revision of the manuscript. AM contributed to data interpretation, writing and critical revision of the manuscript. All authors read and approved the final manuscript.

Competing interests

The authors declare that they have no competing interests.

References

1. Helgstrand F, Rosenberg J, Kehlet H, Bisgaard T. Outcomes after emergency versus elective ventral hernia repair: a prospective nationwide study. World J Surg. 2013;37(10):2273–9. doi:10.1007/s00268-013-2123-5.1.
2. Sartelli M, Coccolini F, Ramshorst G, et al. WSES guidelines for emergency repair of complicated abdominal wall hernias. World J Emerg Surg. 2013;8: 50. doi:10.1186/1749-7922-8-.
3. Luijendijk RW, Hop WC, van den Tol MP. A comparison of suture repair with mesh repair for incisional hernia. N Engl J Med. 2000;343:392. doi:10.1056/ NEJM200008103430603.
4. Korenkov M, Sauerland S, Arndt M, Bograd L, Neugebauer EA: Troidl H Randomized clinical trial of suture repair, polypropylene mesh or autodermal hernioplasty for incisional hernia. Br J Surg. 2002, 89 (1): 50-56. 10.1046/j.0007-1323.2001.01974.x
5. Dunne JR, Malone DL, Tracy JK, Napolitano LM. Abdominal wall hernias: risk factors for infection and resource utilization. J Surg Res. 2003;111(1):78–84. doi:10.1016/S0022-4804(03)00077-5.
6. Finan KR, Vick CC, Kiefe CI, Neumayer L, Hawn MT. Predictors of wound infection in ventral hernia repair. Am J Surg. 2005;190(5):676–81. doi:10. 1016/j.amjsurg.2005.06.041.
7. Choi JJ, Palaniappa NC, Dallas KB, Rudich TB, Colon MJ, Divino CM. Use of mesh during ventral hernia repair in clean-contaminated and contaminated cases: outcomes of 33,832 cases. Ann Surg. 2012;255(1):176–80. doi:10.1097/ SLA.0b013e31822518e6.
8. Xourafas D, Lipsitz S, Negro P. Impact of mesh use on morbidity following ventral hernia repair with a simultaneous bowel resection. Arch Surg. 2010; 145(8):739–44. doi:10.1001/archsurg.2010.144.
9. Health Protection Agency. Surveillance of Surgical Site Infection in England: October 1997–September 2005. London: Health Protection Agency; 2006.
10. Baucom RB, Ousley J, Oyefule OO, Stewart MK, Phillips SE, Browman KK, et al. Evaluation of long-term surgical site occurrences in ventral hernia repair: implications of preoperative site independent MRSA infection. Hernia. 2016; 20(5):701–10. doi:10.1007/s10029-016-1523-5.
11. Malik AM, Jawaid A, Talpur AH, Laghari AA, Khan A. Mesh versus non-mesh repair of ventral abdominal hernias. J Ayub Med Coll Abbottabad. 2008;20(3): 54–56.
12. Burger JWA, Luijendijk RW, Hop WCJ, Halm JA, Verdaasdonk EGG, Jeekel J. Long-term follow-up of a randomized controlled trial of suture versus mesh repair of incisional hernia. Ann Surg. 2004;240(4):578–85. doi:10.1097/01.sla. 0000141193.08524.e7.
13. Bedewi MA, El-Sharkawy MS, Al Boukai AA, Al-Nakshabandi N. Prevalence of adult paraumbilical hernia. Assessment by high-resolution sonography: a hospital-based study. Hernia. 2012;16(1):59–62. doi:10.1007/s10029-011-0863-4.
14. Aguirre DA, Santosa AC, Casola G, Sirlin CB. Abdominal wall hernias: imaging features, complications, and diagnostic pitfalls at multi-detector row CT. Radiographics. 2005;25(6):1501–20.
15. Abdel-Baki NA, Bessa SS, Abdel-Razek AH. Comparison of prosthetic mesh repair and tissue repair in the emergency management of incarcerated para-umbilical hernia: a prospective randomized study. Hernia. 2007;11(2): 163–7.
16. Nieuwenhuizen J, van Ramshorst GH, ten Brinke JG, de Wit T, van der Harst E, Hop WC, Jeekel J, Lange JF. The use of mesh in acute hernia: frequency and outcome in 99 cases. Hernia. 2011;15(3):297–300. doi:10.1007/s10029-010-0779-4.
17. Bessa SS, Abdel-Razek AH. Results of prosthetic mesh repair in the emergency management of the acutely incarcerated and/orstrangulated ventral hernias: a seven years study. Hernia. 2013;17(1):59–65. doi:10.1007/ s10029-012-0938-x.
18. Nieuwenhuizen J, van Ramshorst GH, ten Brinke JG, et al. The use of mesh in acute hernia: frequency and outcome in 99 cases. Hernia. 2011;15(3):297–300. doi:10.1007/s10029-010-0779-4.
19. Abd Ellatif ME, Negm A, Elmorsy G, Al-Katary M, Yousef Ael-A, Ellaithy R. Feasibility of mesh repair for strangulated abdominal wall hernias. Int J Surg. 2012;10(3):153-6. Doi: 10.1016/j.ijsu.2012.02.004. Epub 2012 Feb 16.
20. Carbonell AM, Criss CN, Cobb WS, Novitsky YW, Rosen MJ. Outcomes of synthetic mesh in contaminated ventral hernia repairs. J Am Coll Surg. 2013; 217(6):991–8. doi:10.1016/j.jamcollsurg.2013.07.382. Epub 2013 Sep 14.
21. Geisler DJ, Reilly JC, Vaughan SG, Glennon EJ, Kondylis PD. Safety and outcome of use of nonabsorbable mesh for repair of fascial defects in the presence of open bowel. Dis Colon Rectum. 2003;46:1118–23. doi:10.1007/ s10350-004-7290-x.
22. Campanelli G, Nicolosi FM, Pettinari D, Avesani EC. Prosthetic repair, intestinal resection, and potentially contaminated areas: safe and feasible? Hernia. 2004;8:190–2.
23. Falagas ME, Kasiakou SK. Mesh-related infections after hernia repair surgery. Clin Microbiol Infect. 2005;11:3–8. doi:10.1111/j.1469-0691.2004.01014.x.
24. Casqueiro J, Casqueiro J, Alves C. Infections in patients with diabetes mellitus: a review of pathogenesis. Indian J Endocrinol Metab. 2012; 16(Suppl1):S27–36. doi:10.4103/2230-8210.94253.
25. Holihan JL, Nguyen DH, Nguyen MT, Mo J, Kao LS, Liang MK. Mesh location in open ventral hernia repair: a systematic review and network meta-analysis. World J Surg. 2016;40(1):89–99. doi:10.1007/s00268-015-3252-9.
26. Smart NJ, Marshall M, Daniels IR. Biological meshes: a review of their use in abdominal wall hernia repairs. Surgeon. 2012;10(3):159–71. doi:10.1016/j. surge.2012.02.006.
27. Rosen MJ, Bauer JJ, Harmaty M, Carbonell AM, Cobb WS, Matthews B, et al. Multicenter, prospective, longitudinal study of the recurrence, surgical site infection, and quality of life after contaminated ventral hernia repair using biosynthetic absorbable mesh: the COBRA study. Ann Surg. 2017;265(1): 205–11. doi:10.1097/SLA.0000000000001601.

Laparoscopic cholecystectomy for acute calculous cholecystitis: a retrospective study assessing risk factors for conversion and complications

Petra Maria Terho[1], Ari Kalevi Leppäniemi[2] and Panu Juhani Mentula[2*]

Abstract

Background: The purpose of the study was to identify risk factors for conversion of laparoscopic cholecystectomy and risk factors for postoperative complications in acute calculous cholecystitis. The most common complications arising from cholecystectomy were also to be identified.

Methods: A total of 499 consecutive patients, who had undergone emergent cholecystectomy with diagnosis of cholecystitis in Meilahti Hospital in 2013–2014, were identified from the hospital database. Of the identified patients, 400 had acute calculous cholecystitis of which 27 patients with surgery initiated as open cholecystectomy were excluded, resulting in 373 patients for the final analysis. The Clavien-Dindo classification of surgical complications was used.

Results: Laparoscopic cholecystectomy was initiated in 373 patients of which 84 (22.5%) were converted to open surgery. Multivariate logistic regression identified C-reactive protein (CRP) over 150 mg/l, age over 65 years, diabetes, gangrene of the gallbladder and an abscess as risk factors for conversion. Complications were experienced by 67 (18.0%) patients. Multivariate logistic regression identified age over 65 years, male gender, impaired renal function and conversion as risk factors for complications.

Conclusions: Advanced cholecystitis with high CRP, gangrene or an abscess increase the risk of conversion. The risk of postoperative complications is higher after conversion. Early identification and treatment of acute calculous cholecystitis might reduce the number of patients with advanced cholecystitis and thus improve outcomes.

Keywords: Acute cholecystitis, Laparoscopic cholecystectomy, Open cholecystectomy, Conversion

Background

Laparoscopic cholecystectomy (LC) is the standard treatment for acute cholecystitis [1, 2]. LC has been linked to a lower complication rate and shorter postoperative hospital stay compared with open cholecystectomy (OC) [3, 4]. Performing early cholecystectomy on patients admitted for acute cholecystitis is preferable to postponing the operation to be performed when the acute phase is over, since an early procedure has been recognized to shorten postoperative hospital stay and lower hospital care expenses [5, 6].

Gallbladder disease is among the leading causes for hospital admission for acute abdomen among adults and the most common indication for abdominal surgery in the elderly [7, 8]. In situations when LC is unsafe the surgeon might have to convert to an open procedure. The risk of conversion is higher in LC for acute cholecystitis than it is in an elective procedure [9]. The risk of conversion for patients undergoing LC for acute cholecystitis has been linked to male gender, age, previous endoscopic retrograde cholangiopancreatography (ERCP), a non-palpable gallbladder, elevated C-reactive protein (CRP) and white blood cell count (WBCC), gangrenous inflammation and the

* Correspondence: panu.mentula@hus.fi
[2]Department of Abdominal Surgery, Helsinki University Central Hospital, P.O.Box 340, 00029 HUS Helsinki, Finland
Full list of author information is available at the end of the article

experience of the operating surgeon [10–13]. Conservative treatment with antibiotics and delaying the procedure to be performed after the acute phase has shown no change in conversion and complication rates [5, 14]. Patients who have had to undergo conversion have had more complications, which have led to further operations and a longer postoperative hospital stay [10].

Accounting for risk factors for conversion and complications is important when planning the procedure and deciding on whom to assign to perform the cholecystectomy. Experienced surgeons have been shown to have a lower complication rate for LC compared with surgeons in training [11]. Informing the patient about the procedure and the risk of complications is likewise important.

The aim of this study was to identify risk factors associated with conversion in patients with acute calculous cholecystitis. The risk factors for postoperative complications and the most common complications were also to be identified.

Methods

Patients and data collection

The study was a retrospective analysis of consecutive patients who had undergone emergent cholecystectomy in Meilahti Hospital, a university teaching hospital, from January 2013 till December 2014. A total of 499 patients were identified from the operating room database by procedure codes for LC and OC and International Classification of Diseases codes for acute cholecystitis. Fifty-four patients were excluded due to acalculous cholecystitis, and 33 due to missing signs of acute inflammation on the removed gallbladder described by the operating surgeon. Nine excluded patients received cholecystectomy during the treatment of another disease that required hospital care and three patients were excluded due to gallbladder malignancy. Twenty-seven patients received OC and were excluded. The remaining 373 patients with acute calculous cholecystitis were included into analysis. Acute calculous cholecystitis was defined as stones visible on preoperative imaging or during gallbladder removal and signs of acute cholecystitis described by the surgeon during the operation.

The preoperative diagnosis of acute cholecystitis had been reached by clinical assessment (tenderness in right upper quadrant, Murphy's sign, fever), laboratory findings (elevated CRP and WBCC) and radiological signs of acute cholecystitis on imaging (thickened gallbladder wall, stones, enlarged gallbladder, edema, abscess).

More than 70 variables concerning personal data, clinical, laboratory, radiographic and intraoperative findings, the procedure and possible complications were collected directly or manually from the patient records. Complications were rated according to the Clavien-Dindo classification and the comprehensive complication index was calculated [15]. It was also specified what the complications were and how they were treated. Appropriate permissions to conduct the study were obtained from the hospital review board.

Statistical analysis

The analysis of the data was conducted by SPSS Statistics v.22 for Mac OS X (IBM, Armonk, NY). Proportions were reported for categorical variables. Median, interquartile range and range was reported for continuous variables. P value was obtained using either Chi-square test or Fischer's exact test for categorical variables and Mann-Whitney U test for continuous variables. Continuous variables used for multivariate analysis (CRP, WBCC, age, duration of surgery) were made categorical using cut off values determined from receiver operating characteristic (ROC) curves (Additional files 1: Figures S1, Additional files 2: Figures S2, Additional files 3: Figures S3 and Additional files 4: Figures S4). Optimal cut off values were defined as the values showing the highest sum of sensitivity and specificity on the ROC curves. Variables with a P value of <0.05 were considered statistically significant and were considered for inclusion in the multivariate analysis. A stepwise forward conditional approach of binary logistic regression was used to identify both risk factors for conversion and complications at a 0.05 significance level.

Results

LC was initiated in 373 patients of which 84 (22.5%) were converted. Ultrasound ($n = 301$, 80.7%) was the main choice of imaging in patients with clinical suspicion of acute cholecystitis. Computed tomography ($n - 127$, 34.0% was mainly used in patients who presented with severe or diffuse symptoms, and magnetic resonance imaging ($n = 93$, 24.9%) was mainly used in patients with suspicion of bile duct stones in addition to cholecystitis. There were signs of acute calculous cholecystitis on imaging in 314 patients (84.2%) and of acute cholecystitis without radiologically visible stones in 46 patients (12.3%). Gallstones without signs of inflammation were visible in 12 patients (3.2%), and one patient did not undergo any preoperative imaging since the patient was in line for an elective cholecystectomy due to symptomatic gallstones and there was a strong suspicion of acute cholecystitis based on clinical and laboratory findings. On histopathological examination acute cholecystitis was found in 181 (48.5%), gangrenous cholecystitis in 98 (26.3%), acute on chronic cholecystitis in 48 (12.9%) and chronic cholecystitis in 46 (12.3%) patients.

Conversion

Univariate analysis was performed in order to identify risk factors for conversion (Table 1). A multivariate analysis was conducted separately for preoperative risk factors only

Table 1 Univariate analysis of risk factors for conversion

	Conversion (n = 84 22.5 %)[a]	LC (n = 289)	Total (n = 373)	OR (95% CI)	P
Gender; Male	48 (25.4%)	141 (48.8%)	189 (50.7%)	1.4 (0.9–2.3)	0.178
Age in years, median (range)	70 (30–92)	61 (20–94)	63(20–94)	NA	<0.001
Heart failure	7 (29.2%)	17 (5.9%)	24 (6.4%)	1.5 (0.6–3.6)	0.420
Impaired renal function	2 (18.2%)	9 (3.1%)	11 (2.9%)	0.8 (0.2–3.6)	1.000
Diabetes	23 (33.8%)	45 (15.6%)	68 (18.2%)	2.0 (1.2–3.6)	0.014
Previous laparotomy on the upper abdomen	8 (40.0%)	12 (4.2%)	20 (5.4%)	2.4 (1.0–6.2)	0.054
Previous laparotomy on the lower abdomen[b]	21 (23.9%)	67 (24.3%)	88 (24.6%)	1.1 (0.6–1.9)	0.805
Previous laparoscopic surgery on the abdomen[b]	7 (29.2%)	17 (6.2%)	24 (6.7%)	1.4 (0.6–3.6)	0.450
No previous surgeries	52 (21.3%)	192 (66.4%)	244 (65.4%)	0.8 (0.5–1.4)	0.442
Duration of symptoms before admission[c]					
< 24 h	18 (14.4%)	106 (40.2%)	124 (36.9%)	0.5 (0.3–0.9)	0.018
24 h – 48 h	13 (27.1%)	35 (13.3%)	48 (14.3%)	1.4 (0.7–2.9)	0.302
48 h – 72 h	16 (25.0%)	48 (18.2%)	64 (19.0%)	1.3 (0.7–2.4)	0.439
> 72 h	25 (25.3%)	75 (28.4%)	100 (29.8%)	1.3 (0.8–2.3)	0.299
Hours from admission to surgery, median (range, interquartile range)	26 (3–109, 18–42)	29 (3–144, 20–48)	29 (3–144, 20–47)	NA	0.156
Total duration from symptoms onset to surgery[c]					
< 24 h	12 (21.4%)	44 (16.7%)	56 (16.7%)	1.0 (0.5–2.0)	1.000
24 h - 48 h	8 (16.3%)	41 (15.5%)	49 (14.6%)	0.7 (0.3–1.5)	0.346
48 h - 72 h	16 (21.3%)	59 (22.3%)	75 (22.3%)	1.0 (0.5–1.9)	0.982
> 72 h	35 (22.6%)	120 (45.5%)	155 (46.3%)	1.2 (0.7–2.0)	0.564
Clinical findings					
Pain in right upper quadrant	82 (23.1%)	273 (94.5%)	355 (95.2%)	2.4 (0.5–10.7)	0.235
Guarding	41 (25.6%)	119 (41.2%)	160 (42.9%)	1.4 (0.8–2.2)	0.213
Signs of generalized peritonitis	1 (50.0%)	1 (0.3%)	2 (0.5%)	3.5 (0.2–56.0)	0.400
Palpable gallbladder	6 (30.0%)	14 (4.8%)	20 (5.4%)	1.5 (0.6–4.1)	0.410
Preoperative laboratory data, median of highest results (range, interquartile range)[d]					
CRP (mg/l)	215 (3–471, 128–299)	123 (3–524, 58–214)	145 (3–524, 66–244)	NA	<0.001
WBCC (10^9/l)	14 (7–38, 12–18)	13 (2.5–32, 10–16)	13 (2.5–38, 10–17)	NA	0.018
ALAT (U/l)	27 (5–222, 17–48)	30 (4–705, 18–63)	29 (4–705, 18–57)	NA	0.214
AFOS (U/l)	85 (48–371, 66–126)	80 (24–621, 61–112)	81 (24–621, 62–113)	NA	0.075
Bilirubin (μmol/l)	15 (4–121, 9–27)	15 (2–230, 9–24)	15 (2–230, 9–24)	NA	0.668
Radiographic findings[e]					
Abscess	1 (100.0%)	0	1 (0.3%)	NA	0.226
Free fluid	9 (36.0%)	16 (5.6%)	25 (6.7%)	2.0 (0.9–4.8)	0.097
Thickened gallbladder wall	72 (23.2%)	239 (83.0%)	311 (83.6%)	1.2 (0.6–2.4)	0.552
Preoperative ERCP	3 (17.6%)	14 (4.8%)	17 (4.6%)	0.7 (0.2–2.6)	0.773
Surgical findings					
Abscess	10 (66.7%)	5 (1.7%)	15 (4.0%)	7.7 (2.5–23.1)	<0.001
Perforated gallbladder	12 (33.3%)	24 (8.3%)	36 (9.7%)	1.8 (0.9–3.9)	0.102
Gallbladder perforation during surgery	43 (23.0%)	144 (49.8%)	187 (50.1%)	1.1 (0.7–1.7)	0.826
Gangrene of the gallbladder identified by surgeon	58 (43.0%)	77 (26.6%)	135 (36.2%)	6.4 (3.6–10.4)	<0.001

Table 1 Univariate analysis of risk factors for conversion *(Continued)*

Removal of stones from common bile duct	0	0	0	NA	NA
Lead surgeon specialist	32 (25.2%)	94 (32.5%)	126 (33.8%)	1.3 (0.8–2.1)	0.342
Assistant present	53 (29.9%)[f]	124 (42.9%)	177 (48.1%)	2.7 (1.6–4.6)	<0.001

NA Not applicable, *LC* Laparoscopic cholecystectomy, *OR* Odds ratio, *CRP* C-reactive protein, *WBCC* White blood cell count, *ERCP* Endoscopic retrograde cholangiopancretography, *ALAT* Alanine transferase, *AFOS* Alkaline phosphatase

[a]percentages show the proportion of patients with specified risk factor

[b]Fifteen patients had mentions of an appendectomy in their patient journals, but it was not specified whether the procedure was laparoscopic or open

[c]Duration of symptoms missing from 25 patients in LC and 12 in conversion

[d]CRP missing from one patient, ALAT missing from seven patients, AFOS missing from eight patients, bilirubin missing from 18 patients

[e]A total of 239 patients had an ultrasound, 65 had computed tomography (CT) and 62 had both. Magnetic resonance cholangiopancreatography (MRCP) was used in 93 patients. One patient did not undergo any imaging

[f]Assistant present prior to conversion, info on timing of assistant arrival missing in five cases

and for all risk factors for conversion, and the results are presented in Table 2. The most common reasons for conversion were severe inflammation reported in 47 patients (56.0%) and difficulty with identification of anatomy in 17 patients (20.2%).

Complications

A univariate analysis of risk factors for postoperative complications is presented in Table 3. Risk factors for complications identified by multivariate analysis are presented in Table 4. Sixty-seven (18.0%) patients experienced an overall of 83 complications. The complication rates were 14.5 and 29.8% for LC and conversion respectively ($p < 0.001$). The 67 patients are grouped in Table 5 according to their most serious complication. The median comprehensive complication index for all patients with complications was 22.6 with an interquartile range of 20.9–26.2 and a range of 8.7–100. Twenty (5.4%) patients experienced complications that required surgical, endoscopic or radiological intervention. Three patients (0.8%) experienced a life threatening complication (grade IV) and five (1.3%) deaths (grade V) occurred.

Of the total number of 83 complications, the most common complications were pneumonia, which occurred in 14 patients (3.8%), a superficial surgical site infection (SSI) in seven patients (1.9%) and a retained common bile duct stone in five patients (1.3%). A bile leak occurred in four patients (1.1%). Two of the bile leaks were from the cystic duct, one from the main bile duct and one was undefined. None of the bile leaks occurred in patients who had undergone LC. The patients who died had a mean age of 81 years (range 70–92) and they all had at least two comorbidities of which one was a cardiovascular comorbidity. The American Society of Anesthesiologists (ASA) classification was IV for four patients and III for one patient. Of the three deaths in the LC group one was from the worsening of heart failure, another from the worsening of renal failure and the third from sepsis. The two deaths among converted patients were caused by postoperative pneumonia and failure of intubation during the induction of anaesthesia, leading to an anoxic brain injury.

Table 2 Independent risk factors for conversion based on stepwise forward logistic regression

Risk factor	OR (95% CI)	*P*
Analysis of preoperative risk factors only		
CRP over 150 mg/ml	3.0 (1.8–5.0)	<0.001
Diabetes	1.8 (1.0–3.3)	0.045
Analysis including both preoperative and intraoperative risk factors		
Abscess	9.2 (2.7–31.1)	<0.001
Age over 65 years	1.9 (1.1–3.3)	0.023
Gangrene of the gallbladder	5.9 (3.4–10.2)	<0.001

The following preoperative findings were included in the stepwise forward logistic regression analysis of risk factors for conversion: age over 65 years, previous laparotomy on the upper abdomen, diabetes, CRP over 150 mg/ml and WBCC over 13×10^9/l. Gangrene of the gallbladder and abscess were added for the stepwise analysis of all risk factors. CRP C-reactive protein, WBCC white blood cell count

Discussion

LC has become the standard procedure for managing acute calculous cholecystitis. The main concerns are with safety and feasibility as reflected in the risk of conversion to open cholecystectomy as well as the risk of postoperative complications, especially bile duct injuries. Our study focused on the risk factors for conversion and postoperative complications.

Conversion

Age over 65 years, diabetes and CRP over 150 mg/l were identified as independent preoperative risk factors for conversion. Complications of severe inflammation like gangrene of the gallbladder and an abscess identified by the surgeon were also recognized as risk factors in the multivariate analysis including both preoperative and intraoperative findings (Table 2). Diabetes and CRP over 150 mg/l were however not of significant value in this analysis, which might speak for a correlation between diabetes and the development of gangrene and an abscess leading to high CRP levels. Studies have indeed found that diabetes increases the risk of development of gangrenous cholecystitis and that gangrene increases the risk of conversion [13, 16, 17]. Gangrene and an abscess

Table 3 Univariate analysis of risk factors for complications

Risk factor	One or more postoperative complications $n = 67$ (18.0%)[a]	Patients without complications $n = 306$	OR (95% CI)	*P*
Gender: Male	44 (23.3%)	145	2.1 (1.2–3.7)	0.007
Age in years, median (range)	70 (30–92)	61 (20–94)	NA	0.001
Heart failure	7 (29.2%)	17	2.0 (0.8–5.0)	0.139
Impaired renal function	6 (54.5%)	5	5.9 (1.8–20.0)	0.006
Diabetes	18 (26.5%)	50	1.9 (1.0–3.5)	0.043
Previous laparotomy on the upper abdomen	8 (40.0%)	12	3.3 (1.3–8.5)	0.008
Previous laparotomy on the lower abdomen[b]	16 (18.2%)	72	1.0 (0.5–1.8)	0.944
Previous laparoscopic surgery on the abdomen[b]	2 (8.3%)	22	0.4 (0.1–1.7)	0.276
No previous surgeries	43 (17.7%)	200	1.0 (0.5–1.6)	0.854
Duration of symptoms before admission[c]				
< 24 h	18 (14.5%)	106	0.8 (0.4–1.4)	0.360
24 h - 48 h	11 (22.9%)	37	1.6 (0.7–3.3)	0.235
48 h - 72 h	10 (15.6%)	54	0.9 (0.4–1.9)	0.751
> 72 h	18 (18.0%)	82	1.1 (0.6–2.1)	0.742
Hours from admission to surgery, median (range, interquartile range)	26 (3–92, 16–43)	29 (4–144, 20–48)	NA	0.141
Duration from symptoms onset to surgery[c]				
< 24 h	9 (16.1%)	47	0.9 (0.4–2.0)	0.845
24 h - 48 h	9 (18.4%)	40	1.1 (0.5–2.5)	0.777
48 h - 72 h	14 (18.7%)	61	1.2 (0.6–2.3)	0.656
> 72 h	24 (15.5%)	131	0.8 (0.5–1.5)	0.575
Clinical findings				
Pain in right upper quadrant	65 (18.3%)	290	1.8 (0.4–8.0)	0.438
Guarding	33 (20.6%)	127	1.4 (0.8–2.3)	0.246
Signs of generalized peritonitis	0	2	NA	1.000
Palpable gallbladder	4 (20.0%)	16	1.2 (0.4–3.6)	0.767
Preoperative laboratory data, median of the highest results (range, interquartile range)[d]				
CRP (mg/l)	209 (4–477, 114–303)	131 (3–524, 62–232)	NA	<0.001
WBCC (10^9/l)	14.4 (5.4–37.4, 10.8–18.5)	12.7 (2.5–38, 10–16.5)	NA	0.069
ALAT (U/l)	31 (5–473, 18–74)	28 (4–705, 18–51)	NA	0.439
AFOS (U/l)	91 (24–314, 68–118)	79 (26–621, 61–113)	NA	0.105
Bilirubin (μmol/l)	19 (4–92, 11–25)	14 (2–230, 9–24)	NA	0.139
Radiographic findings[e]				
Abscess	0	1	NA	1.000
Free fluid	7 (28.0%)	18	1.9 (0.7–4.7)	0.182
Thickened gallbladder wall	61 (19.6%)	250	2.2 (0.9–5.4)	0.069
Surgical findings and procedures				
Preoperative ERCP	3 (17.6%)	14	1.0 (0.3–3.5)	1.000
Abscess	5 (33.3%)	10	2.4 (0.8–7.2)	0.160
Perforated gallbladder	9 (25.0%)	27	1.6 (0.7–3.6)	0.234
Gallbladder perforation during surgery	38 (20.3%)	149	1.4 (0.8–2.4)	0.452
Gangrene of the gallbladder identified by surgeon	31 (23.0%)	104	1.7 (1.0–2.9)	0.058
	0	0	NA	NA

Table 3 Univariate analysis of risk factors for complications *(Continued)*

Removal of stones from the common bile duct				
Duration of surgery in minutes, median (range, interquartile range)	110 (60–196, 83–138)	98 (34–240, 74–123)	NA	0.023
Lead surgeon specialist	24 (19.0%)	102	1.1 (0.6–1.9)	0.697
Assistant present[f]	34 (19.2%)	143	1.2 (0.7–2.0)	0.540
Conversion	25 (29.8%)	59	2.5 (1.4–4.4)	0.001

NA Not applicable, *LC* Laparoscopic cholecystectomy, *OR* Odds ratio, *CRP* C-reactive protein, *WBCC* White blood cell count, *ERCP* Endoscopic retrograde cholangiopancretography, *ALAT* Alanine transferase, *AFOS* Alkaline phosphatase
[a]percentages show the proportion of patients with specified risk factor
[b]Fifteen patients had mentions of an appendectomy in their patient journals, but it was not specified whether the procedure was laparoscopic or open
[c]Duration of symptoms missing from 25 patients in LC and 12 in conversion
[d]CRP missing from one patient, ALAT missing from seven patients, AFOS missing from eight patients, bilirubin missing from 18 patients
[e]A total of 239 patients had an ultrasound, 65 had computed tomography (CT) and 62 had both. Magnetic resonance cholangiopancreatography (MRCP) was used in 93 patients. One patient did not undergo any imaging
[f]Assistant present prior to conversion, info on timing of assistant arrival missing in five cases

might however be hard to recognize prior to the operation and therefore CRP levels and history of diabetes might be of better use when estimating the difficulty of the planned procedure.

High age, diabetes and CRP have been recognized as risk factors for conversion by other studies as well [10, 12, 13, 18]. Age as a risk factor has been speculated to be related to a longer history of gallbladder disease, masked symptoms and patient delay [12, 18]. History of previous abdominal surgeries and male gender have also been linked to conversion [18]. Seven (8.3%) patients were converted due to adhesions from previous surgeries, but history of previous abdominal surgeries was not recognized as a risk factor in this study and neither was male gender. The presence of an assistant was associated with conversion in the univariate analysis, which is probably a result from assistants being called to particularly challenging surgeries. Hence we did not consider the presence of an assistant as a risk factor for conversion.

Early cholecystectomy is recommended over conservative treatment followed by delayed cholecystectomy [14, 19]. The optimal time point for cholecystectomy resulting in the lowest conversion and complication rates is still under debate [2]. Some have found that surgery within 48 h from admission lowers the complication rate, whilst others have concluded that cholecystectomy within 5 days of admission yields as good as results in conversion and complications as surgery performed as soon as scheduling allows [20, 21]. Also, a recent randomized trial found that early LC results in lower morbidity and hospital stay compared to delayed cholecystectomy even in acute cholecystitis with symptoms over 72 h prior to admission [22].

No correlation between the time from admission to surgery or the total duration of symptoms and conversion or complications was however documented in this study. This might have been caused by a selection bias resulting from patients with a clinically more severe condition being operated on earlier. Also the initial onset of symptoms might have been hard to notice by elderly patients with several comorbidities. After diagnosis of cholecystitis antibiotics were initiated, which might have slowed down the progression of cholecystitis. Prehospital delay of less than 24 h from symptoms onset was associated with the lowest conversion rate, which might tell us that cholecystitis without any treatment is of higher significance than the in-hospital delay. It is also possible that the inflammation progresses individually and that time does not seemingly have a great impact on the development of the inflammatory process.

Table 4 Independent risk factors for complications based on stepwise forward logistic regression

Risk factor	OR (95% CI)	*P*
Age over 65 years	2.1 (1.2–3.6)	0.012
Male gender	2.1 (1.2–3.7)	0.013
Impaired renal function	4.8 (1.4–17.0)	0.015
Conversion	2.3 (1.3–4.1)	0.006

Variables included in the stepwise forward logistic regression analysis of risk factors for complications were age over 65 years, male gender, C-reactive protein over 150 mg/ml, diabetes, impaired renal function, previous laparotomy on the upper abdomen, duration of surgery over 90 min and conversion

Complications

Age over 65 years, male gender, impaired renal function and surgery finished as open cholecystectomy were identified as independent risk factors for complications. The overall complication rate of 18.0% falls within complication rates of 9 – 20% reported by other studies [12, 13]. The complication rate after conversion was significantly higher than after LC. Since higher age, diabetes and advanced infection were associated with conversion it is possible that these factors also contribute to increased postoperative complications. Furthermore, wound complications like wound infections and ruptures were more common after conversion to open surgery. Age, male gender and gangrene have been recognized as risk factors for complications by

Table 5 Classification of complications that occurred within 30 days from surgery according to the Clavien-Dindo classification and their treatment

Clavien-Dindo classification	LC ($n = 289$)	Conversion ($n = 84$)	Total ($n = 373$)	Treatment
Grade I-II	24 (8.3%)	15 (17.9%)	39 (10.5%)	
Infections				Antimicrobial medication
Pneumonia	8	4	12	
Superficial SSI	4	2	6[a]	
Urinary tract infection	1		1	
Other infection	1	2	3	
Arrhythmias	4		4	Antiarrhythmic medication
High blood pressure		2	2	Blood pressure medication
Perioperative MI	2		2	Medication
Respiratory insufficiency	1	1	2	Medication
Congestion	1	1	2	Medication
Urinary retention		1	1	Catheterisation
Postoperative delirium	1		1	Medication
Nausea		1	1	Antiemetic medication
Perihepatic hematoma		1	1	Follow-up
Wound hematoma	1		1	Change of dressings
Grade III a-b	13 (4.5%)	7 (8.3%)	20 (5.4%)	
Common bile duct stone	5		5	ERCP
Surgical site effusion	4		4	Drainage
Bile leak		3	3[a]	ERCP, stenting
Deep SSI; abscess	2	1	3	Drainage
Wound dehiscence		2	2	Re-suturation
Bleeding from urinary catheter	1		1	Bladder washout
Intra-abdominal bleeding	1		1	Laparotomy
Pneumonia; pleural effusion		1	1	Thoracocentesis
Grade IV a-b	2 (0.7%)	1 (1.2%)	3 (0.8%)	
Respiratory failure	2	1	3	Intubation, CPAP
Grade V	3 (1.0%)	2 (2.4%)	5 (1.3%)	
Sepsis	1		1	
Pneumonia		1	1	
Heart failure	1		1	
Anoxic brain injury during induction of anaesthesia		1	1	
Renal failure	1		1	
Total	42 (14.5%)	25 (29.8%)	67 (18.0%)	

The most serious complication was classified in patients who experienced multiple complications *LC* Laparoscopic cholecystectomy, *SSI* Surgical site infection, *ERCP* Endoscopic retrograde cholangiopancreatography, *CPAP* Continuous positive airway pressure, *MI* Myocardial infarction

[a]The numbers of superficial SSIs and bile leaks are reported lower here than in the text (seven respectively four), since only the most serious complication in patients with multiple complications was categorised in this table. The most serious complication in the fourth patient with a bile leak was a wound dehiscence (Clavien-Dindo grade IIIb)

other studies on acute cholecystitis [12, 13, 17]. Studies with patients operated on both electively and emergently have also recognized age, male gender and conversion as risk factors for complications [23, 24].

The overall bile duct injury (BDI) rate in this study was 1.1%, with a rate of 4.8% for cholecystectomies finished as open surgeries. However, most bile duct injuries were Strasberg classification type A, and all injuries were managed endoscopically [25]. None of the BDIs in this study occurred in patients who received LC, which reflects on the safety of LC, but might also be a result from difficult procedures being converted before BDIs could occur. This is supported by the rather high conversion rate in our study. Other studies have reported BDI rates of 0.62–0.9% for LC and 0.38–1.24% for OC [26–28]. These studies were however not homogenous for acute cholecystitis for which the risk of BDI has been reported as twice as high compared with patients who undergo cholecystectomy electively [29].

It was predicted that the BDI rates after LC would become lower as the procedure became more common, but according to some studies this prediction has not yet been fulfilled [30]. There are also results on the opposite trend – BDI injuries having become more common after OC – which raises concern on surgeons in training not learning appropriate technique for OC in the laparoscopic era [27]. Patients chosen for conversion or direct OC are however often suffering from a more severe inflammation that makes the tissues more prone to rupture and hence patients who have their surgery finished as an open procedure might be at risk for BDI due to inflamed, rupture-prone tissues rather than inadequate surgical technique. Some studies comparing the results on surgeons in training versus specialists performing cholecystectomy have concluded that the overall complication rate is higher for surgeons in training [11]. Our study did not show such a correlation, but this might be due to a bias resulting from clinically more severe cases being assigned to specialists. Prospective randomized trials are naturally unethical to perform since patients should always be offered the best care available.

Mortality (1.3%) in the present study was somewhat higher than mortality rates of 0.7–1.1% reported by other studies [12, 31]. The patients who suffered a mortal complication in this study had several comorbidities and were clinically considered high risk surgical patients. Treatment options for severe acute cholecystitis apart from cholecystectomy consist of antibiotics and interval cholecystectomy or the use of percutaneous transhepatic cholecystostomy (PTHC) possibly followed by cholecystectomy. Currently there are no results on the impact of interval cholecystectomy or PTHC for subgroups of high risk surgical patients. To determine the best treatment in such patients a randomized controlled trial has been initiated in the Netherlands where the use of LC and PTHC in high risk patients are to be compared [32].

Limitations

Like all retrospective review studies this study has its limits. Data concerning body mass index, which might have been associated with conversion, was missing from many patients and was not included in the study. Data on symptoms duration was also missing from many patients and hence it was not included in the multivariate analysis. The study is also limited by its sample size. Different risk factors might correlate with different complications and the severity of complications, but such a correlation cannot be evaluated with a limited sample size.

Conclusions

Early LC is safe and feasible in the treatment of acute calculous cholecystitis. The risk of postoperative complications is increased by risk factors like male gender, high age and impaired renal function and conversion to open surgery. Of these factors the only one that can be influenced is conversion. Manifestations of advanced cholecystitis like high CRP, gangrene of the gallbladder or abscess formation increase the risk of conversion to open cholecystectomy. Early identification and treatment of acute calculous cholecystitis might lower the number of patients with advanced cholecystitis and thus reduce the amount of converted patients and postoperative complications. When LC cannot be performed safely conversion should be initiated to minimize the risk of bile duct injuries. Also enough attention should be paid to surgeons in training learning appropriate technique for performing open cholecystectomy.

Additional files

Additional file 1: Figure S1. a) Receiver operating characteristic (ROC) curve for C-reactive protein (CRP) in converted patients. CRP level of 150 mg/ml yields sensitivity of 0.69 and specificity of 0.58. Area under the curve (AUC) 0.67. **b**) ROC curve for CRP in patients with complications. CRP level of 150 mg/ml yields sensitivity of 0.64 and specificity of 0.55. AUC 0.64. (PDF 113 kb)

Additional file 2: Figure S2. a) Receiver operating characteristic (ROC) curve for age in converted patients. Age of 65 years yields sensitivity of 0.58 and specifity of 0.57. Area under the curve (AUC) 0.63. **b**) ROC curve for age in patients with complications. Age of 65 years yields sensitivity of 0.63 and specificity of 0.59. AUC 0.63. (PDF 131 kb)

Additional file 3: Figure S3. Receiver operating characteristic (ROC) curve for white blood cell count (WBCC) in converted patients. WBCC of 13x10^9/l yields a sensitivity of 0.62 and specificity of 0.54. Area under the curve (AUC) 0.59. (PDF 106 kb)

Additional file 4: Figure S4. Receiver operating characteristic (ROC) curve for duration of surgery in patients with complications. Surgery duration of 90 min yields a sensitivity of 0.72 and specificity of 0.40. Area under the curve (AUC) 0.59. (PDF 88 kb)

Abbreviations

BDI: Bile duct injury; CRP: C-reactive protein; ERCP: Endoscopic retrograde cholangiopancreatography; LC: Laparoscopic cholecystectomy; OC: Open cholecystectomy; PTHC: Percutaneous transhepatic cholecystostomy; ROC: Receiver operating characteristic; SSI: Surgical site infection; WBCC: White blood cell count

Acknowledgements

Not applicable.

Funding

The study was funded by Governmental Competitive Funds (EVO).

Authors' contributions

PT acquired, analysed and interpreted the data and drafted the article. AL contributed substantially to study design and revised the article critically. PM designed the study, contributed to data analysis and interpretation and revised the article critically. All authors read and approved the final version of the article.

Competing interests

The authors declare that they have no competing interests.

Author details

[1]Institute of Clinical Medicine, Faculty of Medicine, University of Helsinki, Haartmaninkatu 8, 00014 Helsinki, Finland. [2]Department of Abdominal Surgery, Helsinki University Central Hospital, P.O.Box 340, 00029 HUS Helsinki, Finland.

References

1. Coccolini F, Catena F, Pisano M, Gheza F, Fagiuoli S, Di Saverio S, et al. Open versus laparoscopic cholecystectomy in acute cholecystitis. Systematic review and meta-analysis. Int J Surg. 2015;18:196–204.
2. Ansaloni L, Pisano M, Coccolini F, Peitzmann AB, Fingerhut A, Catena F, et al. 2016 WSES guidelines on acute calculous cholecystitis. World J Emerg Surg. 2016;11:25.
3. Kiviluoto T, Sirén J, Luukkonen P, Kivilaakso E. Randomised trial of laparoscopic versus open cholecystectomy for acute and gangrenous cholecystitis. Lancet. 1998;351:321–5.
4. Boo YJ, Kim WB, Kim J, Song TJ, Choi SY, Kim YC, et al. Systemic immune response after open versus laparoscopic cholecystectomy in acute cholecystitis: A prospective randomized study. Scand J Clin Lab Invest. 2007;67:207–14.
5. Gurusamy K, Samraj K, Gluud C, Wilson E, Davidson BR. Meta-analysis of randomized controlled trials on the safety and effectiveness of early versus delayed laparoscopic cholecystectomy for acute cholecystitis. Br J Surg. 2010;97:141–50.
6. Wilson E, Gurusamy K, Gluud C, Davidson BR. Cost-utility and value-of-information analysis of early versus delayed laparoscopic cholecystectomy for acute cholecystitis. Br J Surg. 2010;97:210–9.
7. Miettinen P, Pasanen P, Lahtinen J, Alhava E. Acute abdominal pain in adults. Ann Chir Gynaecol. 1996;85:5–9.
8. Ukkonen M, Kivivuori A, Rantanen T, Paajanen H. Emergency Abdominal Operations in the Elderly: A Multivariate Regression Analysis of 430 Consecutive Patients with Acute Abdomen. World J Surg. 2015;39:2854–61.
9. Giger UF, Michel J-M, Opitz I, Th Inderbitzin D, Kocher T, Krahenbuhl L. Risk factors for perioperative complications in patients undergoing laparoscopic cholecystectomy: analysis of 22,953 consecutive cases from the Swiss Association of Laparoscopic and Thoracoscopic Surgery database. J Am Coll Surg. 2006;203:723–8.
10. Dominguez LC, Rivera A, Bermudez C, Herrera W. Analysis of factors for conversion of laparoscopic to open cholecystectomy: a prospective study of 703 patients with acute cholecystitis. Cir Esp. 2011;89:300–6.
11. Hobbs MS, Mai Q, Knuiman MW, Fletcher DR, Ridout SC. Surgeon experience and trends in intraoperative complications in laparoscopic cholecystectomy. Br J Surg. 2006;93:844–53.
12. Wevers KP, van Westreenen HL, Patijn GA. Laparoscopic cholecystectomy in acute cholecystitis: C-reactive protein level combined with age predicts conversion. Surg Laparosc Endosc Percutan Tech. 2013;23:163–6.
13. Eldar S, Sabo E, Nash E, Abrahamson J, Matter I. Laparoscopic Cholecystectomy for Acute Cholecystitis: Prospective Trial. World J Surg. 1997;21:540–5.
14. Gutt CN, Encke J, Koninger J, Harnoss J-C, Weigand K, Kipfmuller K, et al. Acute cholecystitis: early versus delayed cholecystectomy, a multicenter randomized trial (ACDC study, NCT00447304). Ann Surg. 2013;258:385–93.
15. Dindo D, Demartines N, Clavien P-A. Classification of surgical complications: a new proposal with evaluation in a cohort of 6336 patients and results of a survey. Ann Surg. 2004;240:205–13.
16. Bourikian S, Anand RJ, Aboutanos M, Wolfe LG, Ferrada P. Risk factors for acute gangrenous cholecystitis in emergency general surgery patients. Am J Surg. 2015;210:730–3.
17. Ganapathi AM, Speicher PJ, Englum BR, Perez A, Tyler DS, Zani S. Gangrenous cholecystitis: a contemporary review. J Surg Res. 2015;197:18–24.
18. Simopoulos C, Botaitis S, Polychronidis A, Tripsianis G, Karayiannakis AJ. Risk factors for conversion of laparoscopic cholecystectomy to open cholecystectomy. Surg Endosc. 2005;19:905–9.
19. Lo CM, Liu CL, Fan ST, Lai EC, Wong J. Prospective randomized study of early versus delayed laparoscopic cholecystectomy for acute cholecystitis. Ann Surg. 1998;227:461–7.
20. Banz V, Gsponer T, Candinas D, Guller U. Population-based analysis of 4113 patients with acute cholecystitis: defining the optimal time-point for laparoscopic cholecystectomy. Ann Surg. 2011;254:964–70.
21. Chandler CF, Lane JS, Ferguson P, Thompson JE, Ashley SW. Prospective evaluation of early versus delayed laparoscopic cholecystectomy for treatment of acute cholecystitis. Am Surg. 2000;66:896–900.
22. Roulin D, Saadi A, Di Mare L, Demartines N, Halkic N. Early Versus Delayed Cholecystectomy for Acute Cholecystitis, Are the 72 hours Still the Rule? A Randomized Trial Ann Surg. 2016;264:717–22.
23. Murphy MM, Ng S-C, Simons JP, Csikesz NG, Shah SA, Tseng JF. Predictors of Major Complications after Laparoscopic Cholecystectomy: Surgeon, Hospital, or Patient? J Am Coll Surg. 2010;211:73–80.
24. Roslyn JJ, Binns GS, Hughes EF, Saunders-Kirkwood K, Zinner MJ, Cates JA. Open cholecystectomy. A contemporary analysis of 42,474 patients. Ann Surg. 1993;218:129–37.
25. Strasberg SM, Hertl M, Soper NJ. An analysis of the problem of biliary injury during laparoscopic cholecystectomy. J Am Coll Surg. 1995;180:101–25.
26. Diamantis T, Tsigris C, Kiriakopoulos A, Papalambros E, Bramis J, Michail P, et al. Bile duct injuries associated with laparoscopic and open cholecystectomy: an 11-year experience in one institute. Surg Today. 2005;35:841–5.
27. Karvonen J, Salminen P, Grönroos JM. Bile duct injuries during open and laparoscopic cholecystectomy in the laparoscopic era: alarming trends. Surg Endosc. 2011;25:2906–10.
28. Viste A, Horn A, Ovrebo K, Christensen B, Angelsen J-H, Hoem D. Bile duct injuries following laparoscopic cholecystectomy. Scand J Surg. 2015;104:233–7.
29. Tornqvist B, Waage A, Zheng Z, Ye W, Nilsson M. Severity of Acute Cholecystitis and Risk of Iatrogenic Bile Duct Injury During Cholecystectomy, a Population-Based Case-Control Study. World J Surg. 2016;40:1060–7.
30. Slater K, Strong RW, Wall DR, Lynch SV. Iatrogenic bile duct injury: the scourge of laparoscopic cholecystectomy. ANZ J Surg. 2002;72:83–8.
31. Scollay JM, Mullen R, McPhillips G, Thompson AM. Mortality associated with the treatment of gallstone disease: a 10-year contemporary national experience. World J Surg. 2011;35:643–7.
32. Kortram K, van Ramshorst B, Bollen TL, Besselink MGH, Gouma DJ, Karsten T, et al. Acute cholecystitis in high risk surgical patients: percutaneous cholecystostomy versus laparoscopic cholecystectomy (CHOCOLATE trial): study protocol for a randomized controlled trial. Trials. 2012;13:7.

28

Vacuum-assisted closure (VAC®) systems and microbiological isolation of infected wounds

Valerio Cozza[1,3*], Gilda Pepe[1], Marco Cintoni[1], Flavio De Maio[2], Giuseppe Tropeano[1], Sabina Magalini[1], Gabriele Sganga[1], Giovanni Delogu[2] and Daniele Gui[1]

Abstract

Background: Negative pressure wound therapy is now largely used to treat infected wounds. The prevention and reduction of healthcare-associated infections is a high priority for any Department of Health and great efforts are spent to improve infection control systems. It is assumed that vacuum-assisted closure (VAC®) dressings should be watertight and that all the secretions are gathered in a single container but there is no consistent data on air leakage and possible dispersion of bacteria from the machine.

Methods: We have conducted a prospective experimental study on 10 patients with diagnosis of wound infection to verify whether the filtration process is microbiologically efficient. We compared the bacteria population present in the wound to the one present in the air discharged by the VAC® machine.

Results: This study shows that the contamination of the VAC® machine is considerably lower than the environment or wound contamination.

Conclusions: Negative pressure wound therapy system does not represent a risk factor for healthcare-associated infections.

Keywords: Negative pressure wound therapy, Infection control, Wound infection, Wound contamination

Introduction

Vacuum-assisted closure (VAC®) therapy is a system which promotes open wound healing through the application of negative pressure (negative pressure wound therapy, NPWT) [1–3], especially in infected tissues [4–7]. When applying negative pressure onto the bed of the wound, fluid material is removed, formation of granulation tissue is promoted, and wound edge approximation is helped [8]. These mechanisms are effective in promoting the healing process which would be otherwise difficult to treat, leading not only to economic advantages, but especially to a noticeably improved patients' health [9].

It is assumed that VAC® dressings should be watertight and that all the secretions are gathered in a single container. Actually, a minimum leakage of air cannot be avoided completely. The air is vacuumed, filtrated, and discharged from the machine into the environment. Moreover, filters used in this process cannot be replaced by medical staff.

The object of this study is to verify whether the filtration process is microbiologically efficient. We compared the bacteria population present in the wound to the one present in the air discharged by the unit.

* Correspondence: Valerio.cozza@policlinicogemelli.it
[1]Emergency Surgery Department, Università Cattolica del Sacro Cuore, Fondazione Policlinico A. Gemelli IRCCS, Rome, Italy
[3]Istituto di Clinica Chirurgica (9B) Catholic University of Sacred Heart, Largo Francesco Vito, 1, 00168 Rome, Italy
Full list of author information is available at the end of the article

Materials and methods

For this study, we enrolled 10 patients with abdominal wound or soft tissue infections (see Table 1), all treated with VAC® therapy. All the patients considered in the study were adult, hospitalised from February 2016 to April 2017 in the Emergency Surgery Unit at University Hospital "A. Gemelli", Rome. The inclusion criteria were as follows: full thickness wound (involving subcutaneous fat down to fascia without extension to muscles or

Table 1 All the microbiological results

Study no.	Age	Male/ female	LOS (days)	Site of VAC application	Inner machine plate		Injury swab		Environmental plate		Machine swab	
					P/N	Identified microorganisms	P/N	Identified microorganisms	P/N	Identified microorganisms	P/N	Identified microorganisms
1	27	M	74	Thigh abscesses	Y	*S. hominis*	Y	*C. striatum* *A. baumannii*	Y	*S. hominis* *S. haemolyticus* *A. baumannii*	Y	*E. faecium* *A. baumannii* *(1 colonia)*
2	27	M	74	Thigh abscesses	Y	*S. hominis*	Y	*E. coli (1 colonia)*	Y	*S. hominis*	Y	*S. hominis*
3	65	F	26	Sacral pressure ulcers	N		Y	*A. baumannii* *P. mirabilis* *P. stuartii*	Y	*S. epidermidis* *(1 colonia)*	N	
4	67	F	45	Necrotizing fasciitis	N		N		Y	*B. pumilus* *E. faecalis* *S. hominis*	N	
5	72	F	13	Sacral pressure ulcers	N		Y	*A. baumannii* *P. mirabilis* *E. faecium*	Y	*B. pumilus* *S. aureus* *P. mirabilis*	Y	*A. baumannii* *(1 colonia)*
6	48	M	62	Median laparotomy	N		Y	*A. baumannii*	Y	*S. hominis* *S. epidermidis* *B. simplex*	N	
7	70	M	21	Median laparotomy	N		Y	*A. baumannii*	Y	*A. baumannii* *S. hominis*	N	
8	66	M	37	Median laparotomy	N		Y	*A. baumannii*	Y	*S. haemolyticus* *S. hominis* *S. aureus*	N	
9	79	F	11	Median laparotomy	N		N		Y	*S. hominis* *E. faecalis*	N	
10	58	F	15	Enterocutaneous fistula	N		Y	*S. epidermidis*	Y	*S. hominis* *B. megaterium* *E. faecalis*	N	

A. baumanii Acinetobacter baumanii, *B. megaterium* Bacillus megaterium, *B. pumilus* Bacillus pumilus, *B. simplex* Bacillus simplex, *C. striatum* Corynebacterium striatum, *E. coli* Escherichia coli, *E. faecalis* Enterococcus faecalis, *E. faecium* Enterococcus faecium, *P. mirabilis* Proteus mirabilis, *P. stuartii* Providencia stuartii, *S. aureus* Staphylococcus aureus, *S. epidermidis* Staphylococcus epidermidis, *S. haemolyticus* Staphylococcus haemolyticus, *S. hominis* Staphylococcus hominis

intra-abdominal organs), larger than 10 cm and producing at least 200 ml/day of exudate (in 7/10 cases), and with a verified positivity of bacterial culture (from the wound) [10].

Study population description

Our study population was composed of 10 people, 5 males and 5 females. The average age was 57.9 years (median age 65.5 years, 27–79). VAC® was used in different types of wounds: 2 thigh abscesses, 2 sacral pressure ulcers, 4 infected median laparotomy, 1 necrotizing fasciitis, and 1 enterocutaneous fistula. As the majority of the patients admitted in our service, even among this study population, many were affected by multiple comorbidities (both acute and chronic). The most frequent were found to be cardiovascular and metabolic diseases, followed by malnourishment and bedridden syndrome. All of these promote bacterial superinfection, the infection persistence, delaying, consequently, the healing process. Two patients were otherwise healthy. Table 1 reports the demographics of the patients.

Methodology of VAC® application and microbiological assays

The machine used was the VAC Ulta™ with standard GranuFoam™ dressing (different sizes) which was usually changed every 48/72 hours (h).

In order to assess the eventual microbiological contamination of the air discharged from the VAC® unit, the following experimental study was designed: a sterile plastic bag was closed around the VAC® unit in a loose manner. As we can see from Fig. 1, the bag was sealed around the VAC® suction tube and the power cable. Data were collected through the microbiological examination of four different samples in a single 12-h span period (see Fig. 1): a specimen from a Petri dish in the patient room—usually at the head of the bed (to sample the environmental contamination) (a); a specimen collected from patient's wound at the time of dressing change (b); a specimen scrubbed from the VAC® unit bodywork, i.e. the screen and the handle of the machine (c); and a specimen from a Petri dish collocated inside the bag (d).

The environmental plate was positioned on a shelf over the patient's bed, high above the head. The machine swab was obtained rubbing a swab on the *canister* attached to

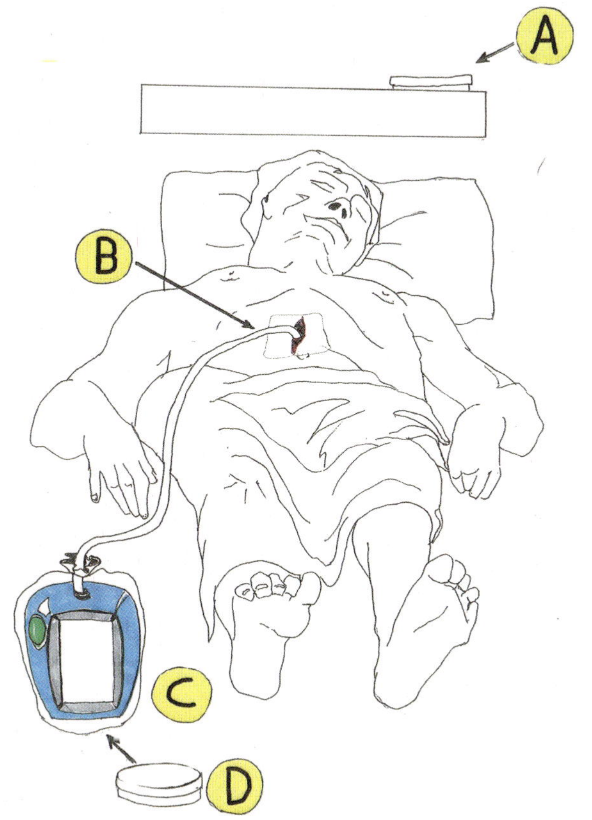

Fig. 1 The four different specimens taken for the study. **a** Environment sample, a petri dish on the shelf. **b** Specimen collected from patient's wound at the time of dressing change. **c** Specimen scrubbed from the VAC® unit *bodywork*. **d** Specimen from a Petri dish collocated inside the bag

the unit, as well as on the screen and handle of the device (considered to be the parts of the machine most frequently touched).

During the study, all the machines have worked correctly and no air leak was detected.

Specimens of the wound and the machine bodywork were plated on Trypcase Soy Agar (TSS, bioMérieux) and MacConkey agar (bioMérieux) and incubated overnight at 37 °C, supplemented with 5% CO_2. Plates arising from the bag and from the environment were incubated in the same growth condition. Finally, single colonies of the positive specimens were identified using MALDI-TOF instrument (Bruker Daltonics) according to the manufacturer's procedure.

To verify the object of the study, the bacterial growth from a swab of the wound was compared with the isolated colonies derived from the Petri dishes inserted in the bag next to the machine.

Results

Table 1 shows the results. The injury swab (i.e. the swab taken from the wound) was positive in 80% of patients. In three patients, Gram-positive bacteria were isolated (*Corynebacterium striatum*, *Enterococcus faecium* and *Staphylococcus epidermidis*), whereas in seven patients Gram-negative bacteria were isolated. In particular, six out of seven patients were positive for *Acinetobacter baumannii;* of these, three presented a co-infection with *C. striatum*, *Proteus mirabilis* and *Providencia stuartii*, and *P. mirabilis* and *E. faecium* respectively.

The inner machine plate (i.e. taken inside the bag) resulted positive in 20% of patients, and Gram-positive bacteria were isolated in two patients (*Staphylococcus hominis*).

All environmental plates resulted positive. Gram-positive bacteria were present in the plates derived from all 10 patients and the most represented bacteria were *S. hominis* (70%), followed by *Enterococcus faecalis* (30%), *S. epidermidis*, *Staphylococcus aureus* and *Staphylococcus haemolyticus* (20%). Eighty percent of the patients had co-infection. Among these, the most frequent was *S. hominis* and *Streptococcus faecalis* (30%). Conversely, Gram-negative bacteria were isolated in 20% of our population (*A. baumannii*).

Machine swab (i.e. taken on the machine case) resulted positive in 30% of patients. Gram-positive bacteria were identified in two patients (*S. hominis* and *E. faecium*), as well as Gram-negative bacteria (*A. baumannii*).

Discussion

Infections carry a heavy weight of intra-hospital deaths and costs, and there is a high level of attention towards aspects such as limitation of cross-contamination and reducing antibiotic treatments. A worldwide campaign has been conducted in many hospitals, including ours, to raise the attention on handwashing, which has shown to be one of the few very effective means to reduce nosocomial infections due to multi-resistant strains [11–13].

Extending the use of negative pressure wound therapy could potentially help in this sense: secreting wounds, in particular if infected, require multiple dressing changes, sometimes daily, whereas a NPWT dressing change can last for even more than 48 h. Furthermore, suction in the NPWT reduces pooling of fluid, which can itself facilitate bacterial growth. The dressing film is waterproof and therefore it does not allow pathogens from the skin to enter the wound. Additionally, some studies have shown that the NPWT could stop pathogens such as *S. aureus* from creating their biofilm [14].

The VAC® machine tolerates a minimal air leak before the alarm sets off; however, the amount of this leak is not known. The machine has a filter, which cannot be replaced by the medical staff; likely, it is replaced during the revision process that all the machines undergo periodically.

The rationale of this study is that the filter itself could represent a risk factor for environment or interhuman contamination. In fact, a large amount of infected fluid remains inside the canister and inside the system and potentially could be spread inside the environment. If so, we should radically change our approach to VAC® dressing changes to avoid potential contamination.

Our study shows that contamination in the air inside the bag containing the VAC® machine and the VAC® is considerably lower than the environment or wound contamination. This means that the cleaning work of the filter is successful, as shown by the fact that just 20% of the "inner machine plate" were positive.

The change of wound dressing represents a risk for environment contamination as well as the interhuman one [15–17]. Some of the pathogens isolated in the wounds are probably only contaminating bacteria; however, the percentages would suggest that this kind of dressing is not a risk factor for healthcare-associated infections.

This is a small study, and a larger group of patients is needed for a more significant statistical analysis. A larger study, better if multicentric, considering the heterogeneity of clinical practice (materials and methods used for wound treatment and dressing change) would indicate results reflecting different hospital realities. Anyway, this would require many resources and an excessively long time for the results' publication which, in our case, seem to be very interesting from a microbiological point of view and promising from a clinical perspective as well. Furthermore, this data can be interpreted as a demonstration that the advanced wound dressing in our service is effective.

Conclusions

The negative pressure wound therapy (NPWT), as analysed in our study, does not increase the risk of infection transmission: in fact, the contamination of the VAC® machine is considerably lower than the environment or wound contamination.

Abbreviations

NPWT: Negative pressure wound therapy; VAC®: Vacuum-assisted closure

Acknowledgements

Not applicable.

Funding

No funding

Authors' contributions

MC and GP carried out the experiment and swabs. FDM and GD performed the microbiological tests. VC and GT drafted the manuscript. SM and GS participated in the design of the study. DG conceived the study, participated in its design and coordination and helped to draft the manuscript.
All authors read and approved the final manuscript.

Competing interests

The authors declare that they have no competing interests.

Author details

[1]Emergency Surgery Department, Università Cattolica del Sacro Cuore, Fondazione Policlinico A. Gemelli IRCCS, Rome, Italy. [2]Microbiology Department, Università Cattolica del Sacro Cuore, Fondazione Policlinico A. Gemelli IRCCS, Rome, Italy. [3]Istituto di Clinica Chirurgica (9B) Catholic University of Sacred Heart, Largo Francesco Vito, 1, 00168 Rome, Italy.

References

1. Arundel C, Buckley H, Clarke E, et al. Negative pressure wound therapy versus usual care for surgical wounds healing by secondary intention (SWHSI trial): study protocol for a randomised controlled pilot trial. Trials. 2016;17:535.
2. Huang C, Leavitt T, Bayer LR, Orgill DP. Effect of negative pressure wound therapy on wound healing. Curr Probl Surg. 2014;51(7):301–31.
3. Itani HE. Reviewing the benefits and harm of NPWT in the management of closed surgical incisions. Br J Community Nurs. 2015; 20(Suppl 6):S28–34.
4. Zaidi A, El-Masry S. Closed incision negative pressure therapy in high-risk general surgery patients following laparotomy: a retrospective study. Color Dis. 2016;353(87).
5. Zhou M, Yu A, Wu G, Xia C, Hu X, Qi B. Role of different negative pressure values in the process of infected wounds treated by vacuum-assisted closure: an experimental study. Int Wound J. 2013;10:508–15.
6. Baharestani MM, Gabriel A. Use of negative pressure wound therapy in the management of infected abdominal wounds containing mesh: an analysis of outcomes. Int Wound J. 2011;8:118–25.
7. Gabriel A, Shores J, Berntein B, de Leon J, Kamepalli R, Wolvos T, Baharestani MM, Gupta S. A clinical review of infected wound treatment with vacuum assisted closure® (VAC®) therapy: experience and case series. Int Wound J. 2009;6:1–25.
8. Ciliberti M. The effect of a Bacteria and Fungi binding mesh dressing on the bacterial load of pressure ulcers treated with negative pressure wound therapy (NPWT). Wounds. 2016;28(11):408–20.
9. Janssen AHJ, Mommers EHH, Notter J, de Reilingh TS, Wegdam JA. Negative pressure wound therapy versus standard wound care on quality of life: a systematic review. J Wound Care. 2016;25(3):154–9.
10. Horan TC, Gaynes RP, Martone WJ, et al. CDC definitions of nosocomial surgical site infections, 1992: a modification of CDC definitions of surgical wound infections. Infect Control Hosp Epidemiol. 1992;13:606–8.
11. Luongo JC, Fennelly KP, Keen JA, Zhai ZJ, Jones BW, Miller SL. Role of mechanical ventilation in the airborne transmission of infectious agents in buildings. Indoor Air. 2015:1–13.
12. Russotto V, Cortegiani A, Raineri SM, Giarratano A. Bacterial contamination of inanimate surfaces and equipment in the intensive care unit. J Intensive Care. 2015;3(1):54.
13. Sergent AP, Slekovec C, Pauchot J, et al. Bacterial contamination of the hospital environment during wound dressing change. Orthop Traumatol Surg Res. 2012;98(4):441–5.
14. Li T, Zhang L, Han L, et al. Early application of negative pressure wound therapy to acute wounds contaminated with Staphylococcus aureus: an effective approach to preventing biofilm formation. Exp Ther Med. 2016; 11(3):769–76.
15. Bache SE, Maclean M, Gettinby G, Anderson JG, Macgregor SJ, Taggart I. Airborne bacterial dispersal during and after dressing and bed changes on burns patients. Burns. 2015;41(1):39–48.
16. Bache SE, MacLean M, Gettinby G, Anderson JG, MacGregor SJ, Taggart I. Quantifying bacterial transfer from patients to staff during burns dressing and bed changes: implications for infection control. Burns. 2013;39(2):220–8.
17. King MF, Noakes CJ, Sleigh PA. Modeling environmental contamination in hospital single- and four-bed rooms. Indoor Air. 2015;25(6):694–707.

Urine flow rate monitoring in hypovolemic multiple trauma patients

Evgeni Brotfain[2*†], Yoram Klein[1†], Ronen Toledano[3], Leonid Koyfman[2], Dmitry Frank[2], Micha Y. Shamir[4] and Moti Klein[2]

Abstract

Background: The urine output is an important clinical parameter of renal function and blood volume status, especially in critically ill multiple trauma patients. In the present study, the minute-to-minute urine flow rate and its variability were analyzed in hypotensive multiple trauma patients during the first 6 h of their ICU (intensive care unit) stay. These parameters have not been previously reported.

Methods: The study was retrospective and observational. Demographic and clinical data were extracted from the computerized Register Information Systems. A total of 59 patients were included in the study. The patients were divided into two study groups. Group 1 consisted of 29 multiple trauma patients whose systolic blood pressure was greater than 90 mmHg on admission to the ICU and who were consequently deemed to be hemodynamically compromised. Group 2 consisted of 30 patients whose systolic blood pressure was less than 90 mmHg on admission to the ICU and who were therefore regarded as hemodynamically uncompromised.

Results: The urine output and urine flow rate variability during the first 6 h of the patients' ICU stay was significantly lower in group 2 than in group 1 ($p < 0.001$ and 0.006 respectively). Statistical analysis by the Pearson method demonstrated a strong direct correlation between decreased urine flow rate variability and decreased urine output per hour ($R = 0.17$; $P = 0.009$), decreased mean arterial blood pressure ($R = 0.24$; $p = 0.001$), and increased heart rate ($R = 0.205$; $p = 0.001$).

Conclusion: These findings suggest that minute-to-minute urine flow rate variability is a reliable incipient marker of hypovolemia and that it should therefore take its place among the parameters used to monitor the hemodynamic status of critically ill multiple trauma patients.

Keywords: Minute-to-minute urine flow rate, Urine flow rate variability, Monitoring, Multiple trauma

Background

Trauma-associated acute hemorrhage is a leading cause of intravascular volume depletion [1–3] ranging from mild hypovolemia to hemorrhagic shock [1, 2]. The foremost priorities in acute trauma are hemorrhage control and hemodynamic resuscitation [1]. The urine output is a vital clinical parameter of renal function and blood volume status, especially in critically ill multiple trauma patients during their hospital admission and ICU (intensive care unit) stay [3, 4]. It is typically measured hourly and expressed in milliliters per hour. However, the blood volume status and the renal function of multiple trauma patients change more rapidly, especially during the first 24 h of ICU admission [5]. In previously published animal and human studies [6, 7], the use of a continuous minute-to-minute urine flow rate monitoring system (URINFO™, FlowSense Medical, Misgav, Israel) has been shown to detect hypovolemia earlier than other standard parameters. The minute-to-minute UFR was found to be a dynamic variable, which significantly decreases during acute bleeding and is restored after rehydration [6]. Furthermore, an animal model of the minute-to-minute UFR demonstrated that during euvolemia there is variation in the flow rate and that this parameter decreases and eventually disappears during acute hemorrhage. This

* Correspondence: bem1975@gmail.com
†Equal contributors
[2]Department of Anesthesiology and Critical Care, General Intensive Care Unit, Soroka Medical Center, Ben-Gurion University of the Negev, Beer Sheva, Israel
Full list of author information is available at the end of the article

variability has also been shown to decrease and eventually disappear during acute gradual hemorrhage [7].

This study analyzed minute-to-minute UFR and its variability in hypotensive multiple trauma patients during the first 6 h of their admission to the intensive care unit (ICU). This is the first such study of the significance of these parameters.

Methods

Soroka Medical Center is a University Level I trauma center with approximately 2500–3000 trauma admissions per year. About 10% of those trauma patients have an Injury Severity Score (ISS) of 16 or above (severe trauma). The study was retrospective and observational. Clinical and laboratory data were collected retrospectively from the records of all multiple trauma patients hospitalized in the Soroka Medical Center general intensive care unit (GICU) between January 2013 and January 2014. All the clinical data were extracted from the computerized Register Information Systems (MetaVision® and iMDsoft®, Israel). The Human Research and Ethics Committee at Soroka Medical Center in Beer Sheva, Israel, approved this study (RN-SOR-0158-14). The patients' concern has not been needed because of retrospective nature of the study. Patients were not involved in the design or recruitment of the study.

Inclusion criteria

All multiple trauma patients over the age of 18 who were admitted to the GICU for more than 24 h were considered eligible for inclusion in the study.

Exclusion criteria

Patients who stayed in the GICU for less than 24 h were excluded from the study. Also, anuric patients on admission to the GICU as well as patients previously known to have chronic renal failure or kidney disease were excluded from the study. Lastly, patients were excluded if their medical record data were incomplete.

Variables and measurements

The following data were collected: demographic data (age, gender, weight); minute-to-minute UFR (see below; urine output per hour; total fluid balance per hour; heart rate; arterial blood pressure; body temperature; central venous pressure (CVP); arterial blood pH and lactate and bicarbonate levels, serum urea, creatinine, sodium and chloride levels; hemoglobin level; admission trauma diagnosis; and the APACHE-II score on admission to the ICU. Clinical data was collected for the first 6 h of ICU stay. Data on significant therapeutic measures (administration of intravenous fluids, blood products, and vasopressors) and clinical parameters (vital signs) were collected for the first 6 h of the patients' ICU stay.

Scores

Severity of critical illness and multiorgan failure were evaluated by the APACHE II (Acute Physiology and Chronic Health Evaluation II) score within 24 h of admission to the GICU.

URINFO2000™ (FlowSense Medical, Misgav, Israel)

All multiple trauma patients admitted to the GICU underwent insertion of a Foley catheter which was routinely connected to a URINFO 2000™ device. URINFO 2000™ (FlowSense Medical, Misgav, Israel) is a novel urine collecting and urine flow measurement system that uses an optical drop detector to measure urine flow every 3 min through a measuring chamber. The detector enables the reliable calculation of the UFR at varying flow rates and urine osmolarities. The system was connected to the computerized patients' record system of the GICU.

UFR variability

The minute-to-minute UFR variability was defined and calculated as the variance of UFR changes from minute to minute [7]. The URINFO 2000™ (Flow Sense Medical, Misgav, Israel) is a novel urine collecting and urine flow measurement system that uses an optical drop detector to measure urine flow every 3 min through a measuring chamber. The difference between two consecutive values (total 6 min), divided by the first value, multiplied by 100. The result of the formula represents the percentage of change from the measured value every 3 min.

Study groups

The patients were divided into two study groups. Group 1 consisted of 29 multiple trauma patients and who were consequently deemed hemodynamically stable on admission to ICU (systolic blood pressure (SBP) was greater than 90 mmHg, mean arterial pressure more than 65 mmHg, central venous pressure more than 8 cmH_2O) on admission to the ICU. Group 2 consisted of 30 patients and who regarded as hemodynamically unstable (SBP was less than 90 mmHg, mean arterial pressure less than 65 mmHg, central venous pressure less than 8 cmH_2O, elevated blood lactate level) at admission to the ICU.

Statistical analysis

The two study groups ("compromised" and "uncompromised") were compared for UFR variability which was the primary parameter under study.

The patients' characteristics and outcomes were compared using chi-square or Fisher's exact tests for categorical variables. Continuous variables were analyzed with a Student's t test or the Mann-Whitney Test, depending on the validity of the normality assumption.

For comparison of minute-to-minute urine rate variability, the coefficient of variation was calculated and analyzed with a Student's t test. The Pearson method was used to analyze statistical correlation between different vital parameters.

Dynamic changes of UFR variability during the first 6 h of ICU stay were demonstrated by the LOESS curves non-parametric regression method. A p value of less than 0.05 represents a statistically significant finding. Statistical analyses were performed using IBM SPSS Statistics 20 (IBM Corp.).

Results

Initially, the clinical and laboratory data of 120 critically ill multiple trauma patients admitted to the ICU during the study period were analyzed. Of these, 59 patients were eventually included in the study (Table 1).The remaining 61 patients were excluded on the basis of the exclusion criteria (of them, 30 patients were oligo-anuric on admission to ICU have chronic renal failure or kidney disease or had previously documented chronic renal failure or kidney disease, 9 patients had incomplete medical record data and 22 patients were hospitalized in our ICU less than 24 h). The patients' epidemiological and clinical characteristics are summarized in Table 1. The two groups ("uncompromised" and "compromised") were similar in age, gender, weight, APACHE score, and length of ICU stay.

The patients in group 2 had significantly lower systemic and mean arterial pressures and higher heart rates on admission to the ICU compared to the patients in group 1 ($p < 0.001$, Table 2).

The UO and the UFR variability during the first 6 h of the patients' ICU stay were significantly lower in the group 2 patients than in the group 1 patients ($p < 0.001$ and 0.006 respectively).

The CVP and arterial blood pH were also significantly lower in the group 2 patients than in the group 1 patients ($p < 0.001$; Table 3). The laboratory parameters and body temperatures of the patients in both groups were similar during the first 6 h of their ICU stay (Table 3).

Statistical analysis by the Pearson method demonstrated strong direct correlation between decreased UFR variability and the following parameters: decreased urine output per hour ($R = 0.17$; $p = 0.009$); decreased mean arterial blood pressure (MAP) ($R = 0.24$, $p = 0.001$); and increased heart rate ($R = 0.205$, $p = 0.001$). No correlation with systolic blood pressure ($R = 0.11$, $p = 0.073$).

The dynamic changes in UFR variability are graphically presented in Fig. 1. In contrast to the wide UFR variability found in the group 1 (uncompromised) patients, we demonstrated a significant trend towards decreased UFR variability in the group 2 (compromised) patients during the first 6 h of their ICU stay (Fig. 1).

Discussion

The American College of Surgeons Committee on Trauma guidelines define hypotension as a systolic blood pressure (SBP) of less than 90 mmHg [1]. This threshold is often used as a marker of hemodynamic instability in adult patients with multiple trauma [8–10]. The cornerstone of appropriate management of multiple trauma patients is the early evaluation of their hemodynamic status to detect potential hemorrhage or subacute ("occult") hypoperfusion [11–13]. The initial assessment of these patients and decisions regarding further administration of resuscitatory fluid or blood products are accomplished by monitoring the patients' vital signs, especially blood pressure, heart rate, and urine output. However, there are cases in which the clinical picture is difficult to interpret because of the presence of pain, hyper/hypothermia, neurogenic or cardiogenic shock, or other factors [14]. An ideal monitoring device for such patients would be noninvasive, small in size, transportable, and easy to use and understand. It should be able to provide early assessment of even a very minor degree of hypoperfusion and as well as information on the adequacy of blood volume resuscitation [15].

Optimal and adequate treatment of hypoperfusion is crucial in preventing the development of reperfusion injury, the systemic inflammatory response syndrome (SIRS) and further progression to irreversible multiple organ failure [11]. Despite "normalization of vital signs", including maintenance of a urine output of 0.5–1 cm^3/kg/h, occult hypoperfusion can still be present in multiple trauma patients [11–13]. In the last two decades, a large variety of noninvasive continuous hemodynamic monitoring devices have been introduced into trauma centers

Table 1 Patients' demographic data, clinical outcome and underlying condition

	Group 1 ($n = 29$)	Group 2 ($n = 30$)	p value (95%CI)*
Age, years (mean ± SD)	35.34 ± 11.71	36.66 ± 13.27	0.68
Male gender (%)	27 (93.1)	26 (86.7)	0.67
Weight, kg (mean ± SD)	76.65 ± 14.75	70.4 ± 12.32	0.72
APACHE II, units (mean ± SD)	24 (24–27.5)	24.5 (22–27.25)	0.41
ICU stay, days (mean ± SD)	7.3 ± 2.9	7.91 ± 1.8	0.2

*P values less than 0.05 considered to be statistically significant

Table 2 Vital signs (mean ± SD)

	Group 1 (*n* = 29)	Group 2 (*n* = 30)	*p* value (95%CI)*
Systolic blood pressure (SBP) (mmHg)[a]	121.58 ± 21.2	82.6 ± 5.28	< 0.001
Mean arterial blood pressure (MAP) (mmHg)[a]	81.13 ± 16.32	55.33 ± 5.59	< 0.001
Heart rate (beat/min)[a]	100.78 ± 1.80	118.86 ± 23.71	< 0.001
Urine output per hour (ml)[b]	151.75 ± 29.22	63.58 ± 3.04	< 0.001
Urine flow rate variability (mean, ml)[b]	4.29 ± 1.3	3.78 ± 1.46	0.006

*P values less than 0.05 considered to be statistically significant
[a]Vital signs at admission to ICU (mean ± SD)
[b]Mean of urine output and urine flow rate variability per hour during first 6 h of ICU stay

worldwide. However, UO is the single important clinical parameter that is not monitored electronically in most centers. Early recognition of renal dysfunction in multiple trauma patients is extremely important in the prevention of further kidney injury, a complication which often adversely affects the clinical outcome [16]. In recent years, Urinfo, a new digital continuous minute-to-minute UFR monitoring device (URINFO™, FlowSense Medical, Misgav, Israel) has been shown to be significantly superior to manual nurse-handled urinometers in terms of accuracy of measurement, ease of handling, and staff satisfaction [4].

In a previous study, Shamir et al. [6] described the successful use of continuous minute-to-minute UFR monitoring in 11 patients who underwent elective spine surgery. They demonstrated that the kidneys show rhythmic variation in the minute-to-minute UFR, a phenomenon which is probably mediated by pacemaker activity located in the proximal portion of the upper urinary tract and influenced by prostaglandins and sensory nerves [17]. A decrease in the variability of the minute-to-minute UFR was an early sign of bleeding or hypovolemia in these previously healthy patients during their elective spinal surgical procedures [6]. Moreover, these authors [6] showed that the UFR variability not only decreased during the bleeding process but also returned to baseline after rehydration. In animal models, Klein et al. [7] demonstrated a strong correlation between the decrease in URF variability and the onset of hypovolemia induced by controlled bleeding.

In the present study, we analyzed clinical data describing minute-to-minute UFR and urine flow variability in multiple trauma patients. We found a significant decrease in minute-to-minute UFR and urine flow variability in multiple trauma patients who presented to the ICU with hemodynamic compromise (SBP less than 90 mmHg) compared to trauma patients who were hemodynamically normal. In both study groups, minute-to-minute UFR and urine flow variability decreased during the first 6 h of ICU admission in parallel with decreases in SBP and MAP and increases in heart rate and arterial blood lactate levels. Importantly, trauma patients in both study groups had an "adequate" (about 1 cm^3/kg/h) urine output. We found a strong clinical correlation between decreased UFR variability and decreased urine output per hour, decreased mean arterial pressure and increased heart rate in the group 2 (unstable) trauma patients. Thus, the minute-to-minute UFR/urine flow variability as a continuous, sensitive measurement has a significant clinical advantage and superior to other vital parameters as an early diagnosis of hypovolemia in multiple trauma patients.

Our study has a number of limitations. The main limitations are its retrospective design and the small number of patients included in the study. Also, there is no sample size calculation. Furthermore, because our study is retrospective, the influence of directed, active control of SBP on the minute-to-minute UFR, and urine flow variability could not be estimated or taken into account.

Finally, it seems that low minute-to-minute UFR variability correlate with hypovolemia and that means it occur in opposite. Future investigations in a new prospective

Table 3 Clinical and laboratory data of study group patients (mean ± SD)

	Group 1 (*n* = 29)	Group 2 (*n* = 30)	*p* value (95%CI)*
Hemoglobin (g\dL)	11.91 ± 2.04	11.36 ± 2.0	0.31
Serum sodium (mmol/L)	137.03 ± 3.26	137.93 ± 2.56	0.24
Serum chloride (mmol/L)	106.2 ± 4.44	106.56 ± 4.51	0.76
Arterial blood pH	7.33 ± 0.05	7.24 ± 0.07	< 0.001*
Arterial blood bicarbonate (mmol/L)	22.45 ± 2.31	20.54 ± 2.31	0.002
Arterial blood lactate (mmol/L)	1.77 ± 0.88	2.41 ± 1.06	0.015
CVP (mmHg)	10.03 ± 1.76	2.26 ± 1.59	< 0.001
Body temperature (°C)	36.63 ± 0.63	35.53 ± 0.82	0.09

*P values less than 0.05 considered to be statistically significant

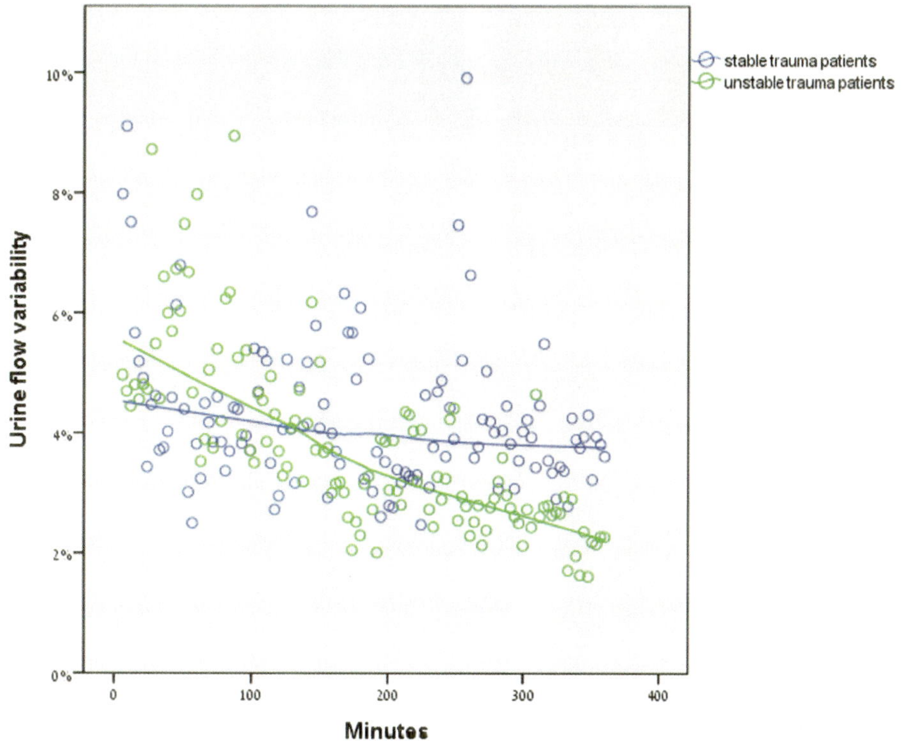

Fig. 1 Dynamic changes in urine flow rate variability during the first 6 h of ICU stay. (Variability and time) (Note: blue—group 1 [compromised trauma patients]; green—group 2 [uncompromised trauma patients])

design setup with control of all resuscitative parameters need to be provided to clarify that.

Conclusions

We suggest that UFR variability can serve as a reliable incipient marker of occult hypovolemia and also as an indicator of the end-point of blood volume resuscitation. We therefore propose that it should be one of the parameters used to monitor the hemodynamic status of critically ill multiple trauma patients. Furthermore, in view of our findings, we suggest that more comprehensive randomized and prospective studies should be undertaken to evaluate the potential clinical role of UFR variability and its influence on the ICU outcome of multiple trauma patients.

Abbreviation

UFR: Urine flow rate

Acknowledgements

There are no acknowledgements.

Funding

This research did not receive any specific grant from any funding agency in the public, commercial or not-for-profit sectors.

Authors' contributions

Dr. EB participated in study design, data collection, data analysis, data interpretation, writing. Dr. YK participated in literature search, study design, data collection, data analysis, data interpretation. Dr. RT participated in data collection, performed the statistical analysis, data interpretation. Dr. LK participated in the design of the study, performed the statistical analysis and helped to revise the manuscript. Dr. DF participated in the design of the study, performed the statistical analysis and helped to revise the manuscript. Dr. MYS participated in the sequence alignment and drafted the manuscript. Dr. MK participated in the design of the study, coordination and helped to draft the manuscript. All authors read and approved the manuscript. The manuscript has not been submitted to more than one journal for simultaneous consideration.

Competing interests

The authors declare that they have no competing interests.

Author details

[1]Trauma unit, Sheba Medical Center, Tel Aviv University, Tel Aviv, Israel. [2]Department of Anesthesiology and Critical Care, General Intensive Care Unit, Soroka Medical Center, Ben-Gurion University of the Negev, Beer Sheva, Israel. [3]Clinical Research Center, Soroka Medical Center, Ben-Gurion University of the Negev, Beer Sheva, Israel. [4]Department of Anesthesiology, Hadassah-Hebrew University Medical Center, Jerusalem, Israel.

References

1. Committee on Trauma, American College of Surgeons. ATLS: advanced trauma life support program for doctors. 8th ed. Chicago: American College of Surgeons; 2008.
2. Søreide E, Deakin CD. Pre-hospital fluid therapy in the critically injured patient-a clinical update. Injury. Int J Care Injured. 2005;36:1001–10.
3. Shackelford SA, Colton K, Stansbury LG, Galvagno SM, Anazodo AN, DuBose JJ, et al. Early identification of uncontrolled hemorrhage after trauma: current status and future direction. J Trauma Acute Care Surg. 2014;77:222–7.
4. Hersch M, Einav S, Izbicki G. Accuracy and ease of use of a novel electronic urine output-monitoring device compared with standard manual urinometer in the intensive care unit. J Crit Care. 2009;24(629):13–7.
5. Gutierrez G, Reines HD, Wulf-Gutierrez ME. Clinical review: hemorrhagic shock. Crit Care. 2004;8:373–81.
6. Shamir MY. MD, Kaplan L., Marans R.S., Willner D., Klein Y. Urine flow is a novel hemodynamic monitoring tool for the detection of Hypovolemia. Anesth Analg. 2011;112:593–6.
7. Klein Y, Grinstein M, Cohn SM, Silverman J, Klein M, Kashtan H, et al. Minute-to-minute urine flow rate variability: a new renal physiology variable. Anesth Analg. 2012;115:843–7.
8. Parks JK, Elliott AC, Gentilello LM, Shafi S. Systemic hypotension is a late marker of shock after trauma: a validation study of advanced trauma life support principles in a large national sample. Am J Surg. 2006;192:727–31.
9. American College of Surgeons Committee on Trauma. FAQ for resources for optimal Care of the Injured Patient: 2006. Chicago, IL: American College of Surgeons; 2006. Available at: www.facs.org/trauma/faq_answers.html. Accessed May 20, 2008
10. Wiencek RG, Wilson RF, Demaeo P. Outcome of trauma patients who present to the operating room with hypotension. Am Surg. 1989;55:338–42.
11. Schulman AM, Claridge JA, Carr G, Diesen DL, Young JS. Predictors of patients who will develop prolonged occult Hypoperfusion following blunt trauma. J Trauma. 2004;57:795–800.
12. Drucker W, Pearce F, Glass-Heidenreich L, et al. Subcutaneous tissue oxygen pressure: a reliable index of peripheral perfusion in humans after injury. J Trauma. 1996;40:116–22.
13. Moore FA, Haenel JB, Moore EE, Whitehill TA. Incommensurate oxygen consumption in response to maximal oxygen availability predicts postinjury multiple organ failure. J Trauma. 1992;33:58–65.
14. Kuster M, Exadaktylos A, Schnürige B. Non-invasive hemodynamic monitoring in trauma patients. World J Emerg Surg. 2015;10:11.
15. Moore FA, McKinley BA, Moore EE. The next generation in shock resuscitation. Lancet. 2004;363:1988–96.
16. Costantini TW, Fraga G, Fortlage D, Wynn S, Fraga A, Lee J, et al. Redefining renal dysfunction in trauma: implementation of the acute kidney injury network staging system. J Trauma. 2009;67:283–8.
17. Weiss RM, Tamarkin FJ, Wheeler MA, M.A. Pacemaker activity in the upper urinary tract. J Smooth Muscle Res. 2006;42(4):103–15.

Role of intraoperative cholangiography for detecting residual stones after biliary pancreatitis: still useful?

Abdelrahman Abdelaal[1], Moamena El-Matbouly[1], Ibnouf Sulieman[1], Ahmad Elfaki[1], Tamer El-Bakary[1], Sherif Abdelaziem[1], Salahdin Gehani[1], Adriana Toro[2] and Isidoro Di Carlo[1,3*]

Abstract

Background: Intraoperative cholangiography (IOC) may detect residual stones in the common bile duct (CBD) after acute biliary pancreatitis (ABP). The aim of the present study is to analyze the utility of IOC in detecting residual stones in patients undergoing cholecystectomy for ABP and if complications are related with this procedure.

Methods: Demographic and clinical factors were assessed in patients with mild ABP who underwent IOC during laparoscopic cholecystectomy. Factors assessed included preoperative size of the CBD on ultrasonography, presence of stones in the gallbladder and the CBD, and IOC results. For the statistical analysis, χ^2 or Fisher's exact tests to compare proportions and the nonparametric Mann–Whitney *U* test for analysis of values with abnormal distribution were used.

Results: The study included 113 patients, 82 males (72.6%) and 31 females (27.4%), of mean age 46.9 ± 14.7 years (range 18–86 years). All preoperative laboratory indicators were elevated. The group of the patients with stones in the CBD diagnosed by IOC was divided in patients with diameters <0.8 mm and with diameters ≥0.8 mm of the CBD diagnosed preoperatively with ultrasound. The laboratory tests do not demonstrate difference statistically significative between these two groups. The group of the patients without stones in the CBD diagnosed by IOC was also divided in patients with diameters <0.8 mm and with diameters ≥0.8 mm of the CBD. Also in these two groups, the statistical analysis of the laboratory tests does not demonstrate significative difference. Most procedures were performed by specialists (64.6%), and all patients underwent IOC. IOC showed stones in 84/113 patients (74.3%). A comparison of patients with and without stones at IOC showed similar mean times from hospitalization to surgery (5.9 days [range 2–12 days] vs. 6.1 days [range 2–23 days]), from surgery until hospital discharge (2.0 days [range 0–4 days] vs. 2.2 days [range 0–11 days]), and overall length of stay (7.9 days [range 3–19 days] vs. 8.3 days [range 3–23 days]) ($P > 0.001$).

Conclusions: IOC is useful to diagnose residual CBD stones, without increasing complications related to the procedure itself.

Keywords: Acute biliary pancreatitis, Intraoperative cholangiography, Common bile duct, Laparoscopic cholecystectomy, Intraoperative common bile duct exploration

* Correspondence: idicarlo@unict.it
[1]Department of General Surgery, Hamad General Hospital, Al Rayyan Road, 3050 Doha, Qatar
[3]Department of Surgical Sciences and Advanced Technologies "G.F. Ingrassia", University of Catania, Via Santa Sofia 78, 95100 Catania, Italy
Full list of author information is available at the end of the article

Background

One of the consequences of gallbladder stones is acute biliary pancreatitis (ABP), present worldwide in 40% of patients diagnosed with pancreatitis [1]. Mild ABP, defined when 2 of the 3 criteria (clinical, laboratory, or imaging) are present, is caused by passage of the stones from the gallbladder to the common bile duct (CBD) [2], by obstruction of the ampulla of Vater, and by the reflux of bile in the pancreatic duct [1]. Most stones are small and pass spontaneously without further clinical consequences. However, stones that persist in the CBD can result in severe complications

Laparoscopic cholecystectomy (LC) is the technique of choice for removing gallbladder stones, but its timing is unclear. Performing LC 6 to 8 weeks after the onset of ABP may reduce both acute inflammation and the conversion rate [3]. In contrast, performing LC 48 h after hospital admission may reduce morbidity rates and hospital expenses [4].

As stones may persist in the CBD after ABP, intraoperative cholangiography (IOC) may be performed during LC to detect these stones [5]. This may allow their removal by CBD exploration or by intra- or postoperative endoscopic retrograde cholangiopancreatography (ERCP) [2]. In many studies, however, IOC has failed to detect stones, suggesting that IOC may not be useful in these patients. Thus, there is little evidence that IOC may be useful to diagnosis residual CBD stones, despite the guidelines recommending the routine performance of IOC in patients undergoing LC after ABP [2]. The aim of the present study is to analyze the utility of IOC in detecting residual stones in patients undergoing cholecystectomy for ABP and if complications are related with this procedure.

Methods

This retrospective study included patients with mild ABP who underwent LC and IOC for residual stones, at the Department of Surgery of Hamad General Hospital, Doha, Qatar, over a 5-year period from 2010 to 2015. The demographic and clinical characteristics of these patients, including age, sex, nationality, abdominal pain, jaundice, fever, and chills before or during admission were recorded. Laboratory tests include preoperative serum concentrations of total bilirubin, alkaline phosphatase (ALP), aspartate aminotransferase (AST), alanine aminotransferase (ALT), gamma glutamyltransferase (GGT), amylase, and lipase were recorded. Only for laboratory tests, median and 25°–75° percentiles were considered for statistical analysis.

Other factors analyzed at preoperative ultrasonography were CBD size (diameters >0.8 mm was considered as dilated) and the presence of gallbladder stones and/or stones in the CBD.

Operative factors included the status of the surgeon (i.e., consultant, specialist, resident), conversion to open surgery, and the presence of stones diagnosed during IOC. Patients who underwent transcystic exploration were evaluated, including the number of stones retrieved and conversion to open surgery.

In-hospital parameters included the number of days from hospitalization to surgery, the number of days from surgery until discharge, and the total length of stay (LOS). Factors were compared in groups of patients with and without stones on IOC and with and without preoperative dilatation of the CBD.

Finally, complications have been considered.

χ^2 or Fisher's exact tests to compare proportions and nonparametric Mann–Whitney U test for analysis of values with a non normal distribution were used for statistical analysis.

Results

Although 268 patients underwent LC for ABP during the study period, complete data were available for only 113 patients. These patients included 82 males (72.6%) and 31 females (27.4%), of mean age 46.9 ± 14.7 years (range 18–86 years). Of these 113 patients, 14 (12.4%) were native Qataris and 99 (87.6%) were natives of other countries.

One hundred twelve patients (99.1%) presented abdominal pain, 19 patients (16.8%) jaundice, 11 patients (9.7%) fever, and 5 patients (4.4%) chills the day before admission.

During clinical examination, 9 patients (8.0%) present fever, 33 patients (29.2%) jaundice, and 90 patients (79.6%) abdominal pain.

These patients had a median total bilirubin concentration of 40.5 (18.9–71.2) mmol/L, a median ALP concentration of 153 (102.0–223.0), a median AST concentration of 174 (82.0–287.0) U/L, a median ALT concentration of 265 (137.3–387.0) U/L, a median amylase concentration of 1095.0 (375.0–2231.0) U/L, and a median lipase concentration of 3109.0 (905.5–47.38.0) U/L. Comparisons of these laboratory tests in patients with and without stones in CBD diagnosed by IOC showed that all median concentrations were higher in patients with those without stones in CBD (Table 1). But no significant differences ($P > 0.001$) between sex, nationality, abdominal pain, fever, jaundice, and chills reported by the patients or identified with clinical examinations were recorded in these two groups.

The group of the patients with stones in the CBD diagnosed by IOC was divided in patients with diameters <0.8 mm and with diameters ≥0.8 mm of the CBD diagnosed preoperatively with ultrasound (US). The laboratory tests reported in Table 2 do not demonstrate difference statistically significative between these two groups.

Table 1 Preoperative serum markers in patients with and without CBD stones intraoperatively diagnosed by IOC

ICO	Without stones CBD (29 patients)				With stones CBD (84 patients)				
	Normal value	Increased value	Median	Percentiles (25°–75°)	Normal value	Increased value	Median	Percentiles (25°–75°)	P
Total bilirubin 3.4–20.5 mmol/L	12	17	30.6	13.3–56.5	16	68	42.9	24.1–129.5	$P > 0.001$
ALP 40–150 U/L	9	20	158	104.5–223.0	31	53	152.5	101.5–229.3	$P > 0.001$
AST 5–34 U/L	1	28	157	62.0–280.0	6	78	181.5	93.3–291.5	$P > 0.001$
ALT 0–55 U/L	4	25	251	80.5–334.0	8	76	273.5	155–400.5	$P > 0.001$
Amylase 30–100 U/L	1	28	867	265.5–2173.0	4	80	1261.0	479.5–2397.3	$P > 0.001$
Lipase 23–300 U/L	4	25	2832	1365.5–4778.5	11	73	3223.0	800.5–4769.3	$P > 0.001$

$P > 0.001$: not significative

The group of the patients without stones in the CBD diagnosed by IOC was also divided in patients with diameters <0.8 mm and with diameters ≥0.8 mm of the CBD. Also in these two groups, the statistical analysis of the laboratory tests reported in Table 3 does not demonstrate significative difference.

Surgical procedures were performed in 33 patients (29.2%) by consultants, in 73 (64.6%) by specialists, and in 7 (6.2%) by residents. None of these 113 patients required conversion to open surgery. IOC showed stones in 84/113 patients (74.3%).

Nine patients (10.7%) on 84 with CBD stones diagnosed by IOC underwent transcystic exploration. Eight patients have their stones retrieved, using Dormia basket with multiple attempts. The clearance of the CBD has been checked using IOC. Other patients were referred to a gastroenterologist for postoperative ERCP. All explorations of the CBD were performed by consultants.

The mean time from hospitalization to surgery was 5.9 days, the mean time from surgery until hospital discharge was 2.1 days, and the mean LOS was 8.0 days. A comparison of patients with and without stones at IOC showed similar mean times from hospitalization to surgery (5.9 days [range 2–12 days] vs. 6.1 days [range 2–23 days]), from surgery until hospital discharge (2.0 days [range 0–4 days] vs. 2.2 days [range 0–11 days]), and overall length of stay (7.9 days [range 3–19 days] vs. 8.3 days [range 3–23 days]) (Table 4). Similar results were observed in patients with and without preoperative dilatation of the CBD. No statistically significant differences were identified in any group ($P > 0.001$)

No complications have been recorded.

Discussion

Gallbladder stones were first correlated with ABP in 1901 [6], with this correlation later confirmed [7]. Between 3 and 7% of patients with gallbladder stones develop pancreatitis [7], especially due to passage of a small calculus (<5 mm). According to the "migratory stone" theory, 63–75% of patients with ABP develop CBD stones within 48 h of admission [7]. Similarly, we observed that 74.3% of patients retained stones at surgery. The mean time from admission to surgery in our study was about 5 days, due to the clinical conditions of the patients and to the long daily waiting list in our hospital. Following the acute episode of pancreatitis, however, only 5% of patients retained stones in the CBD [4, 7].

Table 2 Preoperative serum markers in patients with CBD stones on IOC with and without CBD dilatation on preoperative US

ICO	Patients with stones in CBD								
Preoperative US	CBD <0.8 mm (35 patients)				CBD ≥0.8 mm (49 patients)				
	Normal value	Increased value	Median	Percentiles (25°–75°)	Normal value	Increased value	Median	Percentiles (25°–75°)	P
Total bilirubin 3.4–20.5 mmol/L	9	26	31.9	16.1–69.9	8	41	53.0	30.0–88.5	$P > 0.001$
ALP 40–150 U/L	20	15	139.0	101.0–193.0	20	29	173.0	104.0–280.5	$P > 0.001$
AST 5–34 U/L	2	33	162.0	62.0–263.0	3	46	187.0	103.5–368.0	$P > 0.001$
ALT 0–55 U/L	3	32	244.0	141.0–384.0	3	46	280.0	170.0–440.5	$P > 0.001$
Amylase 30–100 U/L	0	35	819.0	276.0–2647.0	3	46	1390.0	490.0–2283.5	$P > 0.001$
Lipase 23–300 U/L	4	31	1438.0	763.0–4899.0	8	41	3563.0	974.5–4211.5	$P > 0.001$

$P > 0.001$: not significative

Table 3 Preoperative serum markers in patients without CBD stones on IOC with and without CBD dilatation on preoperative US

ICO	Patients without stones in CBD								
Preoperative US	CBD <0.8 mm (7 patients)				CBD ≥0.8 mm (22 patients)				
	Normal value	Increased value	Median	Percentiles (25°–75°)	Normal value	Increased value	Median	Percentiles (25°–75°)	*P*
Total bilirubin 3.4–20.5 mmol/L	1	6	58.8	31.5–118.0	10	12	23.5	12.8–41.1	$P > 0.001$
ALP 40–150 U/L	3	4	158.0	66.0–479.0	11	11	158.0	94.0–176.0	$P > 0.001$
AST 5–34 U/L	1	6	157.0	126.0–212.0	1	21	155.5	57.5–292.3	$P > 0.001$
ALT 0–55 U/L	1	6	273.0	148.0–554.0	5	17	152.5	68.5–319.5	$P > 0.001$
Amylase 30–100 U/L	0	7	1013.0	572.0–2229.0	1	21	662.5	232.8–2146.0	$P > 0.001$
Lipase 23–300 U/L	0	7	3049.0	1514.0–4909.0	3	19	2427.0	1072.8–4819.6	$P > 0.001$

$P > 0.001$: not significative

Stones in the CBD have been observed in patients after ABP and in patients who have never experienced ABP. The latter represents about 4.6% of all patients who undergo LC; in one-third of these patients, stones spontaneously pass 6 weeks after cholecystectomy [8]. However, a small percentage of patients who have retained their stones in the CBD may develop severe complications.

The mean age of our patients was 46 ± 14.7 years, within the range of 37–58 years reported in earlier studies of patients undergoing cholecystectomy for ABP [9]. Although this condition has been reported to occur more frequently in women [7], we observed a male predominance, perhaps due to the admission to our country of many male workers.

The management of ABP has changed, from delayed surgery to immediate cholecystectomy. Following the resolution of pancreatitis to prevent its recurrence or other related complications, including choledocholithiasis and cholangitis, early removal of the gallbladder has been recommended [10]. Patients affected by ABP are at a 30-fold higher risk of a second attack of pancreatitis than the normal population [11]. Surprisingly, however, a longer preoperative interval has been associated with both an increased risk of ABP recurrence and a reduced risk of finding retained stones in the CBD. The likelihood of finding stones in the CBD was found to be 70% at admission, decreasing to 20% after 4 days [12]. Similarly, only 25.6% of our patients presented with stones at the time of surgery. As spontaneous stone migration in most patients is affected by pancreatitis, assessment of the CBD may be unnecessary, with ERCP performed in patients with biliary obstruction or cholangitis and total bilirubin >5 mg/ml not resolving spontaneously [11].

Early LC after ABP is defined as being performed within 1 week of admission and is currently considered the standard of treatment [8, 9]. Many patients discharged after the first episode of ABP who later undergo surgery can experience gallstone-related events (including recurrent ABP), have a prolonged length of stay, and may have adverse postoperative outcomes [13, 14].

Most of our patients underwent LC within 1 week after an episode of ABP, but some did not undergo surgery until 3 weeks after admission. Although 1 week is considered optimal, none of our patients who underwent LC after 3 weeks experienced recurrence, suggesting that the timing of the surgical procedure can be extended. Future studies are needed to determine the maximum length of this extension period.

Table 4 Times from hospital admission to surgery, from surgery to discharge, and from admission to discharge

ICO	Patients without stones in CBD (29 patients)			Patients with stones in CBD (84 patients)		
US	CBD <0.8 mm (7 patients)	CBD ≥0.8 mm (22 patients)	*P*	CBD <0.8 mm (35 patients)	CBD ≥0.8 mm (49 patients)	*P*
Days of length of hospital stay	7.1 (range 5–9 days)	9.1 (range 5–9 days)	$P > 0.001$	7.2 (range 5–9 days)	9.8 (range 5–9 days)	$P > 0.001$
Days from admission to surgery	5.4 (range 5–9 days)	6.7 (range 5–9 days)	$P > 0.001$	5.5 (range 5–9 days)	6.7 (range 5–9 days)	$P > 0.001$
Days after surgery	1.8 (range 5–9 days)	2.5 (range 5–9 days)	$P > 0.001$	1.7 (range 5–9 days)	3.1 (range 5–9 days)	$P > 0.001$

$P > 0.001$: not significative

The efficacy of IOC during cholecystectomy in patients previously affected by ABP is unclear. An intraoperative cholangiogram is usually recommended during LC to detect any retained stones that can be extracted by CBD exploration or by ERCP [9]. However, the usefulness of this procedure has not been determined.

IOC, first described in 1931 [15], is based on cannulation of the cystic duct to visualize the bile duct and has allowed the identification of bile duct stones. IOC can also enable the visualization of anatomic abnormalities, as well as the recognition of very early injuries to the CBD that can occur during surgery. Although the use of IOC is based on surgeon experience and overall preferences, no standardized criteria exist to date [16].

The time required for routine IOC has been reported to range from 8 to 20 min [17] and to depend on the availability of local resources. Other factors associated with the efficacy of routine IOC include the expertise of the specialist who analyzes the data, the exposure to radiation of persons in the operating room, and the cost of the procedure, which can vary from 100 to 700 US dollars [18]. Stone extraction can increase costs, especially if stones are expected to migrate spontaneously.

The success rate of stone extraction has been reported to range from 86–94% [19]. Failures have been reported to result from technical difficulties, especially cannulation of the cystic duct. The sensitivity and specificity of this procedure range between 93%–99%. False-positive results due to air bubbles are inevitable and can affect up to 35% of patients [20].

Postoperative stay has been reported longer in patients who did than did not undergo IOC, although the percentages of patients with retained stones in the CBD following surgery were similar (5.1 vs. 2.8%) [21]. A systematic review of six studies that included 1715 patients at low risk for choledocholithiasis randomized to undergo or not undergo IOC and followed up for 1–8 years found retained stones in only five patients, with no difference in outcomes between the two groups

All patients in our study underwent IOC, but hospitalization times did not differ in the groups of patients with and without stones. Eight patients with stones at IOC underwent stone retrieval during the laparoscopic procedure, but their postoperative LOS was similar to that in patients with stones who were not treated laparoscopically and patients without stones. A small difference in LOS was observed in patients with and without preoperatively dilated CBD (both with and without stones). The advantages of the patients submitted to the IOC, in which the stones have been diagnosed and retrieved, was to completely cure the disease at this step. Furthermore, the procedure does not have complications in relation to the group without IOC. Last, the procedure, when performed, helps young surgeons to familiarize with this intraoperative technique.

To avoid unnecessary IOC, many studies have attempted to identify preoperative factors associated with the need for IOC. Elevated bilirubin, ALP, and ALT concentrations, as well as bile duct dilatation, are considered indications for IOC in patients undergoing LC for ABP [22]. Transient increases in bilirubin, ALP, AST, and ALT concentrations can indicate papillary obstruction, due to the passage of sludge or gallstone or papillary edema. If these indicators fluctuate over a prolonged period, other methods are needed to determine the optimum time for cholecystectomy [23]. Routine intra-operative cholangiogram at the time of cholecystectomy for ABP may be unnecessary, especially if preoperative biochemical and imaging markers do not indicate an increased likelihood of CBD stones.

GGT and ALP concentrations are regarded as sensitive markers for the presence of stones in the CBD. Another study, however, reported that increases in bilirubin and ALP, as well as CBD dilatation, are not associated with abnormal cholangiograms [24]. We found that preoperative bilirubin, ALP, and GGT concentrations were similar in patients with and without stones on IOC.

A study of all patients who underwent cholecystectomy in Uppsala, Sweden, found that elevated ALP and bilirubin concentrations were the best predictors of CBD stone, but IOC yielded false positive (5%) and false negative (1%) results. Normal bilirubin and ALP levels in patients with CBD stones can be due to partial obstruction or migration of the stone before the surgical procedure. In contrast, elevated bilirubin and ALP levels in patients without CBD stones can be due to a secretory hepatic dysfunction, to a migration of stones in the duodenum, and to sludge or to CBD compression caused by other conditions [25].

Diagnosis of remnant stones in the CBD after ABP remains a challenge. Efforts to selectively manage patients with ABP, based on variables, including ultrasound findings and ALP, total bilirubin, and direct bilirubin concentrations, have attempted to identify patients requiring IOC [14]. Stratification was not possible, and the decision to perform IOC was based on the results of magnetic resonance cholangiopancreatography (MRCP). Endoscopic ultrasound can be considered to perform diagnosis of CBD stones, but is not available in all hospitals, and the results of MRCP can be comparable and more safe [26]. Another study reported that some patients positive on IOC were negative on postoperative ERCP, suggesting that IOC is unnecessary [24]. Moreover, only 2–3% of patients with markers indicative of CBD stones who did not undergo IOC were later admitted for CBD stones, again suggesting that IOC is unnecessary [8]. A recent study specifically assessing the impact of IOC on recurrent pancreatitis found that IOC did not improve the outcome after cholecystectomy for gallstone pancreatitis [10].

The limitations of the present work are the small number of the patients analyzed and that is a retrospective study.

Conclusions

IOC is useful to diagnose residual CBD stones, without increasing complications related to the procedure itself. Although not mandatory, IOC may be useful in patients who undergo LC after ABP. Future studies are required to well elucidate this problem.

Abbreviations

ALP: Alkaline phosphatase; ALT: Alanine aminotransferase; AST: Aspartate aminotransferase; ABP: Acute biliary pancreatitis; CBD: Common bile duct; ERCP: Endoscopic retrograde cholangiopancreatography; GGT: Gamma glutamyltransferase; IOC: Intraoperative cholangiography; LC: laparoscopic cholecystectomy; LOS: Length of stay; MRCP: Magnetic resonance cholangiopancreatography

Acknowledgements

Special thanks to Prof. Filippo Palermo University of Catania, Italy, for the statistical analysis.

Funding

None.

Authors' contributions

AA, AT, and IDC contributed to the study conception and design. IS, MEM, and SA contributed to the data acquisition. TEB, SG, and AT contributed to the data analysis and interpretation. AT contributed to the writing of the article. AA and IDC contributed to the editing, reviewing, and final approval of the article. All authors read and approved the final manuscript.

Competing interests

The authors declare that they have no competing interests.

Author details

[1]Department of General Surgery, Hamad General Hospital, Al Rayyan Road, 3050 Doha, Qatar. [2]Department of Surgery, Barone Romeo Hospital, via Mazzini 14, 98066 Patti, (ME), Italy. [3]Department of Surgical Sciences and Advanced Technologies "G.F. Ingrassia", University of Catania, Via Santa Sofia 78, 95100 Catania, Italy.

References

1. Frossard JL, Steer ML, Pastor CM. Acute pancreatitis. Lancet. 2008;37:143–52.
2. WORKING GROUP IAP/APA. IAP/APA evidence-based guidelines for the management of acute pancreatitis. Pancreatology. 2013;13:e1–e15.
3. Murphy PB, Paskar D, Parry NG, Racz J, Vogt KN, Symonette C, Leslie K, Mele TS. Implementation of an acute care surgery service facilitates modern clinical practice guidelines for gallstone pancreatitis. J Am Coll Surg. 2015; 221:975e981.
4. Kelly TR, Wagner DS. Gallstone pancreatitis: a prospective randomized trial of the timing of surgery. Surgery. 1988;104:600–5.
5. Singh G, Gupta PC, Sridar G, Natariya KR. Role of selective intra-operative cholangiography during cholecystectomy. ANZ J Surg. 2000;70:106–9.
6. Opie EL. The etiology of acute hemorrhagic pancreatitis. Bull Johns Hopkins Hosp. 1901;12:182–8.
7. Acosta JM, Ledesma CL. Gallstone migration as a cause of acute pancreatitis. N Engl J Med. 1974;290:484–7.
8. Collins C, Maguire D, Ireland A, Fitzgerald E, O'Sullivan GC. A prospective study of common bile duct calculi in patients undergoing laparoscopic cholecystectomy: natural history of choledocholithiasis revisited. Ann Surg. 2004;239:28–33.
9. Telem DA, Bowman K, Hwang J, Chin EH, Nguyen SQ, Divino CM. Selective management of patients with acute biliary pancreatitis. J Gastrointest Surg. 2009;13:2183–8.
10. Alimoglu O, Ozkan OV, Sahin M, Akcakaya A, Eryilmaz R, Bas G. Timing of cholecystectomy for acute biliary pancreatitis: outcomes of cholecystectomy on first admission and after recurrent biliary pancreatitis. World J Surg. 2003; 27:256–9.
11. Hernandez V, Pascual I, Almela P, Añon R, Herreros B, Sanchiz V, et al. Recurrence of acute gallstone pancreatitis and relationship with cholecystectomy or endoscopic sphincterotomy. Am J Gastroenterol. 2004; 99:2417–23.
12. Schwesinger WH, Page CP, Sirinek KR, Levine BA, Aust JB. Biliary pancreatitis. Operative outcome with a selective approach. Arch Surg. 1991;126:836–9. discussion 839–40.
13. Schwesinger WH, Page CP, Gross GW, Miller JE, Strodel WE, Sirinek KR. Biliary pancreatitis: the era of laparoscopic cholecystectomy. Arch Surg. 1998;133: 1103–6.
14. Ito K, Ito H, Tavakkolizadeh A, Whang EE. Is ductal evaluation always necessary before or during surgery for biliary pancreatitis? Am J Surg. 2008; 195:463–6.
15. Mirizzi PL, Quiroza LC. La exploracion de las vias biliares principals en el curso de la operacion. Proc Third Argent Cong Surg. 1931;1:694.
16. Cuschieri A, Shimi S, Banting S, Nathanson LK, Pietrabissa A. Intraoperative cholangiography during laparoscopic cholecystectomy. Routine vs selective policy. Surg Endosc. 1994;8:302–5.
17. Ludwig K, Bernhardt J, Steffen H, Lorenz D. Contribution of intraoperative cholangiography to incidence and outcome of common bile duct injuries during laparoscopic cholecystectomy. Surg Endosc. 2002;16:1098–104.
18. Buddingh KT, Nieuwenhuijs VB. The critical view of safety and routine intraoperative cholangiography complement each other as safety measures during cholecystectomy. J Gastrointest Surg. 2011;15:1069–70.
19. Strömberg C, Luo J, Enochsson L, Arnelo U, Nilsson M. Endoscopic sphincterotomy and risk of malignancy in the bile ducts, liver, and pancreas. Clin Gastroenterol Hepatol. 2008;6:1049–53.
20. Varadarajulu S, Eloubeidi MA, Wilcox CM, Hawes RH, Cotton PB. Do all patients with abnormal intraopeative cholangiogram merit endoscopic retrograde cholangiopancreatography? Surg Endosc. 2006;20:801–5.
21. Ford JA, Soop M, Du J, Loveday BP, Rodgers M. Systematic review of intraoperative cholangiography in cholecystectomy. Br J Surg. 2012;99:160–7.
22. Shiozawa S, Tsuchiya A, Kim DH, Usui T, Masuda T, Kubota K, et al. Useful predictive factors of common bile duct stones prior to laparoscopic cholecystectomy for gallstones. Hepatogastroenterology. 2005;52:1662–5.
23. Hallal AH, Amortegui JD, Jeroukhimov IM, Casillas J, Schulman CI, Manning RJ, et al. Magnetic resonance cholangiopancreatography accurately detects common bile duct stones in resolving gallstone pancreatitis. J Am Coll Surg. 2005;200:869–75.
24. Tabone LE, Sarker S, Fisichella PM, Conlon M, Fernando E, Yi S, et al. To 'gram or not'? Indications for intraoperative cholangiogram. Surgery. 2011; 150:810–9.
25. Videhult P, Sandblom G, Rudberg C, Rasmussen IC. Are liver function tests, pancreatitis and cholecystitis predictors of common bile duct stones? Results of a prospective, population-based, cohort study of 1171 patients undergoing cholecystectomy. HPB (Oxford). 2011;13:519–27.
26. Jeon TJ, Cho JH, Kim YS, Song SY, Park JY. Diagnostic value of endoscopic ultrasonography in symptomatic patients with high and intermediate probabilities of common bile duct stones and a negative computed tomography scan. Gut Liver. 2017;11:290–7.

Differentiation in an inclusive trauma system: allocation of lower extremity fractures

F. S. Würdemann[1,3*], D. P. J. Smeeing[2,3], S. Ferree[3], F. Nawijn[3], E. J. M. M. Verleisdonk[1], L. P. H. Leenen[3], R. M. Houwert[2,3] and F. Hietbrink[3]

Abstract

Background: Implementation of an inclusive trauma system leads to reduced mortality rates, specifically in polytrauma patients. Field triage is essential in this mortality reduction. Triage systems are developed to identify patients with life-threatening injuries, and trauma mechanisms are important for triaging. Although complex extremity fractures are mostly non-lethal, these injuries are frequently the result of a high-energy trauma mechanism. The aim of this study is to compare injury and patient characteristics, as well as resource demands, of lower extremity fractures between a level (L)1 and level (L)2 trauma centre in a mature inclusive trauma system.

Methods: This is a retrospective cohort study. Patients with below-the-knee joint fractures diagnosed in a L1 or L2 trauma centre between July 2013 and June 2015 were included. Main outcome parameters were patient demographics, trauma mechanism, fracture pattern, and resource demands.

Results: One thousand two hundred sixty-seven patients with 1517 lower extremity fractures were included. Most patients were treated in the L2 centre (L1 = 417; L2 = 859). Complex fractures were more frequently triaged to the L1 centre. Patients in the L1 centre had more concomitant injuries to other body regions and ipsi- or contralateral lower extremity. Patients in the L1 centre were more resource demanding: more surgeries (> 1 surgery; 24.9% L1 vs 1.4% L2), higher immediate admission rates (70.1% L1 vs 37.6% L2), and longer length of stay (mean 13.4 days L1 vs 3.1 days L2).

Conclusion: The majority of patients were treated in the L2 trauma centre, whereas complex lower extremity injuries were mostly treated in the L1 centre, which placed higher demand on resources and labour per patient. This change in allocation is the next step in centralization of low-volume high complex care and high-volume low complex care.

Keywords: Inclusive trauma system, Lower extremity fractures, Level 1, Level 2, Trauma centre, Resource demand, Maturation, Centralization, Triage

Background

Lower extremity injuries have a large impact on the functional outcome after trauma and are frequently seen in both high-energy trauma and polytrauma patients, where the impact of these fractures is even more evident [1–4]. Even more, complex injuries, defined by the severity of the sustained injuries or multiple fractures in the ipsilateral extremity, are important factors that determine long-term functional outcome [2, 5]. Complex extremity injuries might require a different approach compared to non-complex injuries. To optimize outcome in complex lower extremity fractures, 24/7 availability of emergency operating teams, timing of delayed reconstructions, and a multidisciplinary approach are deemed essential. On the other hand, fast tracks, elective procedures, and designated physicians might be factors for patient satisfaction in non-complex cases. Therefore, optimizing

* Correspondence: Franka.wurdemann@gmail.com
[1]Department of Surgery, Diakonessenhuis Utrecht, Utrecht, The Netherlands
[3]Department of Surgery, University Medical Center Utrecht, Heidelberglaan 100, 3584 CX Utrecht, The Netherlands
Full list of author information is available at the end of the article

the distribution of (lower) extremity fractures amongst trauma centres may be beneficial for both patients and trauma systems as a whole.

With improvements in trauma care and the implementation of inclusive trauma systems, mortality rates have declined over the past decades [6, 7]. Allocating patients to the hospital with the most appropriate level of care for their injuries is essential to ensure the best possible outcome and reduce mortality. This applies mostly to patients suffering severe injuries (i.e. polytrauma patients), which is frequently due to high-energy trauma mechanisms. Therefore, trauma mechanism is considered an important factor in field triage systems, in addition to key elements such as the number and severity of sustained injuries and vital signs. Allocation of polytrauma patients to a level 1 (L1) trauma centre is beneficial because of specialized care and in-hospital trauma pathways, as a result of the anticipated high demand on resources and labour intensity [6]. Conversely, less complex injuries tend to require non-urgent, or less urgent interventions, resulting in more efficient use of available resources. Therefore, these injuries are more suitable for treatment in a high-volume level 2–3 (L2) trauma centre.

The allocation of lower extremity fractures within a trauma system has not been described previously. However, volume-outcome relationships have been well established in recent literature [8–11]. Both super-specialisation and logistical arguments might guide differentiation of low complex cases to high-volume centres whilst high complex cases differentiate to specific care facilities such as L1 trauma centres. This is especially the case in a densely populated area with multiple hospitals within a short distance apart [9]. In a mature inclusive trauma system, patients with complex extremity fractures may be preferably allocated to a L1 trauma centre, while a larger number of patients overall may be allocated to a L2 centre. The aim of this study is to compare patients and resource demands of lower extremity fractures between a L1 and L2 trauma centre in a mature inclusive trauma system.

Methods

Setting

A multicentre retrospective cohort study was performed in a level 1 trauma centre hospital (L1) (University Medical Center Utrecht) and a level 2 trauma centre hospital (L2) (Diakonessenhuis Utrecht); both situated in the central region of the Netherlands. Trauma care in the Netherlands is divided into 11 trauma regions. In 2015, the central region covered more than 1.5 million inhabitants and consisted of one L1 trauma centre; the University Medical Center Utrecht (UMCU), plus five L2 hospitals and 12 outpatient clinics, all categorized according to the available resources. This is a mature inclusive trauma system as documented previously [8, 9, 11–13]. The distance between these L1 and L2 centres is 5 km maximum or a 10-min ambulance drive. The L1 has 8 trauma surgeons with 24/7 in-house coverage for initial resuscitation, surgery (general and orthopaedic), and intensive care consultancy. The L2 centre has 3 trauma surgeons on call during shift hours. At the L2 centre, initial resuscitation is delivered by an emergency physician during office hours and by a general surgery house officer during shift hours (5 PM—8 AM during weekdays, plus 24 h on weekends).

Field triage

The ambulance personnel in this region use the nationwide Dutch emergency service protocol to decide the designated level of trauma care [14]. Indications to transport trauma patients to a 1 trauma centre are compromised airway, breathing or circulation; a GCS < 9 or decreasing, anisocoric pupils; neurological deficits (to more than one extremity); and hypothermia (≤ 32 °C). Injury-specific criteria are a penetrating injury to the head, thorax, or abdomen, flail chest, pelvic instability, ≥ 2 fractures (to femur, tibia, and humerus), and amputations proximal to the ankle or wrist. In addition, paramedics may triage a patient after high-energy trauma directly to the L1 trauma centre without immediate identification of any of the aforementioned injuries [15].

Patients

The focus of the current study was on patients with a below-the-knee fracture. All patients, both patients with an isolated fracture below the knee and polytrauma patients, diagnosed with at least one fracture below the knee between July 2013 and June 2015 were included. Inclusion criteria were age ≥ 18 years and initial presentation or referral to the L1 or L2 centre. Exclusion criteria were age < 18 years; ligamentous injuries, including avulsion fractures, Jones fractures, and tibial eminence fractures; isolated phalangeal fractures; pathological or stress fractures; incomplete radiographic imaging; and treatment received elsewhere. Patients who were transferred to or treated in another hospital were regarded as lost to follow-up, but their fracture classification and trauma mechanism were collected. Patients transferred between our L1 and L2 centres due to a capacity issue or patient preference were scored based on the hospital of initial presentation. Patients transferred between our L1 and L2 centres for a medical indication were scored based on the hospital where definitive treatment was performed.

Data extraction

Data were derived from the electronic patient documentation (EPD) and the Dutch National Trauma Database (DNTD) of both hospitals. The DNTD is a prospectively collected database including data on all admitted trauma patients. Prehospital transport, immediate transport to the operation room (OR) or intensive care unit (ICU), and Injury Severity Score (ISS) were collected from the DNTD. Patient characteristics such as gender, age at time of trauma, fracture details, and length of hospital stay in days were collected from the EPD [16, 17].

Trauma mechanisms were categorized as fall from height < 3 or ≥ 3 m, sport-related injury, crush injury, suicide attempt, traffic accident (divided into car, motor, scooter, bicycle, pedestrian), or other. When an isolated trauma mechanism was specified, it was categorized as such: simple sprain, direct impact, or penetrating injury. Trauma mechanism was classified as low-energy trauma (LET) or high-energy trauma (HET) according to the criteria derived from the ATLS guidelines, see Table 1 [18]. Many definitions of polytrauma are used [19]. In this study, polytrauma was defined as an ISS > 15. For patients who did not need clinical admission, an ISS < 15 was noted. The energy of the trauma was classified as 'unknown' in case of insufficient information.

Non-operative and operative treatment was documented for each patient and each fracture. Interventions were categorized as primary, secondary, or complication-related surgery. Open reduction internal fixation, closed reduction internal fixation, and external fixation were considered primary surgeries. Replacing external fixation with internal osteosynthesis, revision or removal of internal osteosynthesis within a year, and flap or split skin surgery for soft tissue damage were categorized as secondary surgeries. Debridement in case of an infection, including vacuum dressing placement or replacement in the operating room (OR), correction of angulation, arthrolysis, fasciotomies, and neurolysis were deemed complication-related surgeries.

To define fracture patterns, the lower leg was divided into eight regions using the rule of squares [20]. The tibial shaft, distal tibia, calcaneus, talus, midfoot, and metatarsals were classified by a simplified OTA-AO (Orthopedic Trauma Association-Arbeitsgemeinschaft für Osteosynthesefragen) system [20]. Ankle fractures were classified using the uni-, bi-, and tri-malleolar Weber classifications, and tibial plateau fractures using the Schatzker classifications [21–23]. Three researchers (FW, DS, and SF) reviewed all radiographic studies and classified the fractures. In case of disagreement, the fractures were classified by two consultant (orthopaedic) trauma surgeons (MH and FH).

The level of soft tissue damage in open fractures was classified using the Gustilo classification system [24, 25]. An extremity was considered mangled when a fracture and 2 of the following criteria were present: nerve, vascular, and/or severe soft tissue damage [20, 26]. Nerve or vascular damage information was retrieved from the physical examination reports in the EPD.

Table 1 Criteria for HET

Fall from height ≥ 3 m or ≥ 3x body length
Car accident - > 65 km/h - Vehicle intrusion passenger compartment > 30 cm - Vehicle rollover - Passenger ejection from vehicle - Fatality in same vehicle
Motor or scooter accident > 32 km/h
Car-pedestrian or car-bicycle impact > 8 km/h
Suicide attempt (any)
Crush injury
Direct impact by blunt object either heavy or at high velocity
Penetrating objects (high velocity)

Data analysis

Statistical analysis was performed with SPSS version 21 for Windows. Parametric tests were used when > 30 items per group were compared. In all other cases, non-parametric tests were used. The χ^2 test was used for categorical variables, and Fisher's exact test was used for categorical variables with a cell volume less than 5. Results were presented according to exact count and percentages of total patients or fractures within a specific trauma centre. Non parametric variables were analysed using the Mann-Whitney test and shown as median and range. The Kruskal-Wallis test was used when two or more groups were combined with a continuous scale. A p value of ≤ 0.05 was considered significant.

Results

Demographics

In this study, 859 patients with a below-the-knee fracture were included in the L2 centre and 417 in the L1 centre (Fig. 1). One thousand five hundred seventeen fractures were analysed: 979 in the L2 centre and 538 in the L1 centre. Two hundred nineteen patients were excluded in the L2 centre and 26 patients in the L1 centre due to avulsion fractures.

Eight patients died during admission, all of which were in the L1 centre. Three died due to their injuries (2 intracranial haemorrhage, 1 hypovolemic shock) and 5 for other reasons (myocardial infarction, cerebral vascular accident, gut ischemia, 2 unknown). Six patients were transferred between the two facilities: 4 patients from the L2 to the L1 and 2 from the L1 to the L2. Patient characteristics are presented in Table 2. In the L1 centre, 32.6% of the patients had injuries due to a high-energy trauma (HET) compared to 3.5% in the L2 centre ($p < 0.001$) (Fig. 2). Of all fractures, 205 patients (218 fractures) were operated on in the L2 centre and 202 patients (259 fractures) in the L1 centre.

Fracture demographics

Ankle and metatarsal fractures were the most prevalent fractures in both centres (Fig. 3), accounting for 70.5%

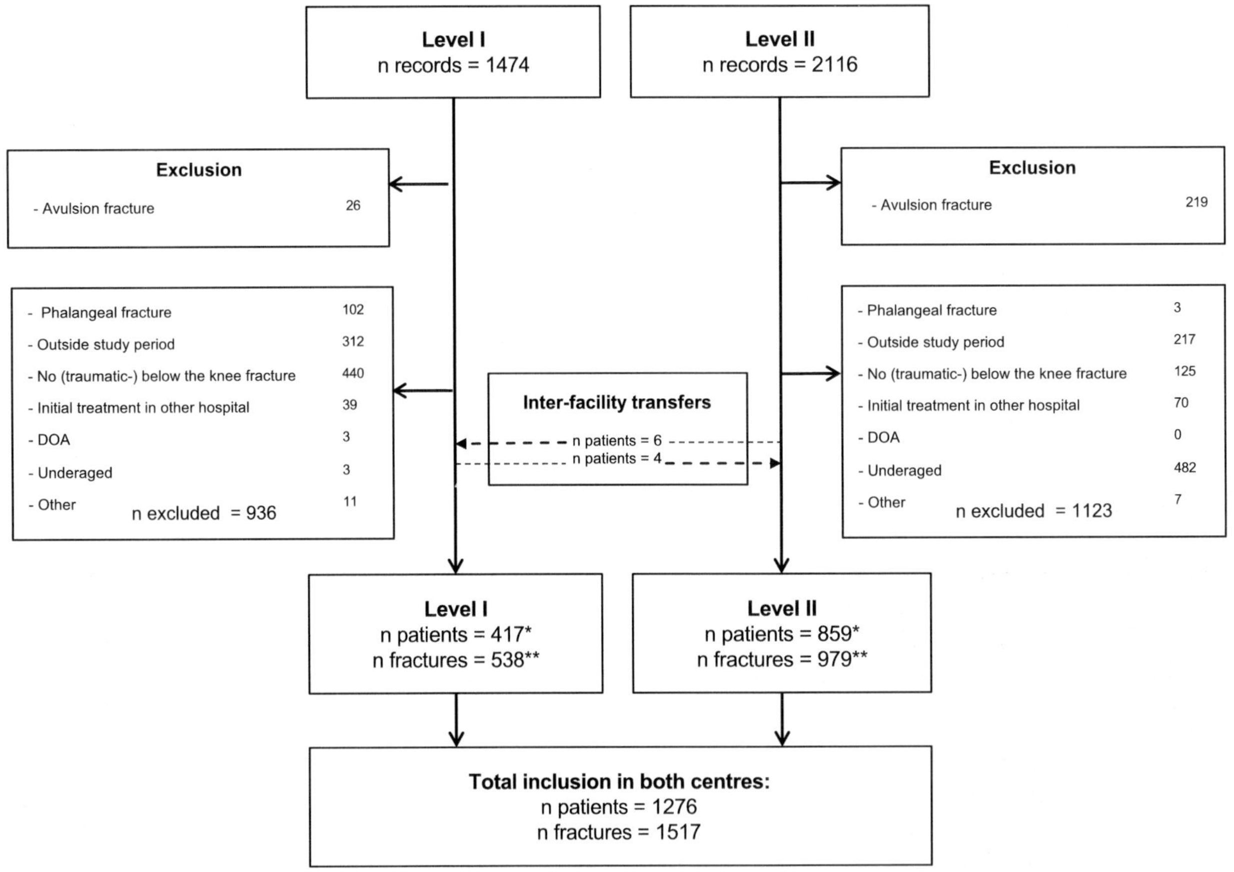

Fig. 1 Inclusion and exclusion scheme. *Patients lost to follow-up: L1 $n = 23$, L2 $n = 56$. **Fractures lost to follow-up: L1 $n = 29$, L2 $n = 65$

Table 2 Patient characteristics per level trauma centre

	Level I		Level II		*p* value
	n patients = 417		*n* patients = 859		
Male gender (*n*, %)	205	(49.2%)	347	(40.4%)	0.005
Age (mean, SD)	47	(19)	51	(20)	< 0.001
Multiple fractures (*n*, %)	67	(16.2%)	70	(8.2%)	< 0.001
Bilateral fractures (*n*, %)	24	(5.8%)	5	(0.6%)	< 0.001
Fractures per patient (mean, SD)	1.3	(0.8)	1.1	(0.5)	< 0.001
ISS > 15 (*n*, %)	55	(13.3%)	1	(0.1%)	< 0.001
HET mechanism (*n*, %)	136	(32.6%)	30	(3.5%)	< 0.001
Out-of-hospital on site medical care delivered by MMT (*n*, %)	17	(4.1%)	0	(0%)	< 0.001
Emergency admission on day of trauma (*n*,% of admittances)	169	(70.1%)	88	(37.6%)	< 0.001
Patients requiring admission for treatment (*n*, %)[1]	241	(61.2%)	234	(29.2%)	< 0.001
Direct transfer to OR and ICU (*n*, %)	33	(7.9%)	0	(0%)	< 0.001
Length of first hospital stay in days (mean, SD)	13.4	(18.9)	3.1	(4.5)	< 0.001
First hospital stay > 1 week (*n*, % of admittances)	126	(52.3%)	40	(17.1%)	< 0.001
Patients surgically treated (*n*, %)	202	(51.3%)	205	(25.6%)	< 0.001
Patients treated with > 1 surgery (*n*, %)	98	(24.9%)	11	(1.4%)	< 0.001
Surgeries on lower extremities per patient (mean, SD)	1.1	(1.7)	0.3	(0.5)	< 0.001

HET high-energy trauma, *MMT* mobile medical team (helicopter)
[1]Both direct admissions and admissions for postponed surgeries

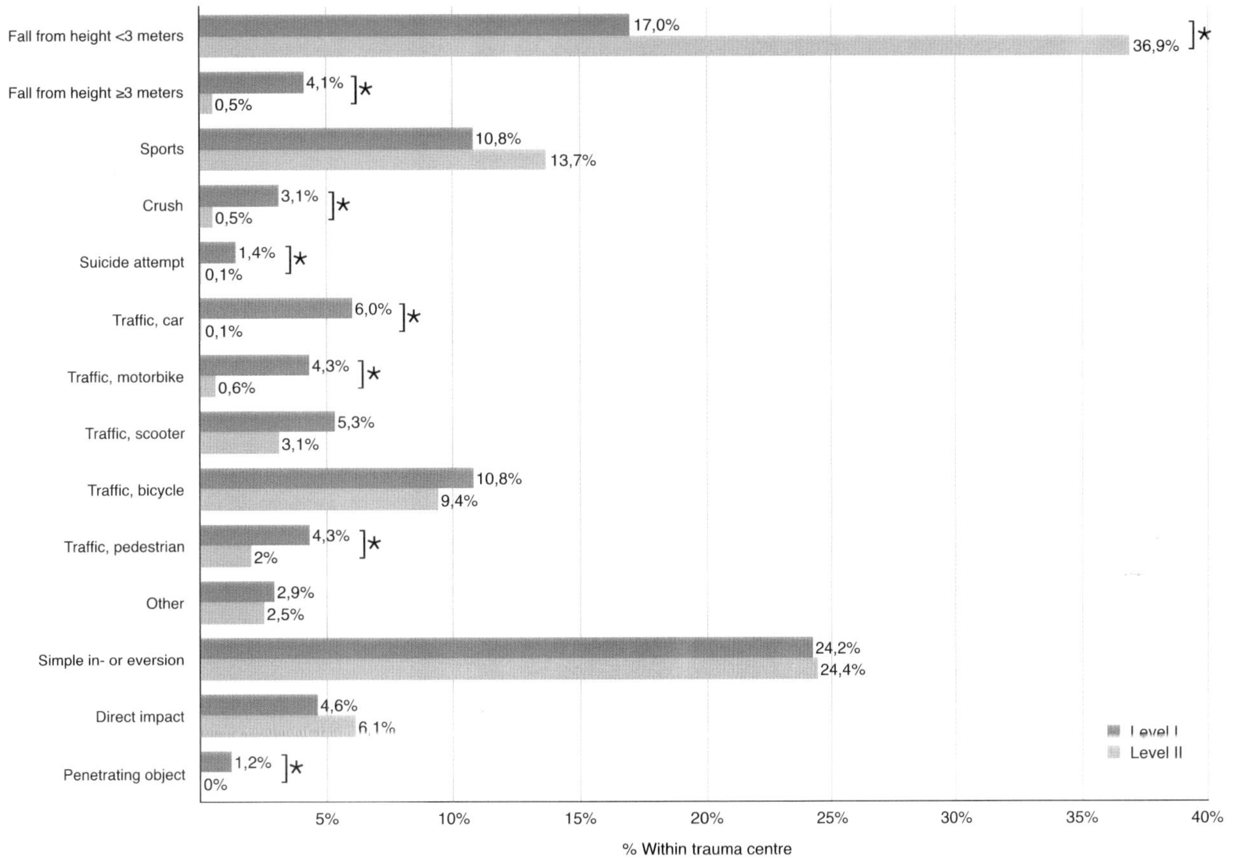

Fig. 2 Trauma mechanism frequencies per level trauma centre. Significant difference: p value of < 0.005

of all fractures (590 ankle fractures and 480 metatarsal fractures total). Most of these were seen in the L2 centre (metatarsal fracture $n = 362$ and ankle fracture $n = 402$). The most infrequent fractures were talus fractures (1.3%) and distal tibia fractures (2.6%). Based on the registry, 219 patients in the L2 and 26 patients in the L1 suffered minor or non-fracture injuries (e.g. avulsion fractures).

Fracture classification

A difference in fracture classification between the L1 and L2 centres was observed for tibial plateau, tibial shaft, ankle, and foot fractures. The presentation of more complex tibial plateau fractures (Schatzker types 4–6), complex tibial shaft fractures, distal tibia fractures, displaced calcaneal fractures, talus fractures, and complex midfoot fractures (Chopart, Lisfranc, and navicular/nutcracker) was significantly greater in the L1 centre.

Ankle fractures were seen more frequently in the L2 centre and accounted for almost half of the total amount of fractures treated ($n = 402$, 41.1%), of which the majority were uni-malleolar fractures (72.4% within L2). Metatarsal fractures were also more often treated in the L2 centre ($n = 362$, 37.0%). A complete overview of the fracture distribution is shown in Table 3.

Fractures were more often associated with concomitant injuries in the L1 centre ($p < 0.001$) (e.g. soft tissue, vascular, and neurological damage). The L1 centre treated more open fractures ($n = 72$ or 13.4% versus $n = 15$ or 1.5%, $p < 0.001$) and more mangled extremities ($n = 15$ or 3% versus $n = 0$ or 0%, $p < 0.001$) than the L2 centre. Fracture characteristics are shown in Table 4.

Resource utilization

Most fractures were seen in the L2 centre, and these were generally treated with cast immobilization. In total, 50.9% of the fractures in the L1 centre were treated surgically compared to 23.9% in the L2. The total number of patients undergoing surgical fixation was comparable for the L1 and L2 ($n = 216$ and $n = 216$). The incidence of secondary surgeries and complication-related surgeries was higher in the L1 centre ($p < 0.001$ and $p < 0.001$). All patients that required soft tissue coverage or primary vascular repair were treated at the L1 centre. More patients were immediately admitted to the L1 centre (70.1% on the day of trauma compared to 37.6% in the L2). The hospital length of stay (HLOS) in the L1 was significantly longer than in the L2 centre, and 52.3% of the patients in the L1 had a HLOS > 1 week (Table 2).

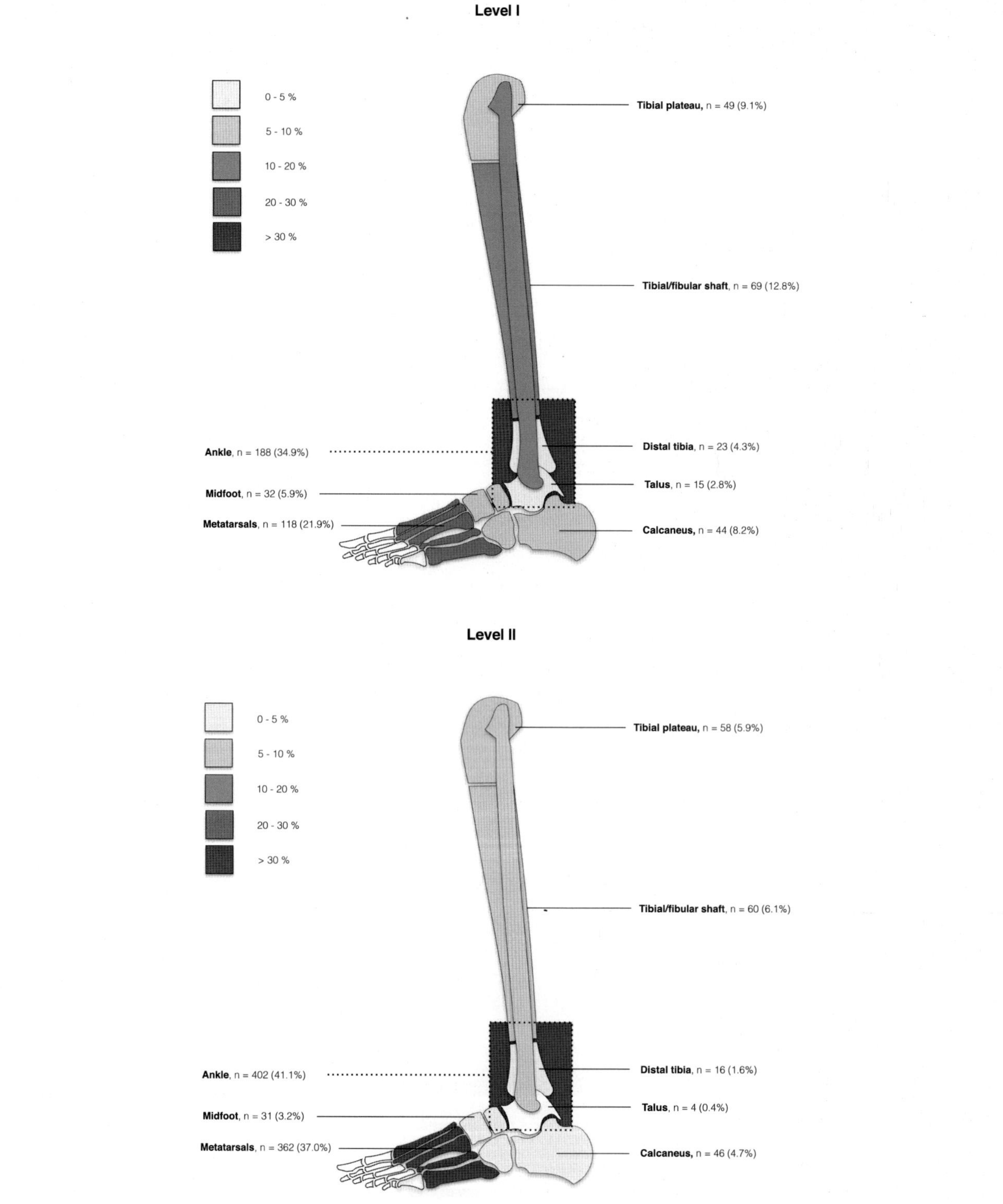

Fig. 3 Fracture frequencies per anatomical region (level 1 and level 2)

Discussion

In this mature inclusive trauma system situated in a densely populated area, most fractures were treated in the L2 centre. The majority of fractures overall (including avulsion fractures) were treated in the L2 centre; the amount of surgical procedures performed per surgeon

Table 3 Fracture classifications and complexity per level trauma centre

		Level I n fractures = 538		Level II n fractures = 979			p-value Simple vs Complex or *total* in level I vs level II
Tibial plateau		49		58			
	Schatzker 1	10	20.4%	15	25.9%	Simple	0.004
	Schatzker 2	3	6.1%	17	29.3%		
	Schatzker 3	5	10.2%	6	10.3%		
	Schatzker 4	11	22.4%	3	5.2%	Complex	
	Schatzker 5	1	2.0%	6	10.3%		
	Schatzker 6	19	38.8%	11	19.0%		
Tibial Shaft / Cruris / Fibula		69		60			
	Simple	20	29.0%	26	43.3%	Simple	0.014
	Wedge	18	26,1%	3	5.0%		
	Isolated fibula	15	21.7%	27	45.0%		
	Complex	16	23.2%	4	6.7%	Complex	
Distal tibia		23		16			*0.002*
	Intra-articular	3	13.0%	3	18.8%		
	Pilon	9	39.1%	5	31.3%		
	Distal cruris	11	47.8%	8	50.0%		
Ankle		188		402			*0.011*
	Unimalleolar - Weber A	37	19.7%	67	16.7%		
	Unimalleolar - Weber B	45	23.9%	160	39.8%		
	Unimalleolar - Weber C	13	6.9%	46	11.4%		
	Isolated medial malleolus	17	9.0%	16	4.0%		
	Isolated tertius	0	0.0%	2	0.5%		
	Bimalleolar - Weber A	2	1.1%	1	0.2%		
	Bimalleolar - Weber B	26	13.8%	50	12.4%		
	Bimalleolar - Weber C	17	9.0%	15	3.7%		
	Medial malleolus + tertius	3	1.6%	1	0.2%		
	Trimalleolar - Weber A	0	0.0%	1	0.2%		
	Trimalleolar - Weber B	20	10.6%	32	8.0%		
	Trimalleolar - Weber C	8	4.3%	11	2.7%		
Talus		15		4			*<0.001*
	Body	11	73.3%	2	50.0%		
	Neck	4	26.7%	2	50.0%		
Calcaneus		44		46			
	Simple nondisplaced	14	31.8%	24	52.2%	Simple	0.006
	Extreme beak	1	2.3%	3	6.5%		
	Sustentacular	0	0.0%	3	6.5%		
	Complex displaced	29	65.9%	16	34.8%	Complex	
Midfoot		32		31			
	Intertarsals	4	12.1%	16	51.6%	Simple	0.002
	Cuboid	3	9.1%	3	9.7%		
	Lisfranc	12	36.4%	3	9.7%	Complex	
	Chopart	7	21.2%	2	6.5%		
	Navicular	6	18.2%	7	22.6%		
Metatarsals		118		362			*<0.001*
	1st - 4th	57	48.3%	173	47.8%		
	5th	61	51.7%	189	52.2%		

was higher in the L2 centre, run by a smaller surgical team. The majority of complex fractures were treated in the L1 centre. This was demonstrated by the number of immediate surgical procedures, late secondary surgeries, a necessary multidisciplinary approach, and utilization of additional resources. Fracture classification supported this

Table 4 Fracture characteristics and treatment per level trauma centre

		Level I		Level II		*p* value
		n fractures = 538		*n* fractures = 979		
Fractures surgically treated (*n*, %)*		259	(50.9%)	218	(23.9%)	< 0.001
ORIF/CRIF (*n*, %)*		216	(42.4%)	216	(23.7%)	< 0.001
Fractures treated with external fixation (*n*, %)*		43	(8.4%)	2	(0.2%)	< 0.001
Fractures requiring secondary surgeries (*n*, %)*		64	(12.6%)	9	(1.0%)	< 0.001
Fractures requiring complication surgeries (*n*, %)*		55	(10.8%)	6	(0.7%)	< 0.001
Open fractures (*n*, %)		72	(13.4%)	15	(1.5%)	< 0.001
Gustilo classification (*n*, %)	1	10	(1.9%)	8	(0.8%)	
	2	18	(3.3%)	2	(0.2%)	
	3a	17	(3.2%)	4	(0.4%)	
	3b	19	(3.5%)	1	(0.1%)	
	3c	8	(1.5%)	0	(0.0%)	
Mangled extremity (*n*, %)		15	(2.7%)	0	(0.0%)	< 0.001
Nerve damage (*n*, %)		11	(2.0%)	3	(0.3%)	< 0.001
Vascular damage (*n*, %)		15	(2.7%)	1	(0.1%)	< 0.001
Fasciotomy (*n*, %)*		13	(2.5%)	0	(0.0%)	< 0.001
Vascular repair needed (*n*, %)*		5	(1.0%)	0	(0.0%)	0.006
Soft tissue coverage (*n*, %)*		16	(3.1%)	0	(0.0%)	< 0.001
Amputations*		11		0	(0.0%)	< 0.001

ORIF open reduction internal fixation, *CRIF* closed reduction internal fixation
*Percentages are based on level I *n* = 509 and level II *n* = 914, excluding fractures lost to follow-up

difference in complexity, as did accompanying soft tissue injury and concomitant injuries to the lower extremity and other body regions.

The presented differentiation in this inclusive trauma system occurred spontaneously, without regional contracts or prehospital guidelines. Several factors may have contributed to this process. First, the prehospital triage guidelines are aimed at the identification of polytrauma patients with potentially lethal injuries and not so much at (isolated) complex lower extremity injuries. These guidelines in combination with some options for the paramedics that allow direct triage to the L1 centre resulted in the allocation of 78% of the polytrauma patients to the L1 centre in our region as demonstrated previously [15]. Trauma mechanism is one of these options in the triage decision making by paramedics in our country, which may have contributed to the described differentiation in allocation of lower extremity fractures. Second, an important factor that may have contributed to this differentiation is the relatively short distance between the L1 and L2 centres, which is applicable not only to the Central Region of the Netherlands, but also to other densely populated areas with multiple established hospitals. This is the case in most large metropolis cities around the world. The geographic localisation might also have contributed to the difference, as the L2 centre is within the centre of the city, while the L1 centre is situated on the edge of the urban area. Last, in a thrive to improve patient care, the L1 and L2 centres optimized their profile and logistics in accordance to their designated role in the inclusive trauma system. The L2 centres implemented fast tracks for specific diagnoses (e.g. ankle fractures/distortion, wrist injuries, hip fractures), with one surgeon responsible for the patient's whole course including clinical care, surgery, post-operative consultation, and outpatient follow-up. In contrast, the L1 centre implemented 24/7 specialist care, emergency operating team availability within minutes, and flexible OR time on a daily basis.

Differentiation and specialisation leads to optimization of care. Although there is a diversity in injury type with regard to the complex injuries, the required treatment regime, necessary resources, and flexible logistics make acute complex care of lower extremity fractures a separate entity that requires its own differentiation. Complex lower extremity fracture types were more frequently treated in the L1 centre. Tibial plateau Schatzker types 4 through 6, complex tibial shaft, displaced calcaneal, and complex midfoot fractures were more prevalent in the L1 compared to the L2 centre (Table 3). It is tempting to speculate that these fractures are more frequently the result of high-energy mechanisms and therefore predisposed to presentation to an L1 centre. This is supported by trauma mechanism analysis, as all high incidence complex fracture types in the L1 were related to HET mechanisms, such as a fall from height (e.g. suicide attempts), traffic, and crush mechanisms [27]. This is further illustrated by a higher incidence of open fractures, an increased need for external fixations, fasciotomies, amputations, and other secondary or complication surgeries in the L1 centre. Open lower extremity fractures have a greater likelihood of infection, which makes early soft tissue coverage within hours to days desirable. Vascular damage and neurological damage ought to be treated urgently [28, 29]. Furthermore, soft tissue damage especially in the case of multiple non-contiguous fractures often requires serial operations [30]. As a result, there is a high demand on multiple resources in the L1 centre. In total, 24.9% of all fractures in the L1 required more than one operation. In contrast, only 1.4% of the patients in the L2 centre underwent multiple procedures. The presence of an in-hospital trauma surgeon as well as a dedicated OR team for complex and severely traumatized patients was initiated to improve outcomes, but adds to the costs incurred per patient [31–33]. Although not all secondary and complication-related surgeries were performed during the initial hospitalization, also in a semi-acute setting, they put pressure on OR capacity and require personnel with a high level of expertise. OR utilization is one of the costliest components in secondary care [34]. As a consequence, treatment of the complex extremity injuries is expensive.

Additionally, the high incidence of immediate admissions on the day of trauma and longer lengths of hospital stay reveal a striking difference between the L1 and L2 centre. The HLOS of patients admitted to the L1 was longer than 1 week in more than 50% of patients. In total, 271 patients (65%) were presented with an isolated injury below the knee in the L1 centre. However, as 50% of the patients required admission over a week, additional injuries (146/417 = 35%) cannot solely explain the difference in HLOS. More likely, the complexity of the injuries explains the difference in admission rate, HLOS, and resources used in the L1 centre. Almost the same number of patients required admission to the L2 centre as the L1 centre, resulting in a high turnover rate in the L2 hospital. Optimization and maturation of this inclusive trauma system is important not only in reducing morbidity and mortality, but also in optimizing management of resources.

Recent studies on fracture epidemiology show an increasing incidence of extremity fractures with a trend towards surgical treatment, possibly due to development in surgical techniques [35–37]. This means a higher demand on resources is to be expected in the near future. A balanced distribution of trauma patients within the inclusive trauma system is of utmost importance in order to optimize logistics, contain costs, and ensure the best clinical outcomes. For specific injuries, official trauma region agreements between centres might prove beneficial, but as this study demonstrated, might not be essential [10].

Limitations of this study are the absence of prehospital triage data which forced assumptions based on ISS scores and trauma mechanisms. Also, surgeon-based considerations in injury management may have influenced type and extent of treatment and are not traceable. Due to the retrospective nature of this study, no data on outcome and fracture union are available. This would have provided additional insight into the outcomes of fractures treated in both trauma centres. Future studies should focus on these subjects.

This is the first study to assess fracture pattern differences in L1 and L2 hospitals in an inclusive trauma system. It provides detailed information on a large number of patients with extensive information on fracture classifications and resource demands. Of great importance is the trauma mechanism, which may have implications on pre- and in-hospital triage. Future studies should investigate factors that influence triage to L1 or L2 trauma centres.

Conclusion

Most patients were treated at the L2 centre, while complex lower extremity injuries were mostly treated at the L1 trauma centre. Treatment of below-the-knee fractures differed, within the mature inclusive trauma system, between the high-volume low complexity L2 trauma centre and low-volume high complexity L1 trauma centre. Patients with complex injuries placed a high demand on available resources. Trauma mechanism may prove important for further differentiation and optimization of resource utilization.

Abbreviations

ATLS: Advance Trauma Life Support; DNTD: Dutch National Trauma Database; EPD: Electronical patient documentation; GCS: Glasgow Coma Scale; HET: High-energy trauma; ICU: Intensive care unit; ISS: Injury Severity Score; L1 or L2: Level 1 or level 2 trauma centre; LET: Low-energy trauma; OR: Operating room; OTA-AO: Orthopaedic Trauma Association-Arbeitsgemeinschaft für Osteosynthesefragen; UMCU: University Medical Center Utrecht

Acknowledgements

We want to thank M. Dijkgraaf for his advice on statistics.

Funding

No funding was received for this project.

Authors' contributions

All authors were involved in the conception and design of the study. FW, FN, DS, and SF performed the acquisition of data. FW, DS, SF, MH, and FH performed the analysis and interpretation of data. FW, DS, and SF drafted the article, and FH, MH, LL, and EV revised it critically. All authors read and approved the final manuscript.

Competing interests

The authors declare that they have no competing interests.

Author details

[1]Department of Surgery, Diakonessenhuis Utrecht, Utrecht, The Netherlands. [2]Traumacenter, University Medical Center Utrecht, Utrecht, The Netherlands. [3]Department of Surgery, University Medical Center Utrecht, Heidelberglaan 100, 3584 CX Utrecht, The Netherlands.

References

1. Fern KT, Smith JT, Zee B, Lee A, Borschneck D, Pichora DR. Trauma patients with multiple extremity injuries: resource utilization and long-term outcome in relation to injury severity scores. J Trauma Acute Care Surg. 1998;45:489–94.
2. Mkandawire NC, Boot DA, Braithwaite IJ, Patterson M, Tscherne H, Molokhia A. Musculoskeletal recovery 5 years after severe injury: long term problems are common. Injury. 2002;33:111–5.
3. Banerjee M, Bouillon B, Shafizadeh S, Paffrath T, Lefering R, Wafaisade A, et al. Epidemiology of extremity injuries in multiple trauma patients. Injury. 2013;44:1015–21.
4. Higgins TF, Klatt JB, Beals TC. Lower Extremity Assessment Project (LEAP)—the best available evidence on limb-threatening lower extremity trauma. Orthop Clin North Am. 2010;41:233–9.
5. Zelle BA, Brown SR, Panzica M, Lohse R, Sittaro NA, Krettek C, et al. The impact of injuries below the knee joint on the long-term functional outcome following polytrauma. Injury. 2005;36:169–77.
6. Peitzman AB, Courcoulas AP, Stinson C, Udekwu AO, Billiar TR, Harbrecht BG. Trauma center maturation: quantification of process and outcome. Ann Surg. 1999;230:87–94.
7. Holtslag HR, van Beeck EF, Lichtveld RA, Leenen LP, Lindeman E, van der Werken C. Individual and population burdens of major trauma in the Netherlands. Bull World Health Organ. 2008;86:111–7.
8. Lansink KWW, Leenen LPH. History, development and future of trauma care for multiple injured patients in the Netherlands. Eur J Trauma Emerg Surg. 2013;39:3–7.
9. Gunning A, Lansink KWW, van Wessem KJP, Balogh Z, Rivara F, Maier R, et al. Demographic patterns and outcomes of patients in level I trauma centers in three international trauma systems. World J Surg. 2015;39:2677–84.
10. van Laarhoven J, van Lammeren GW, Houwert RM, van Laarhoven C, Hietbrink F, Leenen LPH, et al. Isolated hip fracture care in an inclusive trauma system: a trauma system wide evaluation. Injury. 2015;46:1042–6.
11. Lansink KWW, Gunning A, Spijkers ATE, Leenen LPH. Evaluation of trauma care in a mature level I trauma center in the Netherlands: outcomes in a Dutch mature level I trauma center. World J Surg. 2013;37:2353–9.
12. Spijkers ATE, Meylaerts SAG, Leenen LPH. Mortality decreases by implementing a level I trauma center in a Dutch hospital. J Trauma. 2010;69:1138–42.
13. de Knegt C, Meylaerts SAG, Leenen LPH, Busuttil A, Robertson CE. Applicability of the trimodal distribution of trauma deaths in a Level I trauma centre in the Netherlands with a population of mainly blunt trauma. Injury. 2008;39:993–1000.
14. Ambulancezorg Nederland; NVVMMA; V&VN. Landelijk Protocol Ambulancezorg version 8.1. 2016.
15. Voskens FJ, van Rein EAJ, van der Sluijs R, Houwert RM, Lichtveld RA, Verleisdonk EJ, et al. Accuracy of prehospital triage in selecting severely injured trauma patients. JAMA Surg. 2017; https://doi.org/10.1001/jamasurg.2017.4472. [Epub ahead of print]
16. Baker SP, Oneill B. The injury severity score: a method for describing patients with multiple injuries and evaluating emergency care. J Trauma. 1974;14:187–96.
17. Baker SP, Oneill B. The injury severity score: an update. J Trauma. 1976;16:882–5.
18. The ATLS Subcommittee and the International ATLS working group AC of SC on T. Advanced trauma life support (ATLS®): the ninth edition. J Trauma Acute Care Surg. 2013;74:1363–6.
19. Butcher N, Balogh ZJ. The definition of polytrauma: the need for international consensus. Injury. 2009;40(Suppl 4):12–22.
20. Colton C, Krikler S, Schatzker J, Trafton P. AO surgery reference—comprehensive online reference in daily clinical life. https://www2.aofoundation.org/wps/portal/surgery Accessed 21 Jan 2016.
21. Hughes JL, Weber H, Willenegger H, Kuner EH. Evaluation of ankle fractures: non-operative and operative treatment. Clin Orthop Relat Res. 1979;138:111–9.
22. Schatzker JJ, McBroom R, Bruce D. The tibial plateau fracture. The Toronto experience 1968-1975. Clin Orthop Relat Res. 1979;138:94–104.
23. Zeltser DW, Leopold SS. Classifications in brief: Schatzker classification of tibial plateau fractures. Clin Orthop Relat Res. 2013;471:371–4.
24. Gustilo RB, Merkow RL, Templeman D. The management of open fractures. J Bone Jt Surg. 1990;72:299–304.
25. Kim PH, Leopold S. Gustilo-Anderson classification. Clin Orthop Relat Res. 2012;470:3270–4.
26. Tscherne H, Oestern HJ. A new classification of soft-tissue damage in open and closed fractures (author's transl). Unfallheilkunde. 1982;85:111–5.
27. Rockwood CA, Green DP, Bucholz RW. Rockwood and Green's fractures in adults. Philadelphia: Lippincott Williams & Wilkins; 2010.
28. Malhotra AK, Goldberg S, Graham J, Malhotra NR, Willis MC, Mounasamy V, et al. Open extremity fractures: impact of delay in operative debridement and irrigation. J Trauma Acute Care Surg. 2014;76:1201–7.
29. Liu DSH, Sofiadellis F, Ashton M, MacGill K, Webb A. Early soft tissue coverage and negative pressure wound therapy optimises patient outcomes in lower limb trauma. Injury. 2012;43:772–8.
30. Chen AT, Vallier HA. Noncontiguous and open fractures of the lower extremity: epidemiology, complications, and unplanned procedures. Injury. 2016;47:742–7.
31. Luchette F, Kelly B, Davis K, Johanningman J, Heink N, James L, et al. Impact of the in-house trauma surgeon on initial patient care, outcome, and cost. J Trauma. 1997;42:490-5–7.
32. Brasel KJ, Akason J, Weigelt JA. Dedicated operating room for trauma: a costly recommendation. J Trauma. 1998;44:832-6–8.
33. Althausen PL, Kauk JR, Shannon S, Lu M, O'mara TJ, Bray TJ. Operating room efficiency: benefits of an orthopaedic traumatologist at a level II trauma center. J Orthop Trauma. 2014;30(Suppl 5):15–20.
34. Ang WW, Sabharwal S, Johannsson H, Bhattacharya R, Gupte CM. The cost of trauma operating theatre inefficiency. Ann Med Surg. 2016;7:24–9.
35. Polinder S, Haagsma J, Panneman M, Scholten A, Brugmans M, Van Beeck E. The economic burden of injury: health care and productivity costs of injuries in the Netherlands. Accid Anal Prev. 2016;93:92–100.
36. Beerekamp MSH, de Muinck Keizer RJO, Schep NWL, Ubbink DT, Panneman MJM, Goslings JC. Epidemiology of extremity fractures in the Netherlands. Injury. 2017;48:1355–62.
37. Court-Brown CM, Clement ND, Duckworth AD, Biant LC, McQueen MM. The changing epidemiology of fall-related fractures in adults. Injury. 2017;48:819–24.

32

Low values of central venous oxygen saturation ($ScvO_2$) during surgery and anastomotic leak of abdominal trauma patients

Andres Isaza-Restrepo[1,2*], Jose F. Moreno-Mejia[3], Juan S. Martin-Saavedra[4] and Milciades Ibañez-Pinilla[1]

Abstract

Background: There is a well known relationship between hypoperfusion and postoperative complications like anastomotic leak. No studies have been done addressing this relationship in the context of abdominal trauma surgery. Central venous oxygen saturation is an important hypoperfusion marker of potential use in abdominal trauma surgery for identifying the risk of anastomotic leak development. The purpose of this study was to identify the relationship between low values of central venous oxygen saturation and anastomotic leak of gastrointestinal sutures in the postoperative period in abdominal trauma surgery.

Methods: A cross-sectional prospective study was performed. Patients over 14 years old who required surgical gastrointestinal repair secondary to abdominal trauma were included. Anastomotic leak diagnosis was confirmed through clinical manifestations and diagnostic images or secondary surgery when needed. Central venous oxygen blood saturation was measured at the beginning of surgery through a central catheter. Demographic data, trauma mechanism, anatomic site of trauma, hemoglobin levels, abdominal trauma index, and comorbidities were assessed as secondary variables.

Results: Patients who developed anastomotic leak showed lower mean central venous oxygen saturation levels (60.0% ± 2.94%) than those who did not (69.89% ± 7.21%) ($p = 0.010$).

Conclusions: Central venous oxygen saturation <65% was associated with the development of gastrointestinal leak during postoperative time of patients who underwent surgery secondary to abdominal trauma.

Keywords: Abdominal injury, Perfusion, Hypotension, Anastomotic leak, Central venous pressure, Gastrointestinal tract

Background

Perioperative hemodynamic state, usually determined by mean blood pressure, urinary output, and heart rate, is highly related to postoperative (POP) morbidity and mortality [1–3], relationship that has been demonstrated in several studies [4–9]. Evidence has shown that an inadequate tissue perfusion during surgery is associated with anastomotic leak during the postoperative period, which is a major morbid complication [10]. In consequence, objective parameters of tissue perfusion are needed and central venous oxygen saturation ($ScvO_2$) has been studied since the 1980 [4, 5].

Tissue hypoperfusion results from circulatory disturbances during hypoxic and hemorrhagic periods, and evidence suggests that $ScvO_2$ reflects the early stages of hypoperfusion [6, 11–15]. Other hypoperfusion marker is lactic acid, which is elevated during low tissue oxygenation even under normal vital signs. Nevertheless, lactic acid could be elevated by different circumstances like hepatic impairment as well as those treated with Ringer

* Correspondence: andres.isaza@urosario.edu.co
[1]Escuela de Medicina y Ciencias de la Salud, Universidad del Rosario, Bogotá D.C., Colombia
[2]Mederi Hospital Universitario Mayor, Bogotá D.C., Colombia
Full list of author information is available at the end of the article

lactate [15–18]. $ScvO_2$, being an early hypoperfusion marker, could support early and objective decision-making during surgical procedure.

The main purpose of this study was to explore possible associations between tissue hypoperfusion identified through $ScvO_2$ measurement and the development of anastomotic leak during the postoperative period of abdominal trauma patients. Our hypothesis is that low measurements (<65%) may increase the risk of presenting leakages of anastomosis or sutures during POP period.

Methods

Design, setting, and participants

Originally, the study was designed for a case-control study, but in response to the low incidence of cases during the study period, a prospective cross-sectional study approach was preferred. Patients aged 14 years or older, who underwent surgery secondary to abdominal trauma and that required primary gastrointestinal anastomosis, were included in the study. Patients were excluded when they presented hemodynamic or metabolic impairment secondary to previously known pathologies, and patients who died during surgery or in the immediate postsurgical time. As clinical and local conditions for gastrointestinal repair are different after damage control surgery, those that required this procedure before the final repair were also excluded. The study took place at the Hospital Occidente Kennedy, a reference trauma center of high complexity located in Bogotá D.C., Colombia, between 2011 and 2013. Patients underwent surgery according to each surgeon's personal criteria and to the hospital's trauma protocols without taking into account the study objectives.

Variables

The following data was collected for every patient: age, gender, anatomic site of trauma, trauma mechanism, blood pressure, transfusion requirements, hemoglobin levels at arrival, comorbidities, abdominal trauma index (ATI), and the $ScvO_2$ measured during the surgery. $ScvO_2$ was measured through a subclavian venous catheter implanted by the anesthesiologist for central venous pressure measurement. As part of the hospital's protocol, anesthesiologist prepared patients for surgery and implanted the subclavian venous catheter during the first 30 min of entering the surgery room. $ScvO_2$ was measured right after catheter implantation. All remaining data was obtained from clinical records of every patient. Follow-up of patient was done during the hospitalization days until the first postoperative ambulatory control appointment 10 days after discharge or when anastomotic leak was diagnosed.

Anastomotic diagnosis and $ScvO_2$ cut point

Anastomotic leak or suture leakage was diagnosed from clinical manifestations and confirmed through image studies, or surgery during secondary interventions when needed. For this study's main outcome, a $ScvO_2$ cut point was defined as low levels previous to analysis. According to literature, normal levels range between 70 and 75% and levels under 60% suggest an oxidative metabolic disturbance [19]; therefore, the cut point for this study was set at 65%. All patients with $ScvO_2$ at 65% or lower were classified as low levels.

Sample selection and bias assessment

According to literature, incidence for anastomotic leak is ranged between 2.4 and 15.9% [1]. Therefore, considering a risk of 10% to develop anastomotic leak in abdominal trauma patients, a leaked/non-leaked relationship of 1:3; a type I error of 0.05 and type II of 0.010; and an overall final sample of 108 were calculated. Ultimately, due to low incidence of patients during the period of time for the study, an overall sample of 41 patients was reached and an approach for a cross-sectional prospective study was decided.

Selection bias was addressed through sequential and continuous selection of patients until a final sample of 41 patients was achieved taking into account inclusion and exclusion criteria. Hospital's personnel that attended each case were not influenced by the objectives of the study and acted according to usual practice and protocols established in the hospital. Classification bias was addressed by taking into account data obtained from the clinical record of each patient.

Statistical analysis

Qualitative variables were analyzed through descriptive statistics using absolute and relative frequencies. For quantitative variables, central tendency (means and median) and dispersion (rate and standard deviation) measurements were used. For assessing differences in systolic and diastolic arterial pressure, Student's t test was used for two independent groups. Previous analysis of normalized values on arterial pressure and the homogeneity of variants were done using the Shapiro Wilk test and Levene test respectively. If such circumstances were not achieved, an exact non-parametric Mann Whitney test was used.

A Fisher exact test (expected values of <5) was applied for identifying any association between $ScvO_2$ and the development of anastomotic leak. Risk was assessed using relative risk with a Katz exact confidence interval of 95%. Logistic regression and multivariate analysis was done, but due to the low number of patients, it was excluded from the reports.

Results

Participants and descriptive results

A total of 41 patients were analyzed and 4 of those (9.8%) developed an anastomotic leak. The mean age for the study was 32.83 ± 13.77 years (median = 28 years), 32 out of 41 (78%) were male and only 3 of the 41 (7.3%) had any comorbidity (see Table 1). Mean values for systolic blood pressure were 105 ± 14.4 mmHg and diastolic blood pressure were 67 ± 13 mmHg. Patients required red blood cell transfusion in 19.5% ($n = 8$) of the cases, and the mean values for hemoglobin at hospital arrival was 12.14 ± 2.77 (median of 13). Finally, the mean values for $ScvO_2$ were 68.93 ± 7.5 (median of 70). Mean values for ATI was 5.34 ± 4.92 (median of 3) (see Table 2).

The most common site of trauma was the small intestine followed by the stomach and the colon (see Table 3). Main trauma mechanism was sharp weapon injury in 65.9% of the cases ($n = 27$), followed by firearm injury 22% ($n = 9$) and blunt trauma in 12.2% ($n = 5$) of the cases.

Anastomotic leak and $ScvO_2$

Out of the 41 patients, 7 (17.07%) evidenced surgical $ScvO_2$ values <65% and 4 of those 7 patients presented anastomotic leak (see Table 4). Patients that presented anastomotic leak showed significantly lower ($p = 0.010$) values of $ScvO_2$ during surgery (mean value of 60.0 ± 2.94%), compared to those with no anastomotic leak (mean value of 69.89 ± 7.21%). A significant association between values of $ScvO_2$ <65% and the risk of developing an anastomotic leak was identified (RR = 39.8 CI 95%: 2.35, $p < 0.0001$, with a Fisher exact test).

Other variables and $ScvO_2$

No association was found with the presence of comorbidities ($p = 0.729$), gender ($p = 0.204$), age ($p = 0.503$), and systolic and diastolic blood pressure ($p = 0.149$ and $p = 0.260$). A significant association was identified with the requirement of red blood cell transfusion ($p = 0.019$), low values of hemoglobin at arrival ($p = 0.004$), and a greater ATI ($p < 0.001$).

Discussion

An association between low levels of $ScvO_2$ during surgery with anastomotic leak as a complication in the postsurgical period was found. Significant difference was identified between mean values of $ScvO_2$ for patients that developed anastomotic leakages and those who did not (60.0% ± 2.94%, and 69.89% ± 7.21% respectively; $p = 0.010$). A risk of developing an anastomotic leak for patients with low levels of $ScvO_2$ was identified (RR = 39.8 CI 95%: 2.35, $p < 0.0001$, with a Fisher exact test).

These results support the hypothesis that 65% or lower levels of $ScvO_2$ may constitute a risk factor for the development of major complications related to gastrointestinal anastomosis and sutures in abdominal trauma patients. Other authors have found similar results [10, 11, 20–25]. Hoshking et al. showed that levels of 66.5% or lower of $ScvO_2$ are associated with a worst outcome despite a stable hemodynamic state [15]. Pearse et al. described the changes in $ScvO_2$ after mayor surgery finding an independent association between levels of $ScvO_2$ (with a cut point of 65%) and the development of POP complications [11]. Other cases where low values of $ScvO_2$ were associated with a worst prognosis are trauma, acute myocardial infarction [5, 26], severe sepsis, and cardiac failure [11].

In abdominal trauma, anastomotic leak is one of the most morbid complications [1, 27–30] and hypoperfusion is an important factor for its development. Consequently, different strategies have been developed for the prevention and resolution of hypoperfusion such as goal-directed resuscitation [9, 31] and goal-directed fluid replacement [25, 32].

Table 1 Demographic data and red blood cell transfusion requirement

Anastomotic leak	Yes ($n = 4$)	No ($n = 37$)	p value
Gender male	2 (50%)	30 (81%)	0.204
Comorbidities	0 (0%)	3 (8.1%)	0.729
Mean age (SD)	34 (8.36)	32.7 (14.12)	0.503

No significant differences were observed

Table 2 Study outcomes

Anastomotic leak	Yes ($n = 4$)	No ($n = 37$)	p value
Hb (g/dL), mean (SD)	8.55 (2.59)	12.53 (2.52)	0.004*
ATI, mean (SD)	14.75 (5.62)	4.32 (3.66)	<0.001*
SBP (mmHg), mean (SD)	98.25 (16.64)	107.32 (14.20)	0.149
DBP (mmHg), mean (SD)	58.50 (16.66)	66.19 (12.66)	0.260
$ScvO_2$ (%), mean (SD)	60.98 (2.94)	69.89 (7.21)	0.010*
Transfusion requirement, N	3 (75%)	5 (13.51%)	0.019*

SD standard deviation, *N* number of patients, *Hb* hemoglobin, *SBP* systolic blood pressure, *DBP* diastolic blood pressure, *ScvO*$_2$ central venous oxygen saturation, *ATI* abdominal trauma index
*Significant difference

Table 3 Distribution of site of injury by organ

Organ	Frequency	Percent
Stomach	5	12.2
Small intestine	26	63.4
Ascending colon (including hepatic angle)	3	7.3
Tranverse colon (including splenic angle)	2	4.9
Descending colon	2	4.9
Sigmoid colon	3	7.3
Total	41	100

Table 4 Distribution of cases according to $ScvO_2$ saturation

		Anastomotic leak	
		Yes (total)	No (total)
Saturation	<65%	4 (7)	3 (7)
	≥65%	0 (34)	34 (34)
Total		4 (41)	37 (41)

We strongly believe that early and objective hypoperfusion markers can contribute to a supported decision on postponing primary repair. Based on the results from this study, $ScvO_2$ monitoring during surgery could be a potential and easily available hypoperfusion marker. It is important to mention that values of $ScvO_2$ may reflect a low oxygen extraction rate secondary to mitochondrial impairment indicating poor outcomes and limits low levels of $ScvO_2$ sensibility [15, 33, 34].

Another limiting factor is the catheter placement. It has been proved that $ScvO_2$ levels vary according to the catheter's point location [35]; therefore, it is important to note that the sample was taken from the superior vena cava so measurements could be affected by brain metabolism, specially under anesthesia. Other potential marker is serum lactate, but it was not measured for this study as it can vary in different conditions such as fluid replacement with Ringer lactate [15–18], a common practice in trauma patients. Other limitations of this study were the sample size for the study and that $ScvO_2$ values were not measured continuously.

A significant association with the requirement of red blood cell transfusion ($p = 0.019$), low values of hemoglobin at arrival ($p = 0.004$), and a greater ATI ($p < 0.001$) was also found. The first two variables are indirect markers of inadequate perfusion, further supporting its association with anastomotic leak development. This suggests that other markers may also help or may become cofounding factors for $ScvO_2$ efficacy. Measurement of other markers (serum lactate, BE, CO_2 gap, SaO_2, and others), bigger samples, and a proper case-control or randomized controlled trials may be needed for answering these questions. Nonetheless, our results are robust enough to emphasize $ScvO_2$ importance as a hypoperfusion marker and as a risk factor for POP anastomotic leakage in abdominal trauma surgery patients.

Conclusions

Early recognition of hypoperfusion during abdominal trauma surgery is of great importance for adequate decision-making and for identification of patients at risk. This study shows that low $ScvO_2$ levels (<65%) are associated with the development of anastomotic leak during the POP period and that $ScvO_2$ may become an objective and accessible marker of hypoperfusion in patients with abdominal trauma. We consider further studies are required for a better understanding of the relationship between hypoperfusion and anastomotic leak, the use of $ScvO_2$ as an early marker, and its usefulness for decision-making during surgery.

Abbreviations

ATI: Abdominal trauma index; DBP: Diastolic blood pressure; Hb: Hemoglobin; POP: Postoperative; SBP: Systolic blood pressure; $ScvO_2$: Central venous oxygen saturation

Acknowledgements

The authors would like to acknowledge the following:
Miguel Ramirez Gómez, MD. MSc.: Surgical department chief from Hospital Occidente Kennedy
Oscar Geovanni Hernandez, MD. MSc, General Surgeon at Hospital Occidente Kennedy
Sandra Marcela Saade-Lemus, MD and Juan Sebastián Botero-Meneses for the proofreading, grammar, and spelling edition.

Funding

The authors declare that they have not receive any kind of funding for the realization of this paper.

Authors' contributions

AI-R is the main investigator and contributed to the literature research, study design, data analysis, data interpretation, critical revision, and writing of the manuscript. JFM-M contributed to the study design, literature research, data collection, and data interpretation. MI-P contributed to the study design, data interpretation, and statistical analysis. JSM-S contributed to the literature research, data analysis, critical revision, and writing of the manuscript. All authors read and approved the final manuscript.

Competing interests

The authors declare that they have no competing interests.

Author details

[1]Escuela de Medicina y Ciencias de la Salud, Universidad del Rosario, Bogotá D.C., Colombia. [2]Mederi Hospital Universitario Mayor, Bogotá D.C., Colombia. [3]Hospital San Rafael, Tunja, Colombia. [4]Grupo de Investigación Clínica de la Universidad del Rosario, Bogotá, Colombia.

References

1. Kingham TP, Pachter HL. Colonic anastomotic leak: risk factors, diagnosis, and treatment. J Am Coll Surg. 2009;208(2):269–78.
2. Paterno F, Longo WE. The etiology and pathogenesis of vascular disorders of the intestine. Radiol Clin N Am. 2008;46:877–85.
3. Vignali A, Gianotti L, Braga M, Radaelli G, Malvezzi L, Di Carlo V. Altered microperfusion at the rectal stump is predictive for rectal anastomotic leak. Dis Colon Rectum. 2000;43(1):76–82.

4. Scalea TM, Holman M, Fuortes M, Baron BJ, Phillips TF, Goldstein AS, et al. Central venous blood oxygen saturation: an early, accurate measurement of volume during hemorrhage. J Trauma. 1988;28(6):725–32.
5. Scalea TM, Hartnett RW, Duncan AO, Atweh NA, Phillips TF, Sclafani SJ, et al. Central venous oxygen saturation: a useful clinical tool in trauma patients. J Trauma. 1990;30(12):1539–43.
6. Rivers E, Nguyen B, Havstad S, Ressler J, Muzzin A, Knoblich B, et al. Early goal-directed therapy in the treatment of severe sepsis and septic shock. N Engl J Med. 2001;345(19):1368–77.
7. Puyana JC, Pinsky MR. Searching for non-invasive markers of tissue hypoxia. Crit Care. 2007;11(1):116.
8. Teboul JL, Hamzaoui O, Monnet X. SvO2 to monitor resuscitation of septic patients: let's just understand the basic physiology. Crit Care. 2011;15:1005. England.
9. Permpikul C, Sringam P, Tongyoo S. Therapeutic goal achievements during severe sepsis and septic shock resuscitation and their association with patients' outcomes. J Med Assoc Thai. 2014;97 Suppl 3:S176–83.
10. Mohajeri G, Tabatabaei A, Hashemi M, Bistgani MM. Relationship of venous blood gas with cervical esophagogastric anastomotic leak. Asian Cardiovasc Thorac Ann. 2012;20:566–9. England.
11. Pearse R, Dawson D, Fawcett J, Rhodes A, Grounds RM, Bennett ED. Changes in central venous saturation after major surgery, and association with outcome. Crit Care. 2005;9(6):R694–9.
12. Giraud R, Siegenthaler N, Gayet-Ageron A, Combescure C, Romand JA, Bendjelid K. ScvO(2) as a marker to define fluid responsiveness. J Trauma. 2011;70(4):802–7.
13. Reinhart K, Rudolph T, Bredle DL, Hannemann L, Cain SM. Comparison of central-venous to mixed-venous oxygen saturation during changes in oxygen supply/demand. Chest. 1989;95(6):1216–21.
14. Reinhart K, Bloos F. The value of venous oximetry. Curr Opin Crit Care. 2005; 11(3):259–63.
15. Hosking C, Wilander P, Goosen J, Jacobson H, Moeng M, Boffard K, et al. Low central venous oxygen saturation in haemodynamically stabilized trauma patients is associated with poor outcome. Acta Anaesthesiol Scand. 2011;55(6):713–21.
16. Abramson D, Scalea TM, Hitchcock R, Trooskin SZ, Henry SM, Greenspan J. Lactate clearance and survival following injury. J Trauma. 1993;35(4):584–8. discussion 8-9.
17. Husain FA, Martin MJ, Mullenix PS, Steele SR, Elliott DC. Serum lactate and base deficit as predictors of mortality and morbidity. Am J Surg. 2003;185(5): 485–91.
18. Rixen D, Siegel JH. Bench-to-bedside review: oxygen debt and its metabolic correlates as quantifiers of the severity of hemorrhagic and post-traumatic shock. Crit Care. 2005;9(5):441–53.
19. Winters ME, McCurdy MT, Zilberstein J. Monitoring the critically ill emergency department patient. Emerg Med Clin North Am. 2008;26(3):741–57. ix.
20. Kusano C, Baba M, Takao S, Sane S, Shimada M, Shirao K, et al. Oxygen delivery as a factor in the development of fatal postoperative complications after oesophagectomy. Br J Surg. 1997;84(2):252–7.
21. Bland RD, Shoemaker WC, Abraham E, Cobo JC. Hemodynamic and oxygen transport patterns in surviving and nonsurviving postoperative patients. Crit Care Med. 1985;13(2):85–90.
22. Peerless JR, Alexander JJ, Pinchak AC, Piotrowski JJ, Malangoni MA. Oxygen delivery is an important predictor of outcome in patients with ruptured abdominal aortic aneurysms. Ann Surg. 1998;227(5):726–32. discussion 32-4.
23. Poeze M, Ramsay G, Greve JW, Singer M. Prediction of postoperative cardiac surgical morbidity and organ failure within 4 hours of intensive care unit admission using esophageal Doppler ultrasonography. Crit Care Med. 1999; 27(7):1288–94.
24. Shoemaker WC, Montgomery ES, Kaplan E, Elwyn DH. Physiologic patterns in surviving and nonsurviving shock patients. Use of sequential cardiorespiratory variables in defining criteria for therapeutic goals and early warning of death. Arch Surg. 1973;106(5):630–6.
25. Futier E, Constantin JM, Petit A, Chanques G, Kwiatkowski F, Flamein R, et al. Conservative vs restrictive individualized goal-directed fluid replacement strategy in major abdominal surgery: a prospective randomized trial. Arch Surg. 2010;145:1193–200. United States.
26. Schmelzer TM, Perron AD, Thomason MH, Sing RF. A comparison of central venous and arterial base deficit as a predictor of survival in acute trauma. Am J Emerg Med. 2008;26(2):119–23.
27. Hwang RF, Schwartz RW. Enterocutaneous fistulas: current diagnosis and management. Curr Surg. 2000;57(5):443–5.
28. Dudrick SJ, Wilmore DW, Vars HM, Rhoads JE. Long-term total parenteral nutrition with growth, development, and positive nitrogen balance. Surgery. 1968;64(1):134–42.
29. Edmunds Jr LH, Williams GM, Welch CE. External fistulas arising from the gastro-intestinal tract. Ann Surg. 1960;152:445–71.
30. Terzi C, Egeli T, Canda AE, Arslan NC. Management of enteroatmospheric fistulae. Int Wound J. 2014;11 Suppl 1:17–21.
31. Mayorga M. Estrategias para mejorar la sobrevivencia de los pacientes con sepsis severa/Strategies for improving survival in patients with severe sepsis. Lima: Colegio Médico del Perú; 2010. p. 302.
32. Cecconi M, Corredor C, Arulkumaran N, Abuella G, Ball J, Grounds RM, et al. Clinical review: goal-directed therapy-what is the evidence in surgical patients? The effect on different risk groups. Crit Care. 2013;17:209. England.
33. Spronk PE, Zandstra DF, Ince C. Bench-to-bedside review: sepsis is a disease of the microcirculation. Crit Care. 2004;8(6):462–8.
34. Fink MP. Bench-to-bedside review: cytopathic hypoxia. Crit Care. 2002;6(6): 491–9.
35. Pearse RM, Hinds CJ. Should we use central venous saturation to guide management in high-risk surgical patients? Crit Care. 2006;10(6):181.

Permissions

All chapters in this book were first published in WJES, by BioMed Central; hereby published with permission under the Creative Commons Attribution License or equivalent. Every chapter published in this book has been scrutinized by our experts. Their significance has been extensively debated. The topics covered herein carry significant findings which will fuel the growth of the discipline. They may even be implemented as practical applications or may be referred to as a beginning point for another development.

The contributors of this book come from diverse backgrounds, making this book a truly international effort. This book will bring forth new frontiers with its revolutionizing research information and detailed analysis of the nascent developments around the world.

We would like to thank all the contributing authors for lending their expertise to make the book truly unique. They have played a crucial role in the development of this book. Without their invaluable contributions this book wouldn't have been possible. They have made vital efforts to compile up to date information on the varied aspects of this subject to make this book a valuable addition to the collection of many professionals and students.

This book was conceptualized with the vision of imparting up-to-date information and advanced data in this field. To ensure the same, a matchless editorial board was set up. Every individual on the board went through rigorous rounds of assessment to prove their worth. After which they invested a large part of their time researching and compiling the most relevant data for our readers.

The editorial board has been involved in producing this book since its inception. They have spent rigorous hours researching and exploring the diverse topics which have resulted in the successful publishing of this book. They have passed on their knowledge of decades through this book. To expedite this challenging task, the publisher supported the team at every step. A small team of assistant editors was also appointed to further simplify the editing procedure and attain best results for the readers.

Apart from the editorial board, the designing team has also invested a significant amount of their time in understanding the subject and creating the most relevant covers. They scrutinized every image to scout for the most suitable representation of the subject and create an appropriate cover for the book.

The publishing team has been an ardent support to the editorial, designing and production team. Their endless efforts to recruit the best for this project, has resulted in the accomplishment of this book. They are a veteran in the field of academics and their pool of knowledge is as vast as their experience in printing. Their expertise and guidance has proved useful at every step. Their uncompromising quality standards have made this book an exceptional effort. Their encouragement from time to time has been an inspiration for everyone.

The publisher and the editorial board hope that this book will prove to be a valuable piece of knowledge for researchers, students, practitioners and scholars across the globe.

List of Contributors

Suzanne Beecher, Donal Peter O'Leary and Ray McLaughlin
Department of Surgery, Galway University Hospital/ National University of Ireland (NUI), Galway, Republic of Ireland

Frederico Teixeira, Carlos Augusto Metidieri Menegozzo, Sérgio Dias do Couto Netto, Renato S. Poggeti, Francisco de Sales Collet e Silva, Dario Birolini, Celso de Oliveira Bernini and Edivaldo Massazo Utiyama
Departament of Surgery, Division of Surgical Clinic III, University of Sao Paulo School of Medicine, Sao Paulo, Brazil

Yehuda Hershkovitz, Sergei Naveh, Zahar Shapira, Ariel Halevy and Igor Jeroukhimov
Division of Surgery, Assaf Harofeh Medical Center, Zerifin 70300, affiliated to the Sackler Faculty of Medicine, Tel Aviv University, Tel Aviv, Israel

Boris Kessel
Trauma Unit, Hillel Yaffe Medical Center, Hadera 38100, Israel

Dan Crisan and Horia Haragus
I-st Clinic of Orthopedics and Trauma, Pius Brinzeu Emergency Clinical County Hospital, 10 I. Bulbuca Blvd, 300737 Timisoara, Romania

Bogdan Deleanu, Radu Prejbeanu and Dinu Vermesan
I-st Clinic of Orthopedics and Trauma, Pius Brinzeu Emergency Clinical County Hospital, 10 I. Bulbuca Blvd, 300737 Timisoara, Romania
Victor Babes University of Medicine and Pharmacy, 2 Eftimie Murgu Square, 300041 Timişoara, Romania

Florin Birsasteanu
Victor Babes University of Medicine and Pharmacy, 2 Eftimie Murgu Square, 300041 Timişoara, Romania
Department of Radiology, Pius Brinzeu Emergency Clinical County Hospital, 10 I. Bulbuca Blvd, 300737 Timisoara, Romania

Vlad Predescu
St.Pantelimon Clinical Emergency Hospital, 340 - 342 Pantelimon Road, Sector 2, 033092 Bucharest, Romania
Carol Davila University of Medicine and Pharmacy, 8 Eroii Sanitari Blvd, 050474 Bucharest, Romania

Eleftherios Tsiridis
Aristotle University Medical School, 54124 Thessaloniki, Greece

L. Pearce, S. R. Smith, E. Parkin, C. Hall, J. Kennedy and A. Macdonald
Clinical Research Fellow, Department of General Surgery, Central Manchester University Hospitals Foundation Trust, Oxford Road, Manchester M13 9WL, UK

Giulia Montori, Federico Coccolini, Roberto Manfredi, Marco Ceresoli, Luca Campanati, Stefano Magnone, Michele Pisano, Elia Poiasina, Gabriela Nita and Luca Ansaloni
Unit of General and Emergency Surgery, Papa Giovanni XXIII Hospital, P.zza OMS 1, 24128 Bergamo, Italy

Fausto Catena
General surgery department, Ospedale Maggiore, Parma, Italy

Jakub Kenig, Piotr Wałęga, Urszula Olszewska, Aleksander Konturek and Wojciech Nowak
3rd Department of General Surgery, Jagiellonian University Medical College, Pradnicka str. 35-37, 31-202 Kraków, Poland

Marios Papadakis, Peter C. Ambe and Hubert Zirngibl
Helios Klinikum Wuppertal, Department of Surgery II, Witten - Herdecke University, Heusner Str. 40, 42283 Wuppertal, Germany

Yong Hun Kim
Department of Surgery, School of Medicine, Konkuk University, KonkukM University Chungju Hospital, 82, Gugwon-daero, Chungju-si, Chungbuk, Republic of Korea

Woo Surng Lee
Department of Thoracic and Cardiovascular Surgery, School of Medicine, Konkuk University, Konkuk University Chungju Hospital, 82, Gugwon-daero, Chungju-si, Chungbuk, Republic of Korea

Mansur Duran, E. Pohl, K. Grabitz, H. Schelzig, T. A. Sagban and F. Simon
Clinic for Vascular- and Endovascular Surgery, Heinrich-Heine-University, Moorenstr. 5, 40225 Düsseldorf, Germany

Minsu Noh, Song Soo Yang, Yeong Cheol Im and Kyu Yeol Kim
Department of Surgery, Ulsan University Hospital, 290-3 Jeonha-dong, Dong-gu, Ulsan 682-714, Korea

Seok Won Jung and Jae Ho Park
Department of Digestive medicine, Ulsan University Hospital, Ulsan, Korea

Nan-Ping Yang
Department of Surgery and Orthopedics, Keelung Hospital, Ministry of Health and Welfare, Keelung, Taiwan
Faculty of Medicine, School of Medicine, National Yang-Ming University, Taipei, Taiwan
Institute of Public Health and Community Medicine Research Center, National Yang-Ming University, Taipei, Taiwan

Dachen Chu
Faculty of Medicine, School of Medicine, National Yang-Ming University, Taipei, Taiwan
Institute of Public Health and Community Medicine Research Center, National Yang-Ming University, Taipei, Taiwan
Department of Neurosurgery, Taipei City Hospital, Taipei, Taiwan
Department of Health Care Management, National Taipei University of Nursing and Health Sciences, Taipei, Taiwan

Dinh-Van Phan, Ren-Hao Pan and Chien-Lung Chan
Department of Information Management, Yuan Ze University, Taoyuan, Taiwan
Innovation Center for Big Data and Digital Convergence, Yuan Ze University, Taoyuan, Taiwan

Yi-Hui Lee
Department of Nursing, School of Nursing, College of Medicine, Chang-Gang University, Taoyuan, Taiwan

Nien-Tzu Chang
Department of Nursing, School of Nursing, College of Medicine, Chang-Gang University, Taoyuan, Taiwan
School of Nursing, College of Medicine, National Taiwan University, Taipei, Taiwan

Jin-Chyr Hsu
Department of Medicine, Taipei Hospital, Ministry of Health and Welfare, Taipei, Taiwan

Amri Mabewa, Phillipo L. Chalya and Japhet M. Gilyoma
Department of Surgery, Catholic University of Health and Allied Sciences, Mwanza, Tanzania
Department of Surgery, Bugando Medical Centre, Mwanza, Tanzania

Jeremiah Seni and Stephen E.Mshana
Department of Microbiology and Immunology, Catholic University of Health and Allied Sciences, Mwanza, Tanzania

Katrin Stanger
Department of Plastic and Hand Surgery, OKM Orthopädische Klinik Markgröningen gGmbH, Markgröningen, Germany

Raymund E. Horch
Department of Plastic and Hand Surgery, University Hospital of Erlangen, Friedrich-Alexander-University Erlangen-Nürnberg, Erlangen, Germany

Adrian Dragu
Department of Plastic and Hand Surgery, Klinikum St. Georg gGmbH, Leipzig, Germany

Karen Gozel, Patty Reicks and Eric Irwin
North Memorial Medical Center, Robbinsdale, MN, USA

Kaysie Banton and Greg J. Beilman
North Memorial Medical Center, Robbinsdale, MN, USA
Department of Surgery, University of Minnesota Medical Center, Minneapolis, MN, USA

Shrey Modi, Ryan Deisler and Melissa Brunsvold
Department of Surgery, University of Minnesota Medical Center, Minneapolis, MN, USA

Chih-Yuan Fu, Shang-Ju Yang, Chien-Hung Liao, Being-Chuan Lin, Shih-Ching Kang, Shang-Yu Wang and Yu-Pao Hsu
Department of Trauma and Emergency Surgery, Chang Gung Memorial Hospital, Chang Gung University, 5, Fu-Hsing Street, Kwei Shan Township, Taoyuan, Taiwan

Pepijn Krielen, Barend A. van den Beukel, Martijn W. J. Stommel, Harry van Goor, Chema Strik and Richard P. G. ten Broek
Department of Surgery, Radboud University Medical Center, 6500, HB, Nijmegen, The Netherlands

Pinit Noorit
Department of Surgery, Chonburi hospital, Chonburi, Thailand

Boonying Siribumrungwong
Department of Surgery, Faculty of Medicine, Thammasat University Hospital, Pathum thani, Thailand

Ammarin Thakkinstian
Section for Clinical Epidemiology and Biostatistics, Faculty of Medicine, Ramathibodi Hospital, Mahidol University, Rama VI road, Rachatevi, Bangkok 10400, Thailand

Dong Hyuk Shin
Department of Emergency Medicine, Kangbuk Samsung Hospital, Sungkyunkwan University School of Medicine, Seoul, Republic of Korea

Young Suk Cho and Gyu Chong Cho
Department of Emergency Medicine, School of Medicine, Kangdong Sacred Heart Hospital, Hallym University, Seoul, Republic of Korea

Hee Cheol Ahn, Seung Min Park and Seung Wook Lim
Department of Emergency Medicine, Sacred Heart Hospital, Hallym University School of Medicine, Anyang, Republic of Korea

Young Taeck Oh and Young Hwan Lee
Department of Emergency Medicine, Sacred Heart Hospital, Hallym University School of Medicine, Anyang, Republic of Korea
Department of Emergency Medicine, College of Medicine, Kangwon National University, Chuncheon, Gangwon 200-701, Republic of Korea

Ji Woong Cho
Department of Surgery, Kangnam Sacred Heart Hospital, Hallym University Medical Center, Hallym University College of Medicine, Seoul, Republic of Korea

Sang O. Park
Department of Emergency Medicine, School of Medicine, Konkuk University Konkuk University Medical Center, Seoul, Republic of Korea

Jörg Bayer, Jan Kühle, Jörn Zwingmann, Norbert P. Südkamp and Thorsten Hammer
Department of Orthopedics and Trauma Surgery, Medical Center - Albert-Ludwigs-University of Freiburg, Faculty of Medicine, Albert-Ludwigs-University of Freiburg, Hugstetter Str. 55, 79106 Freiburg, Germany

Rolf Lefering
FOM - Institute for Research in Operative Medicine, University Witten/Herdecke, Faculty of Health, Ostmerheimer Str. 200, 51109 Köln, Germany

Sylvia Reinhardt
Department of Orthopedics and Trauma Surgery, Oberschwabenklinik St. Elisabeth, Elisabethenstr. 15, 88212 Ravensburg, Germany

Trauma Register DGU
Committee on Emergency Medicine, Intensive Care and Trauma Management of the German Trauma Society (Sektion NIS), Berlin, Germany

Matti Tolonen
Department of Abdominal Surgery, Abdominal Center, University of Helsinki and Helsinki University Central Hospital, Helsinki, Finland

Federico Coccolini
Emergency and Trauma Surgery Department, Bufalini Hospital, Cesena, Italy

Luca Ansaloni
Unit of General and Emergency Surgery, Bufalini Hospital of Cesena, Cesna, Italy

Jimmy Xiao
Regional Trauma Services, Foothills Medical Centre, Calgary, Canada

Christopher J. Doig
Departments of Critical Care Medicine and Community Health Sciences, Cumming School of Medicine, University of Calgary, Calgary, Canada

Fausto Catena
Emergency Surgery Department, Parma University Hospital, Parma, Italy

Timothy Fabian
University of Tennessee Health Sciences Center, Memphis, TN, USA

Juan G. Posadas-Calleja
Department of Critical Care Medicine, University of Calgary, Calgary, Alberta, Canada

Salomone Di Saverio
Cambridge University Hospitals NHS Foundation Trust, Addenbrooke's Hospital, Cambridge, UK

Patrick B. Murphy, Richard Hilsden and Jennifer Koichopolos
Division of General Surgery, Department of Surgery, Schulich School of Medicine and Dentistry, Western University, London, Canada

Tina S. Mele
Division of General Surgery, Department of Surgery, Schulich School of Medicine and Dentistry, Western University, London, Canada
Divisions of Critical Care, Department of Surgery, Schulich School of Medicine and Dentistry, Western University, London, Canada

Dave Paskar
Divisions of General Surgery Trauma and Critical Care Medicine, University of Toronto, Toronto, Canada

Benoit Gignoux, Marie-Cecile Blanchet and Vincent Frering
Department of General, Visceral and Endocrine Surgery, Clinique de la Sauvegarde, Lyon, France

Thomas Lanz and Alexandre Vulliez
Department of Anesthesiology, Clinique de la Sauvegarde, Lyon, France

Mo Saffarini and Hugo Bothorel
Medical Technology, Re Surg SA, ch. de la Vuarpilliere 35, 1260 Nyon, Switzerland

Maud Robert
Department of Digestive Surgery, University Hospital Edouard Herriot, Lyon, France

Stefan Jansen, Maciej Stodolski and Hubert Zirngibl
Department of Surgery, Helios University Hospital Wuppertal, Witten- Herdecke University, Heusnerstr. 40, 42283 Wuppertal, Germany

Peter C. Ambe
Department of Surgery, Helios University Hospital Wuppertal, Witten- Herdecke University, Heusnerstr. 40, 42283 Wuppertal, Germany
Department of Visceral, Minimally Invasive and Oncologic Surgery, Marien Hospital Düsseldor, Rochusstr. 2, 40479 Düsseldorf, Germany

Daniel Gödde
Department of Pathology and Molecular Pathology, Helios University Hospital Wuppertal, Witten-Herdecke University, Heusnerstr. 40, 42283 Wuppertal, Germany

K. Verhoeff and B. Min
Faculty of Medicine and Dentistry, University of Alberta, 8440-112 St. Edmonton, Edmonton, Alberta T6G 2B7, Canada

P. Glen, A. Taheri B. Tsang, V. Fawcett and S. Widder
Department of Surgery, 2D4.27 Mackenzie Health Sciences Centre, University of Alberta, 8440-112 St. Edmonton, Edmonton, Alberta T6G 2B7, Canada

Sameh Hany Emile, Hesham Elgendy, Ahmad Sakr, Waleed Ahmed Gado, Ahmed Aly Abdelmawla, Mahmoud Abdelnaby and Alaa Magdy
General surgery department, faculty of Medicine, Mansoura University Hospitals, Elgomhuoria Street, Mansoura city, Egypt

Petra Maria Terho
Institute of Clinical Medicine, Faculty of Medicine, University of Helsinki, Haartmaninkatu 8, 00014 Helsinki, Finland

Ari Kalevi Leppäniemi and Panu Juhani Mentula
Department of Abdominal Surgery, Helsinki University Central Hospital, 00029 HUS Helsinki, Finland

Gilda Pepe, Marco Cintoni, Giuseppe Tropeano, Sabina Magalini, Gabriele Sganga and Daniele Gui
Emergency Surgery Department, Università Cattolica del Sacro Cuore, Fondazione Policlinico A. Gemelli IRCCS, Rome, Italy

Valerio Cozza
Emergency Surgery Department, Università Cattolica del Sacro Cuore, Fondazione Policlinico A. Gemelli IRCCS, Rome, Italy
Istituto di Clinica Chirurgica (9B) Catholic University of Sacred Heart, Largo Francesco Vito, 1, 00168 Rome, Italy

Flavio De Maio and Giovanni Delogu
Microbiology Department, Università Cattolica del Sacro Cuore, Fondazione Policlinico A. Gemelli IRCCS, Rome, Italy

Yoram Klein
Trauma unit, Sheba Medical Center, Tel Aviv University, Tel Aviv, Israel

Evgeni Brotfain, Leonid Koyfman, Dmitry Frank and Moti Klein
Department of Anesthesiology and Critical Care, General Intensive Care Unit, Soroka Medical Center, Ben-Gurion University of the Negev, Beer Sheva, Israel

Ronen Toledano
Clinical Research Center, Soroka Medical Center, Ben-Gurion University of the Negev, Beer Sheva, Israel

Micha Y. Shamir
Department of Anesthesiology, Hadassah-Hebrew University Medical Center, Jerusalem, Israel

Abdelrahman Abdelaal, Moamena El-Matbouly, Ibnouf Sulieman, Ahmad Elfaki, Tamer El-Bakary, Sherif Abdelaziem and Salahdin Gehani
Department of General Surgery, Hamad General Hospital, Al Rayyan Road, 3050 Doha, Qatar

Isidoro Di Carlo
Department of General Surgery, Hamad General Hospital, Al Rayyan Road, 3050 Doha, Qatar
Department of Surgical Sciences and Advanced Technologies "G.F. Ingrassia", University of Catania, Via Santa Sofia 78, 95100 Catania, Italy

Adriana Toro
Department of Surgery, Barone Romeo Hospital, via Mazzini 14, 98066 Patti, (ME), Italy

E. J. M. M. Verleisdonk
Department of Surgery, Diakonessenhuis Utrecht, Utrecht, The Netherlands

F. S. Würdemann
Department of Surgery, Diakonessenhuis Utrecht, Utrecht, The Netherlands
Department of Surgery, University Medical Center Utrecht, Heidelberglaan 100, 3584 CX Utrecht, The Netherlands

D. P. J. Smeeing and R. M. Houwert
Traumacenter, University Medical Center Utrecht, Utrecht, The Netherlands
Department of Surgery, University Medical Center Utrecht, Heidelberglaan 100, 3584 CX Utrecht, The Netherlands

Ferree, F. Nawijn, L. P. H. Leenen and F. Hietbrink
Department of Surgery, University Medical Center Utrecht, Heidelberglaan 100, 3584 CX Utrecht, The Netherlands

Milciades Ibañez-Pinilla
Escuela de Medicina y Ciencias de la Salud, Universidad del Rosario, Bogotá D.C., Colombia

Andres Isaza-Restrepo
Escuela de Medicina y Ciencias de la Salud, Universidad del Rosario, Bogotá D.C., Colombia
Mederi Hospital Universitario Mayor, Bogotá D.C., Colombia

Jose F. Moreno-Mejia
Hospital San Rafael, Tunja, Colombia

Juan S. Martin-Saavedra
Grupo de Investigación Clínica de la Universidad del Rosario, Bogotá, Colombia

Index

A

Abdominal Organ Injury, 13

Abdominal Trauma, 13-15, 17-18, 223-226

Abdominal Wall Repair, 30, 32-33, 36

Acute Calculous Cholecystitis, 50, 172, 188-189, 191, 196

Acute Cholecystitis, 39-46, 48-50, 152-153, 155-157, 167-168, 172, 188-189, 193-196

Acute Mesenteric Ischemia, 57, 61-62, 70

Advanced Care Planning, 173-175, 177-178

Ambulatory Appendectomy, 159-160

Appendectomy, 1, 4-5, 51-53, 55-56, 84, 87, 112, 118-121, 124-129, 159-160, 162-166, 191, 193

Appendicitis, 1-5, 31, 51-56, 79, 81, 83-86, 118-130, 140-141, 157, 159-160, 162-166

Appendicolith, 159, 161-166

Avulsion, 24, 88-89, 91-95, 214-215, 217-218

B

Bile Duct Injury, 48, 167, 169, 171, 194-196

Biliary Pancreatitis, 157-158, 207-208, 212

Biological Mesh, 30-31, 35-36

Blunt Trauma, 13-18, 131, 134-135, 138-139, 206, 222, 225

Bowel Obstruction, 110-112, 115-117, 180

C

Care Surgery, 4, 27, 29, 50, 149, 151, 157-158, 212

Cervical Trauma, 6

Chest Injury, 131-132, 138

Cholecystectomy, 38-50, 52, 56, 151-158, 167-168, 171-172, 188-189, 191, 193-196, 207-208, 210-212

Colorectal Surgery, 110-111, 116, 118, 124

Comorbidity, 32-33, 35, 38-39, 41-43, 46, 112, 131, 181, 184, 191, 225

Complex Macroamputation, 88

Cost Effectiveness, 151, 153-154, 156-157

D

Deep Vein Thrombosis, 97-102

Delta Neutrophil Index, 125-129

E

Emergency Surgery, 2-5, 17, 25-26, 28-32, 34, 36-37, 39, 50, 57, 64-66, 68, 87, 103-104, 116, 128, 140-142, 147-148, 157, 159, 179, 197

Empyematous Cholecystitis, 48-49, 168, 172

Endovascular Treatment, 57, 61

Etiology, 69, 71, 81-82, 84-85, 87, 115, 172, 212, 226

F

Frailty, 38-44

Functional Outcome, 88-92, 94, 213

G

Gallbladder Inflammation, 45-50, 167-168, 170-172

Gallstone Pancreatitis, 151-154, 156-158, 211-212

Geriatric Assessment, 38-39, 41-44

Geriatric Trauma, 173-178

H

Hemorrhage, 11, 64, 103-104, 108-109, 201-203, 206, 227

Hypertensive Heart Disease, 47

Hypotension, 64, 108, 142, 203, 206, 223

Hypovolemic Multiple Trauma, 201

I

Imaging Diagnosis, 19, 22

Inclusive Trauma System, 213-214, 218, 220-221

Intra-abdominal Sepsis, 32-33, 35, 140-141, 143, 145, 147-150

Ischemic Colitis, 63, 66, 69-71

Ischemic Heart Disease, 47

L

Laparostomy, 30-31, 35

M

Macrohematuria, 13, 15, 17

Maturation, 213, 221-222

Mesenteric Infarction, 57, 70-71

Mesenteric Ischemia, 57-58, 61-62, 70

Mortality, 1, 4, 6-8, 10, 16, 28, 30, 32-36, 38-42, 44-45, 47-49, 57-59, 61, 63-70, 78, 80-81, 84, 86-87, 103, 105, 108-109, 129, 131-132, 134-150, 170-173, 178, 213-214, 227

Mortality Rate, 6, 30, 35-36, 57, 59, 61, 63, 66, 69, 84, 103, 137, 141, 145-147, 171

Multiple Injuries, 36, 88, 136, 138, 222

Multiple Organ Failure, 70, 131, 133, 139, 141, 147, 206

O

Occult Fracture, 20, 24

Open Abdomen, 30-31, 33, 36-37, 140-141, 149-150

Organ Dysfunction, 131-132, 137-142, 145-147, 150

Organ Failure, 57-59, 63, 66, 68, 70, 81, 131-134, 136, 138-139, 141, 147, 149-150, 169, 203, 206, 227

P

Pediatric, 13-18, 54, 56, 166

Pediatric Trauma Management, 13
Pelvic Fracture, 19, 22, 103-105, 107-109
Penetrating Neck Trauma, 6, 11-12
Peripheral Artery Disease, 47
Polytrauma, 131
Postoperative Morbidity, 10, 38, 40, 42, 44-45, 49, 63, 66
Proximal Femur, 19, 23-24
Pulmonary Embolism, 48, 97, 101-102

R
Replantation, 88-92, 94-95

S
Sacroiliac Joint Disruption, 103
Secondary Peritonitis, 35, 81-86, 140-141, 145-146, 149-150
Septic Shock, 34-35, 58, 63, 65-66, 68, 70, 140-143, 145-150, 227
Severely Injured, 94-95, 131-139, 222
Single-port Laparoscopic Appendectomy, 51, 53, 56
Sternum Fracture, 131
Superior Mesenteric Artery, 57, 62
Surgical Exploration, 6, 8-9, 12
Surgical Management, 45, 48, 50, 70, 86, 153, 155, 158, 171-172
Swine Dermal Collagen, 30-31
Synthetic Mesh, 35, 179-180, 184-187

T
Thoracic Trauma, 131, 133-138
Thoracic Wall, 131
Treatment Outcome, 81, 84, 96

U
Upper Extremity, 78, 88-89, 92-95

V
Vascular Reconstruction, 57
Ventral Hernia, 30, 34-36, 179-182, 184-187

W
Wells Scoring System, 97-101
Wound Contamination, 119, 121, 197, 200
Wound Infection, 34-35, 48, 65-66, 118, 197
Wound Therapy, 33-34, 36, 197, 199-200, 222